D1029185

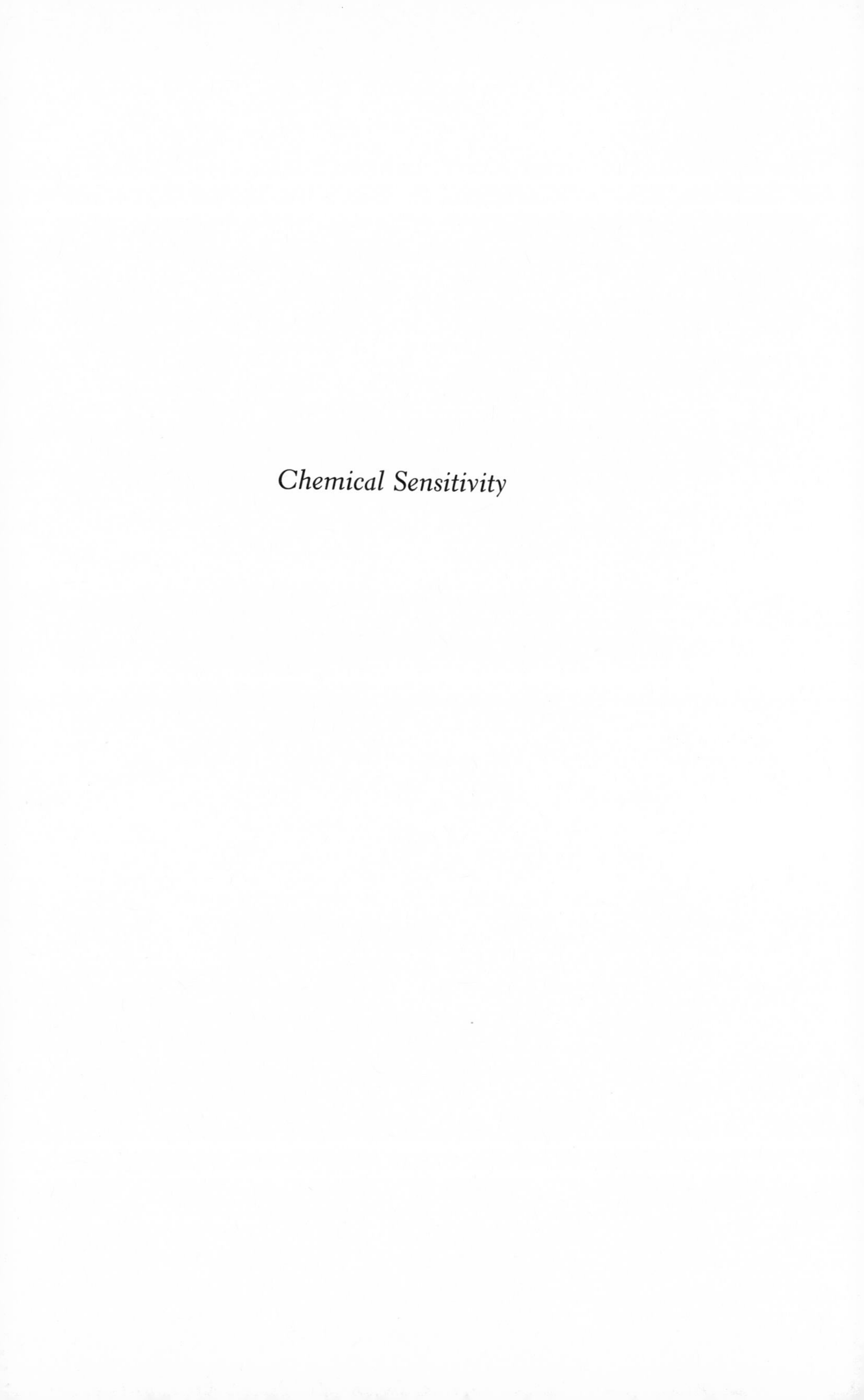

Chemical Sensitivity

Chemical Sensitivity

A GUIDE TO COPING WITH HYPERSENSITIVITY SYNDROME, SICK BUILDING SYNDROME AND OTHER ENVIRONMENTAL ILLNESSES

by

Bonnye L. Matthews

with a foreword by
ROBERT JAMES SINAIKO, M.D.

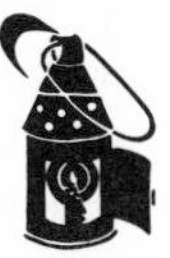

McFarland & Company, Inc., Publishers
Jefferson, North Carolina, and London

British Library Cataloguing-in-Publication data are available

Library of Congress Cataloguing-in-Publication Data

Matthews, Bonnye L., 1943–
Chemical sensitivity : a guide to coping with hypersensitivity syndrome, sick building syndrome and other environmental illnesses / Bonnye L. Matthews.
p. cm.
ISBN 0-89950-731-X (library binding : 50# alk. paper) ♾
1. Environmentally induced diseases. 2. Sick building syndrome. 3. Allergy. I. Title.
[DNLM: 1. Air pollution, Indoor. 2. Drug Hypersensitivity. 3. Environmental Exposure. 4. Occupational Diseases—chemically induced. WA 754 M438c]
RB152.M37 1992
616.9'8—dc20
DNLM/DLC
for Library of Congress 92-54089
CIP

Manufactured in the United States of America

McFarland & Company, Inc., Publishers
Box 611, Jefferson, North Carolina 28640

On July 25, 1989, the United States Congress approved Public Law 101-58 designating the ten years beginning January 1, 1990, the "Decade of the Brain." No group of people has a greater need for real scientific pursuit of the structure and function of the brain than those who have brain impairment, including specifically those chemical sensitives with organic brain syndrome (toxic encephalopathy). This book is dedicated to chemical sensitives and their caregivers. It is written with the hope that before mid-decade CS patients will be afforded the same access to medical treatment and be treated with the same degree of compassion that other individuals receive and expect as basic human rights.

Contents

Foreword

My education in chemical sensitivity began early on a warm summer afternoon in 1976, when I met Dr. Benjamin Feingold, the chairman of the Department of Allergy at Kaiser Foundation Hospital in San Francisco. Feingold had concluded from his own observations that small amounts of certain chemicals in foods could adversely affect behavior and classroom performance of hyperactive children. He welcomed me into his office, and over the next three hours related the story of his discoveries and of his own evolving philosophy of medicine, emphasizing the importance of listening to and learning from patients. With Dr. Feingold's encouragement, I entered the two-year Fellowship Training Program in his department. Under his guidance, I became aware of the profound adverse impact of low levels of chemicals in food, water, and air, on the well-being not only of children with behavioral and learning problems, but on a susceptible group of adults as well. These were patients who had been tossed about from one practitioner to another, with no help for their frustrating and often debilitating symptoms. Virtually all had been told repeatedly that their problems were psychological.

I and many others consider ourselves fortunate to have been guided in the formative years of our careers by physician mentors who had the courage to look deep and reject the posture of convenient skepticism that many in the medical profession adopt when they don't know the answers. Physicians like Benjamin Feingold, Phyllis Saifer, and Joseph McGovern could know about chemical sensitivity because they listened closely to their patients and understood that clinical observation is the cornerstone both of the art and the science of medicine. Building on this foundation, a variety of treatments have been found that help the chemically sensitive patient to live a normal life, and though portions of the serviceable masonry of clinical practice remain unbuttressed by objective data, there is far more scientific corroboration of effective treatments than many doctors currently acknowledge.

The analysis of underlying causes ranges across a spectrum of psychological, psychobiological, and physical phenomena, with the data pointing strongly in the direction of the physical alone or the physical actively interacting with psychological problems which themselves may stem from biochemical factors or illness-related stress. Observations only occasionally support a purely psychological analysis, and psychological treatments by themselves have rarely proven effective.

In this book, Bonnye Matthews focuses on the physical end of the spectrum; for a lay audience, she lucidly amasses the available data in a way that will lift a heavy and lonely burden from those who suffer not only from the symptoms of chemical sensitivity, but from the psychological weight placed upon their shoulders by too many doctors who, failing to treat them, have blamed the victim.

The patients who, like Bonnye Matthews, have the courage to persevere in search of solutions, like the physicians who have taught the rest of us to rely on their insights, are ahead of their time: they will be the lighthouse, illuminating the pathway to recovery that others will follow.

Bonnye Matthews got sick, but she's smart and skilled, and she has found within her illness a silver lining, an opportunity to bring the power of her own being to bear on these questions, not just for herself but for thousands of other chemically sensitive patients in contemporary society. They are the canaries who sing in the mineshafts, warning the rest of us of danger. With the concrete knowledge pulled together in this book, more patients will sing, and the medical profession will increasingly pay attention to their rising chorus.

Robert James Sinaiko, M.D.
Clinical Instructor
Department of Medicine
University of California, San Francisco

Preface

As one who suffers from chemical sensitivity I know what it is to be poisoned by chronic, low level toxic substance; to lose the job I loved; to be ridiculed and harmed by people in the medical profession; to be denied entitlements and civil rights by claims examiners; to be harassed. I also know intelligent, courageous people who have the capacity to be arrested by truth, and the conscience and power to act with wisdom.

There is a medical road to be surveyed and mapped, leveled and paved, and I am proud to know that my name will appear as author of a book on a subject that needs to be addressed. I am deeply in debt to a large number of very special people who have enriched my life as well as contributed to the development and production of this book.

First, I deeply appreciate my devil's advocate, *James M. Vincent, M.D., Pulmonary Specialist.* He asked questions that demanded answers. He still does. Rather than hold a skeptical position, he chose to wait, to observe, and even when he didn't like what he saw, he did not ignore evidence. James Vincent's physician performance rates superlative because of his clinical intellect and drive to research, his capacity to allow himself to feel, and his respect for truth.

Second, there are some other medical professionals who have made significant contributions directly or indirectly to this book. They are:

Rena Hamburger, D.O., Family Practice. This physician has provided my primary medical care for two decades. Quick to listen, not quick to make judgments, aware of developments in the medical world, willing to dig for answers and weigh alternatives, this doctor demonstrates the rare gift of much wisdom. And she remains the same stable, caring, insightful person year after year. Her patients are real people, and she knows them. Her insight and referral significantly reduced the time required in my case to identify the proper diagnosis. Her subsequent care and understanding provide the essential equipment for me to move from CS patient to someone who lives life, despite a disability.

Gordon P. Baker, M.D., Allergist/Immunologist. A physician aware of the work of this doctor has called him "a medical genius who's not afraid of walking into the esoteric and staying there until he finds answers."

Gordon Baker's willingness to tackle the unknown, make sense of it, deal with tremendous disincentives, provide public information, and keep his head when others are losing theirs is testimony to his character. Despite a demanding schedule, he has been extremely helpful in facilitating my understanding of the role of the immune system in CS. His extraordinary staff, long accustomed to a standard practice, has remained intact, despite the incredible demands placed on their time and service by a new set of patients, inquiries from the medical world, demands from attorneys, shifts in the manner in which medical payments are made, and so on.

Joseph C. Ardizzone, D.D.S., Dentist. Having studied immunology in medical school, this dentist provided significant assistance in my early efforts to understand the basics of the immune system from a source external to those involved in my diagnosis and treatment. His help and encouragement provided the framework for my subsequent effort to understand complex medical data and to present those data in appropriate ways.

Eileen McCarty, Clinical Psychologist. It is the unenviable task of Eileen McCarty to administer tests which facilitate the patient's first recognition of the existence and the extent of brain damage or dysfunction that chemicals have caused. She has the compassion and reality focus to enable the CS patient to accept the new knowledge, which can be devastating, during the actual testing, and she provides supportive counseling afterward. Her praises have been sung by psychiatrists who do not recognize chemical sensitivity, for her expertise in identifying the existence of extremely subtle organic brain syndrome symptoms. Her assistance with the difference in functional and organic CS problems was extremely helpful. I depended on her reading of this manuscript for a rigorous, authoritative critique.

George C. Zerr, M.D., Psychiatrist. George Zerr counsels the hundreds of chemical sensitive patients who seek him out, listening to each history and differentiating between organic and functional problems, as well as identifying what is important to address and what is irrelevant. One of his most valuable assets to the CS patient is his honesty. For the patient with organic brain syndrome, George Zerr has the facility to teach with exceptional clarity patients whose ability to learn is compromised. He is responsible for much of what I have learned regarding organic brain syndrome and the concept of chemical intoxication in CS.

Robert (Bob) Sinaiko, M.D., Allergist/Immunologist. I will never forget the feeling I had while placing the telephone receiver in its cradle after spending about two hours talking to this physician. Littering the table before me were many pieces of paper covered with disconnected lines of notes. Somehow Bob Sinaiko had learned that I was writing a book on chemical sensitivity. He had called to ask whether I'd like some help.

He taught me the role of neurotransmitters; the concept of self-quenching and self-perpetuating CS; the potential role for the intestine in immune function; the concepts of learned helplessness, immunomodulation, synchronicity; and the work of Besedovsky, to name a few. His generosity and concern have taught and touched me. He is a specialist with a generalist perspective, a very rare and essential quality.

Richard A. Nelson, M.D., Neurologist/Psychiatrist. In the state of Washington, there is a serious lack of neurologists who understand chemical poisoning with toxic encephalopathy. A chance referral from a CS patient caused me to contact this doctor to see whether he might meet my needs. Since travel is difficult for me, he agreed to travel to see me and other patients who shared the same need. His willingness to answer questions directly and his efforts to provide assistance to those who experienced chemical poisoning require an effort that few would be willing to spare. Yet the quality of patience and level of responsiveness demonstrated by this man are evidence of his attributes.

David Buscher, M.D., Environmental Medicine/Family Practice. David Buscher is devoted to helping patients improve when others might have given up on them or dismissed them to psychiatrists. He enjoys success with patients based not on blind risk-taking but rather on significant study, both with pioneers in the field and on his own, keeping up to date with the amazing amount of literature in the field. His review of this book significantly broadened my level of understanding of the environmental (clinical ecological) treatment. It is my conviction that history will show him to be exceptionally insightful.

Stephen A. Schacher, M.D., and Donald L. Dudley, M.D., of the Washington Institute of Neurosciences, Inc. A single word strikes me when my thoughts turn to these doctors—integrity. Why? They theorized that CS was psychogenic and that they could prove it by using their qEEG and evoked potentials computer equipment. Data gathered, however, convinced them otherwise. Preconceptions melted in understanding.

In addition to being impressed with their integrity I am deeply grateful to these doctors for patiently sharing with me an odyssey into the brain. Without talking to me as if I couldn't possibly understand, they spoke so I could. They showed me and permitted me to videotape the electrical peculiarities of my damaged brain as the mapped images were displayed on the screen. I could see my brain react to glue samples; my ears hearing visual electrical signals; my memory center receiving auditory information too late to be stored; and my hands and feet transmitting signals to the brain properly, where, once there, they bounced all around, never arriving at the motor cortex. No educational excursion, however well planned, could compare to the trip through the working of the brain I've had.

Instead of responding with puffed up pride, these doctors apologize that their technology is far from where it should be in terms of what is available with today's capability. This is ironic, though they fail to see it. Patients and doctors across the nation consider them to be on the cutting edge of understanding where CS is concerned. Because of their knowledge and wisdom thay are aware of what *could be* and are acutely aware of what *is*, and how unacceptable "is" is.

Pharmacists at Manhattan Pharmacy in the Normandy Park area. These patient, kind, helpful people provided assistance on numerous occasions, treating me as courteously as a paying customer, though I was there only for information. Their willingness to share gave me a better perspective on numbers of issues and a broader view of the subject than I would otherwise have had.

Third, there are several volunteers who have done a lot of work required to produce the manuscript. They are:

Ruth A. Matthews. Ruth saw the effect that using the computer was having on me. She offered to take over computer input and output, including editing. Without her early observation and willingness to take over, the manuscript could not have been produced. Ruth also took on the task of developing some of the charts to be used in the book. Her willing constancy through production has been a treasure.

Janet Blessing. At precisely the moment when I began to face the need for extensive library research and the frustration over my own ability to drive to the university medical library or handle the chemicals I could encounter there, Janet asked whether she might be of help in that capacity. Janet understands CS and has the ability not only to do the research I needed but also to do it exceptionally well and in a timely manner. To understand CS requires piecing together data from a number of academic specializations. The Bibliography at the end of the book is largely a result of her excellent effort.

Molly Gerhard. I had the pleasure of meeting Molly in one of the most unique work situations anyone could hope to find. It was called, in 1975, the Training Center of the U.S. Civil Service Commission. The Training Center was composed of wall-to-wall super-professionals whose teamwork had to be experienced to be understood. Becoming part of the Training Center was becoming part of a family, and the relationship continues despite changes in time and space. I've worked in academia, business, and government. Nowhere have I seen any more cohesive group of people with more creative energy, more professionalism, more acutely honed skills, or more capacity to enjoy life.

In writing the first five chapters of this book, I discovered to my horror how chemical poisoning had caused my writing skills to deteriorate. Following a significant toxic exposure and additional brain damage, poor ability to write became inability. The sixth chapter had not been written. I realized that it would be necessary to find a writer. Of all the people I've ever known, I knew immediately where the best writers were: the old Training Center family. I also knew the one I'd choose—Molly, the best. I contacted the Training Center and asked for a volunteer. I couldn't pay. I couldn't work, yet I called on people who were employed and led busy lives. A phone call: Molly had volunteered.

Today Molly is a busy self-employed consultant (Gerhard Consulting Services). She agreed to take on Chapter 6. Molly has excellent ability to listen and absorb technical information, quickly organize that technical information, and communicate it clearly and concisely to a variety of audiences. Molly used her skills and abilities to gather information from my disorganized brain in such a compassionate manner as to make me feel no different from when we worked together. Few could have done what she did in such a supportive manner, expecting nothing in return.

Lois (Patti) Matthews. Patti is my mother. I live in her home. She stood by me and observed as the chronic, low level toxic did its damage; as the toxic reached an intolerable level and exploded; as I sought answers about what had happened; and as I struggled to cope with massive changes in my life. Anyone writing a book today needs a computer. She supplied it. She has spent countless hours poring over my writing, helping me organize distracted thoughts and cut out the extraneous. She will courageously point out from time to time that I need to "defocus" from CS. She can detect the signs of chemical intoxication usually before I am aware of them, and she will discourage my driving under the influence. Her home is a haven from exposure to offending chemicals. As a consequence of her thoughtful, loving caregiving, I have been spared the additional stress experienced by many CS patients of having conflict with loved ones.

My *family* overall. I have a unique family. We are all very close and very different and fiercely mutually supportive. In putting this book together my independent cognitive function has been inadequate to synthesize the many pieces of data I had gathered. Family members consistently pulled together and talked through the information analytically until data began to take form. Acknowledgment and gratitude go to Patti, Ruth, Randy, Dave, and Emelia.

Fourth, there are numbers of individuals who have provided the valuable service of permitting me to perform some formative testing. During the development of the manuscript, I sought people with special areas of expertise and those who had prior knowledge of CS as well as those who knew nothing about it. I sought readers who would feel comfortable providing severe critiques in order to improve the quality of the manuscript.

In addition to many of those already mentioned, the following individuals have made significant contributions in this area: Cynthia Wilson, Philip Dickey, Kimberly Haynie, Mildred Chapman, Katharine Bradley, Emelyn Markwith, Terri Lindhag.

Fifth, there are others who provided critical information and assistance. They are Cha Smith, Ann Liu, Leonard Schacter, John Peard, Stephanie Clough, Dr. Peter Breysse, Dr. Jack Thrasher, Keith Vaughan, Wendy Wendlandt, Will Schroeder, Fred Nelson, Rhonda Burtnett, Ken Campbell, Janiel Edmondson, Carolyn Eichler, Mari Ellingsen, Kathleen George, Richard Knights, Bill Hirzy, Diane Rayner, Debbie Ringman, Georgia Tull, Patricia Way, Robin Wells, Faye Schrum, Billie McCormick, Cheryl Quackenbush, Barry Wise, Steve Erickson, Ellie Sanders, Molly Jensen, Joe Fix, scores of government officials dealing with the effects of low level toxics, various senators and representatives in the U.S. Congress, physicians in the Occupational Medicine Program at Harborview Hospital, and local television and newspaper reporters.

Last but certainly not least, *Matthew S. Sweeting, Attorney at Law.* I spent unbelievable effort to find an attorney willing to take my case, because my worker's compensation entitlements are federal. I could not find one personal injury attorney in Seattle, Washington, who would take my case. Finally, a referral from a Seattle attorney led me to Matthew S. Sweeting in Tacoma. In contrast to the legal experience of numbers of other CS patients, I talk to my attorney, not a paralegal. He knows who I am and the status of my case without having to dig through files. His level of responsiveness is unheard of. I didn't have to ask: When I told him a federal investigator was coming to my house, he told me he would be there, and he was. When he receives information, my copy is in my mailbox the following day. He handles a wide variety of "chemical cases" for those seeking relief through entitlements and litigation. When I asked him why he takes these financially unrewarding cases he gave the same answer as doctors give for why they take CS patients: "Somebody has to do it."

Chemical sensitivity has been an incredible and often bizarre journey for the first couple of years. I'd like very much to return home at this point. Such is the experience with chronic illness. Yet the acknowledgments above are evidence of how all that occurs in life has value. Only a few of the people named above would I have had the opportunity or pleasure to meet had I not become ill. Chances of my coming to learn any of the information presented here would have been virtually nonexistent. The awe in discovery of the amazing structure and function of the human system would not have been open to me. The joy of being able to contribute in any but the most superficial way to other human life would have been denied me in the absence of CS.

1. What Is Chemical Sensitivity?

Chemical sensitivity as used in this book refers to a disease of compromised systemic integrity leaving the individual sensitive to one or more chemicals. This sensitivity appears to have primary effect on the immune, endocrine, and or central nervous systems with secondary effect on many other systems (e.g. respiratory, gastrointestinal, reproductive, and so on). Included in the scope of chemical sensitivity are immune system–related asthma, dermatitis, edema, vasculitis, and other problems. Endocrine-related symptoms may include weight loss or gain, temperature decrease, or sweating problems. Nervous system–related problems consist of organic brain syndromes such as toxic encephalopathy or false neurotransmission or peripheral neuropathy.

Toxic exposure, one of the causes of chemical sensitivity, is not the only cause of these problems, and that fact complicates the medical picture. One may, for example, develop asthma from temperature change (e.g. sudden cold weather) or from exercise. One may also develop asthma from exposure to a toxic chemical. Decreased intellectual function may result from a severe head wound, or the same condition may result from exposure to a toxic. Unless the cause of the medical condition is identified, treatment may make the condition worse. An individual who develops exercise-related asthma may, for example, be able to continue working in the same job. An individual who develops toxic encephalopathy or asthma from working in an office, where the condition is a result of contact with one or more chemicals, may not be able to work in that environment. If the disease progresses, the person may not be able to work in any environment.

Use of the term chemical sensitivity will no doubt raise some eyebrows. Some purists would prefer that the term be reserved for those instances in which a single chemical causes a sensitivity. *Multiple chemical sensitivity syndrome* is preferred by some to illustrate the situation in which more than one chemical causes a set of symptoms and the set of chemicals grows as time passes. Others object to the word *chemical* as too restrictive, failing to account for other elements which may relate to this disease (e.g. environmental stresses, electrical phenomena).

Chemical sensitivity is used in this book because the term does not align with any current specific set of theories and can be used to include all of them. Chemical sensitivity issues have already divided too many people who should be working together. Adding to that division by arguing about terminology is not expedient.

There are four words used by experts to describe medical conditions: *disease, disorder, illness,* and *syndrome. Taber's Cyclopedic Medical Dictionary,* 16th edition, makes the following distinctions:

disease—a pathological condition of the body that presents a group of clinical signs and symptoms and laboratory findings peculiar to it and that sets the condition apart as an abnormal entity differing from other normal or pathological body states (page 513).

disorder—a pathological condition of the mind or body (page 519).

illness—state of being sick (page 892) with sick defined as not well (page 1675).

syndrome—a group of symptoms and signs of disordered function related to one another by means of some anatomic, physiologic or biochemical peculiarity (page 1804).

There are connotations associated with each term. Disease, for example, implies a physical condition resulting from a pathogen (defined on page 1339 as "a microorganism or substance capable of producing disease which causes structural or functional physical change"). Disorder, on the other hand, has come to imply a mental condition such as a personality disorder. The term illness often suggests a prolonged ailment. Syndrome suggests that the cause of an illness is imprecise but provides a framework for investigating it.

These definitions and their connotations are not consistently used. For example, sometimes disease and disorder are used interchangeably. Sometimes illness is used interchangeably with both disease and disorder. Depending on medical practice, the mind and body may be viewed as an integrated entity or as separate elements. A family practitioner may tend to have a more "whole person" view than a cardiologist or psychiatrist. This is not a rule, but rather a tendency.

The term disease is used for CS in this book. For some readers, the choice of the word may provoke a response, depending on one's perspective. In the author's opinion the cause, effect, and treatment of CS are as clear as some other medical conditions which currently meet criteria for classification as disease (as opposed to syndrome). For example, since the 1960s it has been accepted that alcohol is directly toxic to the liver. Alcoholic liver disease is recognized. Compare this with the classic CS disease profile: (1) *cause,* toxic exposure; (2) *effect,* liver damage and impaired mental function; and (3) *treatment,* avoidance of the toxic substance.

One expert has described CS as an illness within an illness. It is the opinion of the author that CS is a *macro-disease* under which numbers of presently identified diseases and disorders may be classified as subordinate elements. This perspective has its roots in systematic organizational analysis principles which have been applied to this medical condition. It compares the organization with the human, a functioning integrated single organism in which mind and body cannot be separated and within which there are numbers of integrated systems and subsystems. In this view some instances of CS have a known causal factor, exposure to one or more toxics. The term macro-disease has been used because there are associated systemic structural and functional effects as a result of toxic exposure. Medical diagnoses of toxic-induced asthma, organic brain syndrome (toxic encephalopathy), neuropathy, skin sensitivity, and so on are subordinate to the macro-disease, not independent elements.

Many of the other terms associated with CS describe sources of toxic exposure, potential mechanisms, and so on:

sick building syndrome
tight building syndrome
20th century disease
chemical poisoning
chronic (toxic substance) inhalation
total allergy syndrome
organic brain syndrome
environmental illness
multiple chemical sensitivity syndrome
environmental hypersensitivity
ecological illness
chemical hypersensitivity
universal reactors (patients)
toxic encephalopathy
chronic immune system activation

The list itself offers a picture of current knowledge. What is known generates opposing views. It is the purpose of this chapter to consolidate what is generally accepted regarding the disease into two parts: first, answers to basic questions for the general reader, and second, a simplified medical overview of the disease for individuals who want a clearer picture of the immune system, an understanding of the mental and emotional aspects, and an idea of the systemic implications of CS.

Chemical sensitivity is a serious disease because it can cause permanent disability. It is serious because less than 2 percent of the medical profession is trained to recognize it.[449]* It is serious because, while it is totally preventable, there is no cure. It is serious because numbers of very sick people are being made sicker through lack of understanding.

A Basic Introduction to CS

When people want to know about a disease, certain questions come to mind: (1) What is it? (2) What causes it? (3) What are the signs and symptoms? (4) How do you find out for certain whether you have it? (5) How do you cure it? These are the same questions doctors ask.

What Is CS?

Chemical sensitivity is an acquired disease characterized by recurrent multi-system symptoms in response to a variety of unrelated chemicals at doses below levels assumed to be safe for the general public. The symptoms recur at increasingly lower levels of exposure over time, and the numbers of substances which trigger the response increase over time. The disease is not new; but it is only now receiving recognition.

Here's an illustration. Bill, age 39, an automotive painter, has recurring headaches on the job, most frequently during the winter months. He develops nausea, occasionally vomits, and becomes disoriented or confused. On weekends he improves. He gets worse during the week. In addition, he becomes infuriated when his wife uses perfume and his daughter sprays her hair. He does not want fabric softener used on clothes he's going to wear. His consumption of alcohol has increased significantly because it seems to be the only way to get rid of the headaches. His family life is deteriorating. After suffering a tough divorce, being fired from his job, and becoming sick from what feels like flu for years, Bill is diagnosed as chemically poisoned with chemical sensitivity as a result.

What Causes CS?

In many (but not all) cases the simple answer to this question is toxic chemicals, often resulting from air pollution. In Bill's case, the cause was chemicals used in his work (paint, solvents, and so on). He became worse in winter because the concentration of chemicals was higher when the doors were closed and the shop was heated. To understand the cause of chemical poisoning, some background is necessary.

**References are to numbered items in the Bibliography.*

First, a word about human need. The average adult can live for five weeks without food, five days without water, five minutes without air. The air we breathe is critical to survival: the average adult human at rest requires 8,640 liters of fresh air a day.

Typically, CS begins with air pollution—both indoors and outside. People come in contact with toxic substances through the air in their homes, their workplaces, their schools, and their vehicles, as well as outdoors. Problems with the air are not new. There are natural sources of air pollution, such as volcanoes, asphalt pits, and naturally occurring fires. However, these sources pale beside the contributions of mankind. Probably the earliest form of human-made air pollution came from heating and cooking with wood fires. The price of warmth included gathering wood, making fire, and breathing smoke.

The discovery and use of coal reduced the smoke, but added carbon monoxide to the air in poorly ventilated places. During the industrial revolution, the use of coal for heating and powering industry brought smoke indoors and outdoors, but sulfur and industrial aerosols were considered minor nuisances in light of enthusiasm for increased productivity. Nothing is different today except that the quantity and variety of pollutants have increased dramatically.

The air in a typical city today includes not only smoke but also a long list of chemicals which are acknowledged as having adverse health effects. To name a few:

arsenic—lung and skin cancer
nitric oxide—bronchitis
cadmium—kidney and lung damage
nickel—lung cancer
lead—brain damage, high blood pressure
chlorine—mucous membrane irritation
nitric acid—respiratory disease
silicon tetrafluoride—lung irritation
sulfur dioxide—obstruction of breathing
hydrogen sulfide—nausea, eye irritation
sulfuric acid—respiratory problems
hydrogen chloride—eye and lung irritation
benzene—leukemia
hydrogen fluoride—eye, skin, mucous membrane irritation
mercury—tremors and behavioral problems
ozone—eye irritation, aggravation of asthma
peroxyacetyl nitrate—eye irritation, aggravation of asthma
carbon monoxide—heart damage
hydrocarbons—nervous system and skin irritation
nitrous acid—respiratory disorders
formaldehyde—eye, nose, skin irritation
manganese—may contribute to Parkinson's disease

These chemicals are routinely found, but by no means are they all the air contains. There are more than 65,000 toxic chemicals in the U.S. Environmental Protection Agency's inventory, with about 1,500 new ones proposed annually.[709] Almost all of these chemicals have unknown effects on human health. Nothing is known regarding the synergistic effects they may have. Testing, when done at all, is done by manufacturers on white male subjects. There are chemicals with extreme toxicity such as dioxins or furans. Dioxins are so toxic that their presence detected at a millionth of a gram is cause for panic among air quality specialists. Where do they originate? The answer is incineration. We contribute by burning garbage and by driving our vehicles.

Concern over air pollution began with odor, not contamination. This is understandable, though insufficient. The sense of smell is an early warning system. People avoid what smells bad. Unfortunately, there are toxic substances which have no odor (odor is added to the natural gas in homes so its presence can be identified) and some which are thought to smell good (perfumes containing neurotoxic substances[454]). Our tendency is to ignore the existence of substances we cannot smell or delight in those with a pleasant scent. That tendency can prove harmful, if not deadly.[451,454]

Outdoor air moves with the wind. One should recognize that indoor air is far more polluted than outdoor air.* In the name of conservation of energy resources, indoor environments are engineered to reduce the entry and exit of air. Unwittingly, people use toxic substances indoors, keeping them over time, which enhances the poisonous effects by accumulation. It's easy to complain about environmentalists crying out doom and gloom, until exposure to toxic carpet glue and perfume cause permanent disability, which prevents the disabled from entering the work environment due to aggravation of symptoms from asthma to brain damage.

Air pollution is not the only pollution problem. The American public likes produce from fields where spraying pesticides is common. Yet those pesticides contaminate those who breathe the spray, get it on their skin, or eat residue; further, in some parts of the country the water supply is being contaminated by water runoff from sprayed fields. Transportation is adding significantly to the pollution of indoor as well as outdoor air. Air intakes for buildings can bring in vehicle exhaust if they are located near roads. Parking garages built under buildings can contribute exhaust and

**The following items in the Bibliography deal with indoor air quality: 30, 84, 91, 96, 111, 156, 169, 186, 194, 209, 216, 224, 225, 230, 238, 241, 242, 252, 255, 288, 328, 339, 346, 360, 399, 401, 410, 411, 414, 417, 431, 432, 433, 451, 452, 453, 455, 456, 459, 490, 501, 510, 563, 582, 595, 596, 601, 625, 631, 647, 659, 660, 698, 699, 705, 706, 707, 708, 710, 726, 728, 729, 730, 731, 732, 733, 734, 735, 737, 741, 755, 756, 757, 758, 761, 763, 781, 791, 798.*

chemicals from cooling vehicles to the building environment. Numbers of homes are built on a split level with bedrooms right over the garage. Occupants of the bedrooms can have difficulty sleeping, develop headaches or sinus trouble, and never connect the problem with the vapors and gasses emitted from their cooling vehicles, until they become so ill that they begin the long task of identifying the cause.

How has our environment become so dangerously polluted? The main cause is not greedy industrialists nor irresponsible governments, but a thought process, common to humankind, *gradualistic deterioration of human reason*. By this distorted thinking, people come to accept problems such as air pollution as inevitable byproducts of progress. Convinced that such problems are insurmountable, they go on to embrace the very dangers that surround them. Who will be the first to stop driving automobiles, or to part willingly with financial resources to build a clean transportation system? Who will spend hours digging weeds instead of spraying them with toxic chemicals?

News of environmental catastrophe, such as the 1986 meltdown at the Chernobyl nuclear reactor, may frighten people out of this thought process for a time—but only for a time. Smaller instances of environmental poisoning are rarely even considered worth mentioning by the news media. A group of children poisoned by a toxic in a small town preschool goes unreported. The retired Smith family whose mobile home formaldehyde emissions caused permanent illness and destroyed a lifetime of financial savings is not newsworthy. Who hears about John, a strong blue-collar worker, who walked down a country lane one afternoon and breathed herbicide sprayed along the roadside, permanently destroying his central nervous system? Nobody hears about the small chronic, low level poisonings.* Yet there is a virtual army of disabled individuals suffering from chemical sensitivity across our nation. One federal estimate[710] put the percentage of such individuals in the United States population at 15. The Census Bureau's 1991 data (Press Release No. CB91-07, *U.S. Population Up Nearly Two-Thirds in 40 Years*) numbers the United States population at 248,709,873. Fifteen percent, if that percent is accurate, would be 37,306,481 people with heightened sensitivity to chemicals.

Coal miners might recognize the value of individuals with chemical sensitivity. They have always been acutely aware of the need for air. They understand the danger of vapors. In times past, before other warning systems were developed, they carried canaries into the mines with them. Canaries have a known susceptibility to toxic inhalants. If a canary died, it was time to get out of the mine. Today's canaries are human. They are

**The following items in the Bibliography explore the subject of low level toxics: 32, 165, 183, 202, 432, 578, 588, 591, 600, 641, 649, 719.*

people who have developed CS through toxic exposure. They serve as today's early warning system in what are thought to be safe environments.

What Are the Signs and Symptoms of CS?

For any disease there are characteristic signs and symptoms. However, unlike measles or mumps, the signs of CS vary from individual to individual. To understand how this is possible, consider two identical houses whose roofs are exposed to heavy rains. Both roofs spring a leak, but the water enters each house in a different way—in one case running across a ceiling beam, in the other traveling down a vertical two-by-four. The results will be different, but both homes will be damaged. In the same way, within the same exposing conditions, one CS patient may suffer from severe gastrointestinal problems and brain damage, while another experiences breathing difficulty, skin rashes, and tremors, and a third is troubled by systemic edema, anxiety, and depression.

As a consequence, it is not possible to say that if a person meets four of a set of five symptom criteria, the diagnosis is chemical sensitivity. Instead, there are some signs and symptoms that point to a diagnosis. Generally, it is expected that more than one body system will be affected, but that expectation is more hypothesis than fact. Some typical initial chemical sensitivity symptoms are:

feeling sick
difficulty sleeping
dizziness or fainting
memory lapses
sore, itchy, burning eyes
running, stopped up, congested, burning nose
dry, burning throat
shortness of breath
asthma
excessive mucus
upset stomach
diarrhea
menstrual problems
muscle aches and pains
swollen extremities
extreme fatigue
poor concentration
ringing ears
headaches
vision problems
nosebleeds

voice problems
pain or burning in chest
cough
vomiting
nausea
cramps
blood in urine
joint pain
irritation, depression, anxiety
organic brain syndrome (includes altered sensory and behavioral function, interference with the integration of normal thought, impaired consciousness, altered motor function)

If a person is suffering from some combination of these symptoms, the next step toward diagnosing CS is to determine whether there has been a possible *toxic exposure.* This event may be a single significant (acute) exposure, such as a massive ammonia leak in an ice cream factory; or it may be chronic low level exposure, such as continuous formaldehyde release from particle board construction in a mobile home. Chronic low level exposure comes from repeated contact with toxics such as are encountered in the workplace or home. The Environmental Protection Agency (EPA) has set levels for indoor toxics on a handful of chemicals. The EPA has known for several years that these levels are not safe for everyone in the population, and they have identified sick building syndromes and chemical sensitivity problems arising at levels much lower than what has been considered safe.[741] Whether the exposure is acute or chronic, toxic substances can reach excessive levels in the human body, resulting in poisoning. *Poisoning* simply means that, somewhere, normal physiological function has been affected by the toxic substance. It is important to recognize that there is a difference between *irritation* and poisoning. Some individuals find certain substances irritating. An irritant may cause a considerable amount of discomfort without causing permanent damage. For example, a person filling an automobile tank may find that skin contact with gasoline causes an irritation which passes in a brief time. A person with chemical sensitivity to gasoline should never fill a tank, because the fumes can cause immediate intoxication, rendering the individual disoriented, unable to see, or unconscious, and increasing the severity of brain damage. Driving afterward would be equivalent to driving while intoxicated.

The poisoned individual may experience the development of an *abnormal, activated immune system.* The immune system is designed to protect the body from bacteria, viruses, fungi, and particulates (small particles such as dust or pollen grains). There are numbers of substances in the body that work to provide protection. These substances are highly activated in the presence of toxic exposure, though the system design leaves some protection lacking in that area. Eventually the activated immune system will become suppressed. This overly active immune system is identified by blood tests, usually ordered because of (1) visible dysfunction in one or more body systems, or (2) appearance of sets of symptoms.

The poisoned individual also may develop *autoantibodies*. This development can result in autoimmunity, a disease in which the antibodies designed to protect the human body fail to recognize parts of the body as self. Essentially, autoimmunity is an attack on the body by substances designed for its protection.

Once an individual has become chemically sensitive, lower and lower levels of contact with the toxic substance will set off the reaction. In addition to the substance(s) responsible for the initial poisoning, the individual may find increasing numbers of substances intolerable. This is the *spreading phenomenon*. These substances, which once could have been tolerated, generate the same symptoms which the initial poisoning caused. For example, Lisa, who was poisoned by formaldehyde in a mobile home, discovers that a number of drugs prescribed for her prior to the poisoning now cause her difficulty. Pharmaceutical research shows her that some drugs contain formaldehyde in minute amounts in the binding substance that holds the medicine together. That accounts for her adverse reactions to medicine containing formaldehyde, but does nothing to explain why she becomes seriously disoriented when in the presence of ammonia.

Chemical sensitive patients experience *compromised systemic integrity*. Any system may be compromised, but the two which receive significant focus in CS research are the immunologic and nervous systems. Patients can be grouped into three large classifications based on these systems: (1) those with immune system–related problems, (2) those with nervous system–related problems, and (3) those with both. Most CS patient symptoms can be tied directly or indirectly to one of these systems. For example, bloodwork during exposure on the patient with chemical-induced asthma will demonstrate an immunologic signature. Positron-emission tomography (PET) scans on a patient suffering memory loss can demonstrate the metabolic anomalies of the toxic encephalopathy in the area of the brain that processes memory activity.

For a diagnosis of CS, then, one would need to have had exposure to toxic chemicals, have signs and symptoms characteristic of chemical poisoning, and have the symptoms recur from reexposure either to a single chemical or a widening array of chemicals. No one but a physician or clinical psychologist, clinical neuropsychologist, or toxicologist can diagnose the disease, and they have to have some form of training to recognize it. A person may have CS and his doctor may not recognize it. Fewer than 2 percent of practicing physicians have formal training to recognize CS.

How Do You Find Out for Certain Whether You Have CS?

Since so few physicians are trained to recognize CS, it is not surprising that some patients report seeing 30 or more doctors prior to diagnosis. Knowledgeable orthodox physicians are hard to find. The experts quoted in Appendix C may be able to direct a person who may be chemically sensitive to a diagnostician.

Telephone directory listings of environmental medicine practitioners, allergists or immunologists, clinical psychologists or neuropsychologists, neurologists, or toxicologists may be helpful. It would be wise in any event for the prospective patient to call the doctor's office and ask for his or her experience with toxic exposure patients prior to making an appointment. Additional useful information can be gleaned from talking to CS patients.

Standard workup for chemical sensitivity involves taking an extensive history. A doctor may have the patient fill out a very lengthy questionnaire.

If the exposure is tied to a place (work environment, home, school) the chemical sensitive should expect trials of putting him in the location and removing him from it, while the doctor observes responses. Blood tests are routinely performed to illustrate the immune system profile, identify possible toxic exposure, and rule out other causes of symptoms. To be effective, blood tests need to be done during exposure. The specific set of symptoms is scrutinized. Neurological and psychological tests may be part of the initial set of exams. It may be necessary to have numerous physical and psychological tests.

After gathering as much data as possible, the doctor will give the diagnosis—that is, his or her opinion of whether CS is indeed the problem.

How Do You Cure CS?

At the present time, there is no cure for chemical sensitivity. The standard treatment for CS is to avoid exposure. For some people that means disability retirement or living on worker's compensation or social security or welfare. For some it means living on the street.

Because of widespread lack of understanding it can be said that the chemical sensitive is often a problem patient with a persistent problem treated by problem physicians and surrounded by problem people.

A Medical Overview of CS

To understand CS more fully, three areas of knowledge are important. The first is an understanding of the immunological response and what can go wrong; the second is a grasp of the difference between functional brain disorders and organic brain syndrome (toxic encephalopathy); and the third is familiarity with some basic information about the systemic implications of CS.

The Normal Immunological Response

In order to understand what happens to a chemical sensitive, it is helpful first to understand the normal immunological response. However, because even the experts know only the rudiments of the complex system that protects us from disease, the following discussion does not pretend to cover every detail. It does reflect current understanding, and it should be kept in mind that as understanding grows, some of this information may be subject to change.

The immune system response is designed to protect the body against invasion by foreign bodies (or *antigens*) such as bacteria, fungi, viruses, and particulates. (Particulates are tiny bodies such as dust or pollen grains.) The immunological response is not designed to protect against man-made toxic chemical substances, despite the fact that it often does so.

The normal immunological response includes three phases, or lines of defense. (See Appendix A for chart.)

• First Line of Defense

The first line of defense is the skin, which protects against penetration, and chemicals in the respiratory, gastrointestinal, and genitourinary tracts which destroy invaders.

When a foreign body, such as pollen or a substance from an insect bite, enters the body, one of the reactions in the first line of defense is that the invading antigen (foreign substance) activates *mast cells* in the connective tissue. Connective tissue is mucous, fibrous, reticular, adipose, cartilage, or bone tissue. Mast cells release *heparin*, which inhibits coagulation. They also release *histamine*, *prostaglandins*, and *leukotrienes*. These highly active chemicals, called *mediators*, have a systemic effect. That means these chemicals affect whole systems (respiratory, gastrointestinal, and so on).

• Second Line of Defense

Once the first line of defense is breached, the next level of defense our bodies provide consists of four components:

1. *Acute phase reactants.* These are chemicals which appear in the blood following an acute event, such as contracting an infectious disease. They are responsible for making us feel the symptoms of flu.

2. *Phagocytic cells. Microphages* eat bacteria. *Macrophages* eat dead tissue, cells, and particulates. *Histiocytes* eat particulates.

3. *Killer cells,* which seek and destroy cancer and cells affected by viruses and bacteria.

4. *Complement.* Proteins that appear in the blood to help burst and phagocytize invaders.

• Third Line of Defense—Full Blown Immune Response

The first and second lines of defense can be breached for two major reasons: (1) the phagocyte cannot grasp the invader, or (2) the foreign body passes undetected by the complement system. If the first and second lines of defense are breached, the body is prepared with two additional defenses: the *humoral immune response,* and the *cellular immune response.*

The humoral immune response originates in bone marrow and lymph. It is generated by the *B lymphocytes,* a type of supply center producing antibodies. Antibodies have three functions: (1) to bind the phagocyte to the invader; (2) to activate the complement system; and (3) to remember the invader, in order to provide life-long immunity.

There are five antibodies:

IgA—prevents invasion through bowel and salivary glands.

IgM—is the first antibody produced after exposure (and it is eventually replaced by IgG). After exposure, IgM may remain in blood for about a year.

IgG—provides long-term protection. After exposure, IgG remains in blood for several years.

IgE—produced in response to antigens, it is the classic allergic reaction. After exposure IgE remains in blood for about two weeks.

IgD—function unknown.

The cellular immune response originates in the thymus, circulates in blood, and settles in the spleen and lymph nodes in this manner:

1. A macrophage captures an antigen and presents it to a *T lymphocyte,* called a *T helper cell.* The macrophage releases a chemical called *interleukin 1.*

2. Interleukin 1 stimulates the T helper cell to produce *interleukin 2.*

3. Interleukin 2 stimulates the production of more T helper cells, which produce more interleukin 2. The T helper cells also produce *lymphokines*. Lymphokines are chemicals that serve a communication function between lymphocytes. That communication function is similar to telephone connections. When lymphokines are generated, the communication is for a full blown immune response.

4. Lymphokines stimulate B cells to change into antibody-producing cells. This is comparable to a call for reinforcements. The immune system is highly activated at this point.

5. Other lymphokines change some of the T lymphocytes into *cytotoxic T cells,* which attack the invader with the aid of complement.

• Cessation of the Immune Response

Chemical poisoning activates the immune response to its full level of activity. The activated immune response is complex, and it would appear that it could go on and on, until the human body was full of internally generated substances. Fortunately, there is a way to turn off the reaction. It is not clear, but the present theory is that either a dying invader or the T helper cells activate a special T cell, called the *T suppressor cell.* The T suppressor cell inhibits the macrophage–T helper cell reaction and turns off the immune response.

What Can Go Wrong with the Normal Immune Response

The immune system can elicit four medically recognized hypersensitive reactions, occurring at any of the three levels of defense. The term *hypersensitive* in some views means extra sensitive; however, when discussing the illness of chemical sensitivity, the terms sensitivity and hypersensitivity are interchangeable. As has already been explained, CS occurs at increasingly lower levels of exposure. There is no line of demarcation for sensitive and hypersensitive reactions. A chemical sensitive could have any of the following reactions:

• Type 1 Hypersensitive Reaction

This is the acute reaction described by various names including immediate type, classic allergy, atopic, reaginic, anaphylactic, or IgE mediated reactions.

Allergy is viewed as (1) antibody-antigen reaction to substances such as pollen, mold, dust, insect stings, and so on, occurring in the third line of defense, and (2) the result of local or systemic release of highly active chemicals called mediators, examples of which are histamine, prostaglandins, and leukotrienes, occurring in the first line of defense. In its attempt to deal with toxic chemical exposure, the human body may initiate this hypersensitive reaction to the chemical.

The release of histamine in the first line of defense can create a number of physical responses:

It dilates capillaries, arteries, and cerebral vessels, leading to a pooling of blood and hypotension.
It increases capillary permeability.
It leads to bronchoconstriction.
It increases gastrointestinal motility, felt as abdominal cramping or pain.
It increases salivary and bronchial gland secretions.
It stimulates catecholamine secretion (epinephrine and norepinephrine), which affects the nervous and cardiovascular systems, metabolic rate, temperature, and smooth muscle.
It causes itching.
It increases heart rate, contractility, and coronary blood flow.
It stimulates gastric acid secretions.

Not only is there substantial immediate response in the first line of defense, but also there is a late phase response that is significant with some conditions such as asthma. (The late phase response should not be confused with the Type 4 Hypersensitive Reaction.) The late phase response is an inflammatory process, influenced by white blood cells called *eosinophils* and *neutrophils*, which may follow the immediate response by 2 to 12 hours and continue on for days, weeks, or months, because it tends to self-perpetuate. The inflammatory process has four stages:

1. *Inflammation*—response to cellular injury marked by capillary dilation, leukocytic (white blood cell) infiltration, redness, heat, and pain for the purpose of eliminating noxious agents and damaged tissue.
2. *Edema*—development of excess fluid accumulation.
3. *Fibrosis*—development of tissue which can be separated into fibers, such as scar tissue.
4. *Necrosis*—death of living tissue.

Release of mediators in the first line of defense includes the following responses: Prostaglandin PGA_1 primarily affects the cardiovascular system; PGE_1, the reproductive system, gastrointestinal tract, respiratory system, and immune system; and leukotrienes, the gastrointestinal tract, skin or the respiratory system.

The most critical reaction is the systemic or anaphylactic reaction. Japanese research in the mid-1980s identified the trigger of almost all of these reactions as the release of leukotrienes from bronchial tissue.[72] Leukotrienes circulate in the blood of patients undergoing asthma attacks, and they are found in lung fluid of patients with chronic bronchitis. Leukotrienes can cause contractile responses.

• Type 2 Hypersensitive Reaction, or Autoimmunity

This reaction is for the destruction of invading bacteria. When it goes wrong, it results in the production of antibodies to the body itself. The reaction may result from the cleanup by macrophages of damaged body cells. It occurs in the second and third lines of defense. A part of a liver or stomach cell, damaged by a toxic, may be mistaken by a macrophage as being foreign. Having autoantibodies is not an indicator of active autoimmune disease. Disease occurs when autoantibodies begin acting on misinformation and destroying parts of the body (autoimmunity), where the body fails to recognize self as self and begins a destructive process. A person who has autoantibodies present should be monitored to determine whether autoimmune disease potential becomes active disease. This hypersensitivity reaction is called cytotoxic, cell-stimulating, antibody-dependent cytotoxicity, or cytolytic complement-dependent cytotoxicity.

• Type 3 Hypersensitive Reaction

This reaction, occurring in the second and third lines of defense, involves the joining of antibody, antigen, and complement (or *immune complexes*). When production exceeds the rate of removal from the body, immune complexes can be deposited in the lung, kidney, eye, and brain. When this occurs, there is immunological disease. Names for this reaction include immune complex–mediated, soluble complex, or toxic complex hypersensitivity reactions.

• Type 4 Hypersensitive Reaction

This reaction is the cellular immune reaction response, usually involving bacterial invaders. It occurs in the third line of defense. Unlike the three above which are mediated by antibodies, it is mediated by T lymphocytes, resulting in delayed hypersensitive reactions. This reaction is called cellular, cell-mediated, delayed, or tuberculin-type hypersensitivity.

Indicators of Chemical Sensitivity

No single test provides conclusive evidence of toxic exposure resulting in an activated immune system. There are medical tests that, taken together, serve as the indicators to demonstrate chemical sensitivity. Any blood test which clearly demonstrates toxic exposure is helpful. There are toxicological studies which can identify poisons from blood or fat. Antibody assays are helpful as a general screen, when the chemical is unknown.

Since chemical sensitives commonly have autoantibodies, an autoantibody profile should be run. This test does not show active disease, but rather the presence of autoantibodies. Demonstrated presence of one or more of these autoantibodies indicates an abnormal, activated immune system, which should be monitored to determine whether disease develops. Finally, study of the white blood cells provides evidence of an activated immune system. Abnormalities such as high white blood cell counts, high interleukin 1 or 2 levels, excessive T helper cells, high B lymphocytes, and high T cells describe a full blown immune system response characteristic of chemical poisoning. A low T cell level may demonstrate chronic, prolonged stress, more than a chronic, activated immune system; or, it could reflect immunosuppression in self-perpetuating CS.[4] One thing should be kept in mind. A CS patient who has been hunting for "the answer" for several years and has carefully avoided exposure through his own trial and error may not show the activated immune system profile in test data. *Lack of evidence does not necessarily signify lack of disease.* The immune system may have been suppressed and the appearance of normality may result from wise action on the part of the patient.

In addition to blood tests, environmental trials, history, etc., there are other tests that CS patients must take. These include magnetic resonance imaging (MRI) of the brain, colonoscopy, abdominal ultrasound, electroencephalogram (EEG), inhalation challenge, PET scan, brain topography (also called brain map or quantitative EEG [qEEG] with evoked potentials), and others. Rarely do the majority of tests show conclusive evidence, because many problems occur at sub-clinical levels. Where individuals have worked around toxic chemicals for a long time prior to removal, some MRIs will show brain atrophy or lesions. Some EEGs will evidence seizure activity. For most CS patients, however, MRIs and EEGs show nothing significant unless read by someone trained to recognize damage caused by toxics. When these fail to provide evidence and a central nervous system (CNS) problem is suspect, a PET scan may provide the metabolic evidence and brain topography is more likely to show electrical evidence. Inhalation challenge, though potentially dangerous, may show asthma symptoms. These tests by themselves do not necessarily indicate CS, but rather parts of the symptom complex. Lack of positive findings is not adequate to rule out CS. Some physicians will fail to diagnose CS if tests demonstrate some other known disease. As a result, the patient and physician end up with only part of the picture, and, if entitlement programs are involved, the CS patient may receive only partial payment or coverage for medical expenses.

A relatively reliable diagnosis of CS may be based on aberrant antibody data and fullblown immune response during exposure plus neuropsychological tests which point to organic brain syndrome secondary to chemical exposure or toxic encephalopathy. These are excellent predictors of metabolic and electrical dysfunction/damage.

Gunnar Heuser[453a] suggests "that appropriate tests of the central nervous system, peripheral nervous system, nose and sinuses, pulmonary function, T-cell subsets, chemical antibodies and autoimmunity be performed. If four of these seven systems show abnormality, the diagnosis of MCS is supported" (page 117). This plan would reduce the high cost of CS diagnosis.

Organic Brain Syndrome

One of the systems frequently affected by poisoning is the nervous system.* Additional exposure to intolerable substances will generate the symptoms. The significance with CNS involvement is that brain cells, unlike other body cells, do not regenerate. Damage to brain cells from toxic exposure causes brain damage and permanent loss of function. This damage, with its symptoms, is called toxic encephalopathy, a form of organic brain syndrome. It is caused by direct poisoning or collateral damage from the toxic. Toxics also affect peripheral nerves, in which case damage is usually detected in arms and legs, and damage such as slowed motor nerve conduction may be found in exposed asymptomatic individuals.

Direct poisoning involves entry of the toxic through the blood-brain barrier. Collateral damage can occur when the toxic breaks the blood-brain barrier by preferentially accumulating in brain endothelial cells (part of the blood-brain barrier). In this manner toxics can disturb normal barrier function, moving plasma into the brain's fluid spaces. Edema increases pressure in the brain, reducing blood flow and, consequently, oxygen and glucose. This action can produce irreversible brain damage and may explain why the number of chemicals causing problems grows. Other microenvironmental brain changes can be caused by toxics. (See Goldstein: "Lead Poisoning and Brain Cell Function." U.S. Health and Human Services *Environmental Health Perspectives*, Vol. 89, pages 91–94.)

The chemical sensitive whose nervous system is compromised may experience a wide variety of sensations (paresthesia) for which there is no clear explanation at present. Tingling in hands and feet, for example, is fairly common. Some people experience a feeling of shock, not as intense but similar to what can result from the release of static electricity when

* *The following items in the Bibliography include discussions of nervous system poisoning: 11, 25, 32, 47, 94, 120, 183, 202, 208, 209, 222, 249, 296, 313, 328, 358, 369, 378, 385, 413, 429, 430, 441, 443, 454, 520, 578, 586, 587, 600, 603, 617, 673, 697, 709, 711, 774, 796.*

crossing a carpet and grasping a door handle. Some people will experience tremors following chemical exposure; others may drop things as if their hands forget they hold something. Some may have difficulty walking.

Where some people with CS experience altered sensory states and motor function, others may react through altered behavioral function. A mature person, for example, who enters a doctor's office for examination, may find the interior of the tight building so offensive that he tries to open windows which cannot be opened or sits in a chair holding his head, using all his willpower not to smash objects he sees. It is easy to see why a physician unfamiliar with CS patients might give such a person a psychological or psychiatric profile reflecting depression, anxiety, and paranoia.

Difficulty integrating normal thought, distractibility, and impaired consciousness are characteristic of large numbers of chemical sensitives, many of whom have no idea that the problem exists, unless something they consider significant, such as fainting, occurs. Delay in recognition results from compensatory behaviors which the chemical sensitive may employ without conscious effort. For example, a person may choose to use a calculator, assuming it is for ease, accuracy, and speed, when the fact is that the ability to do simple math mentally has been compromised. A physician may cue in on observable evidence such as gross behavioral aberrations or significant mental lapses, but miss the subtle problems for which the patient is effectively compensating. Ability to remember short term is often compromised. Forgetting to remember even when calendars are carefully marked and monitored is common. The mind's eye may be temporarily blindfolded or permanently blinded; the mind's ear may be muted or deafened.

Because many of the symptoms above can result from either toxic exposure or a mental or emotional problem, neuropsychological assessment is very important. In fact, it would be wise to perform some of this testing when chemical exposure is suspected and CNS symptoms are not clearly presented. The reason for this testing is to prevent additional brain damage quickly, if it is occurring. Another reason is to identify the patient with functional (mental or emotional) problems as distinct from those with organic problems, because the treatment will be significantly different.

Here's an example of the potential difficulties in separating organic illness from functional problems. In one workplace, there were 35 individuals employed. There was toxic exposure involved in a manufacturing process. Of the 35 individuals, 12 became sick. The diagnosis in each case was flu, reflecting symptoms of headache, nausea, dizziness, and vomiting. Those who got the "flu" had it for months and months, until it was clear that the problem was not flu. After much investigation, a physician finally determined that the cause was toxic chemicals used in the manufacturing process. Thorough examination of the 12 sick employees demonstrated the classic chemical sensitivity profile of toxic exposure, poisoning, and activated immune system/toxic encephalopathy. In time three additional employees became ill. Two of these employees had chemical sensitivity; the third had developed symptoms but was not chemically sensitive. How could this be?

Once an environment has been shown to contain a poison, fear can surface. Fear is a very potent motivator. The individual who developed the symptoms without having the disease exhibited a condition termed *somatization*. The descriptive label for people who develop symptoms without illness is *symptomizer*. An illness of this nature is functional. This behavior is learned through fear motivation and can be unlearned. An individual with functional illness should not be removed from the workplace but rather treated through counseling. An individual with organic brain damage from toxic chemicals should be removed quickly to prevent further irreparable damage. In any environment where people have become poisoned—regardless of whether the levels show a hazard according to the figures issued by EPA—there should be an effort to eliminate the toxic through increasing ventilation or providing safety devices and assuring their use in that environment.

To further complicate the CS picture, it should be kept in mind that just because an individual has chemical sensitivity with toxic encephalopathy, that does not mean that functional mental or emotional illness is not also present. There is nothing to prevent both from occurring simultaneously. Organic brain syndrome can intensify the manifestation of functional illness. Also, chemical sensitives who have no CNS involvement may appear to have organic brain syndrome, when in fact the problem is one of personal history and unresolved problems.

The symptoms of actual organic brain syndrome can be extremely frightening when they begin to occur. Brain fog, a condition similar to what is experienced with anesthesia or alcohol intoxication, is a very common CNS reaction to intolerable chemicals. A person noted for exceptional organizational skills and punctuality may discover suddenly that he has driven his car mindlessly ten blocks beyond the turn-off for an appointment to which he is now late; such a discovery can be devastating. Add to this the rage a chemical sensitive may experience in the presence of perfume, toss in a little paresthesia, and if the individual has no idea what his problem is, chances are he will develop some functional problems. It should be kept in mind that organic brain syndrome can make communication difficult, because integration of normal thought may be a substantial problem. Trying to explain paresthesia to a physician is no easy task, and the simple effort may appear to demonstrate functional illness.

Fortunately, the attempt to sort through functional and organic problems is not as difficult as it may appear. A well-trained neuropsychologist, clinical psychologist, or psychiatrist can administer tests which provide a legitimate basis for medical diagnosis of organic brain syndrome or toxic encephalopathy. A pioneer in this field is Muriel Lezak at the Oregon Health Sciences University Department of Neurology. Her book *Neuropsychological Assessment*[369] deals with study of numbers of chemically exposed individuals and the performance on tests. Proper testing takes a substantial amount of time. It involves:

- Taking a detailed history
- Identifying the subject's reality contact
- Identifying the subject's motivation for performing well
- Determining whether the test scores are probable representations of actual abilities (severe exposure may lower scores; elimination of exposure may render them more accurate)
- Observing for the appearance of depression, anxiety, or symptom focus
- Observing for clues to malingering, if the disorder is a workplace issue
- Identifying whether verbal and math skills are intact
- Testing of:
  - Visuospatial abilities (looking for missing elements in pictures, sequencing pictures logically)
  - Attention and concentration
  - Learning and memory
  - Language
  - Conceptualization
  - Distractibility

To assure that the tests provide the best possible assessment, several may be administered to verify a set of results. Ideally, the testing should be terminated before the CS patient becomes fatigued, and resumed only when the subject is refreshed. No single test provides all required data. Organic brain syndrome is a diagnosis based on the profile generated by the entire set of tests. A battery of tests to diagnose organic brain syndrome (toxic encephalopathy) might include some of the following:

- Wechsler Adult Intelligence Scale—Revised (subtests give clues)
- Wechsler Memory Scale
- Gates-McGinitie reading tests
- Written Calculations
- Hooper Visual Organization Test
- Rey-Osterrieth Complex Figure Drawing Test
- Trail Making Tests A and B
- Sentence Repetition Test
- Visual Search Test
- Symbol Digit Modalities Test
- Digit Sequence Learning Test
- Short Story Recall Tests

Rey-Auditory Verbal Learning Test
Controlled Oral Association Test
Boston Naming Test
Figural Fluency Test
Category Test
Stroop Test (Dodrill)
Symptom Check List–90R
Nonstandardized tests of attention and concentration
Halstead-Reitan Battery
Luria-Nebraska Neuropsychological Battery

Compromised Systemic Integrity

One of the major medical considerations in analyzing disease is the mechanism by which it operates. The mechanism is vital, because it contains the key to treatment, control, and cure, if possible. Experts either deny that the CS mechanism has been identified at this time, or submit potential mechanisms tentatively. Because CS is a macro-disease with a multi-system symptom complex, it must be kept in mind that the mechanism must apply systematically and account for the disparate symptom patterns. In a systemic disease a single cause-effect may not be realistic. On the other hand, because the effects of CS do involve multi-system compromise, a single simple mechanism may be overlooked. Study of CS is hampered by the dilemma of not knowing whether one is involved with "finding a needle in the haystack" or "inability to see the forest for the trees." Whichever is the case, a specialist perspective is likely to inhibit identification of the compromise of systemic integrity.

Systems problems are characteristically solved by systems analysis. From a systems perspective, it can be said that there are diseases which self-quench and those which self-perpetuate. It might be said that measles is a self-quenching disease, whereas lung inflammation is frequently self-perpetuating. Acute illness may be classified as self-quenching, while chronic illness is classified as self-perpetuating.

To understand why one disease self-quenches while another self-perpetuates, an analogy may be helpful. Consider a pendulum: a mild swing causes some movement, but in short order the pendulum returns to the fixed point at rest. Swing the pendulum beyond the critical point while adding an appropriate mechanism, and it will continue to swing in a self-perpetuating manner until the device runs down. It may appear that this principle of physics has no direct application in biochemistry. Yet this very principle serves as the basis for the classification of acute as opposed to chronic illness.

When sensitivity to chemicals is recognized, it is classified as a self-perpetuating (chronic) illness. This book focuses on the chronic aspect of the disease, not the acute type. It is important, however, to recognize that there are certain instances in which sensitivity to chemicals appears in self-quenching form.

• Self-Quenching Sensitivity to Chemicals (Sick Building Syndrome)

It can be argued that sensitivity to chemicals accompanies any instance of immune system activation. It is not an uncommon aspect of the flu for certain foods to have a peculiar taste or for certain odors, normally pleasing or inoffensive, to become temporarily unpleasant. During pregnancy, it is not uncommon for a woman who normally can tolerate cigarette smoke to find suddenly that it causes nausea. Such symptoms disappear when the immune system is no longer activated; they are self-quenching.

Sick building syndrome (SBS) has the following symptoms: irritation of nasal passages, eyes, mucous membranes; lethargy or fatigue; dry skin; headaches.[288] Some lists also include difficulty concentrating, nausea, and dizziness. Sick building syndrome is self-quenching, while CS is self-perpetuating. Remove the worker with SBS from a sick building and he is likely to be able to work elsewhere. Remove a chemical sensitive from a sick building, and he may have difficulty getting home through the traffic exhaust. Sensitivity to chemicals at the self-quenching level is equivalent to a low level of arc in the pendulum swing, followed by the return of the pendulum to rest at the fixed point.

• Self-Perpetuating Sensitivity to Chemicals

Recognizing that sensitivity to chemicals can occur as a self-quenching illness in immune system activation raises a question. Returning to our analogy, what might cause a swing sufficient for the pendulum to reach a critical point of arc and change from self-quenching to self-perpetuating? Drs. Thrasher and Broughton in their book *The Poisoning of Our Homes and Workplaces*[692] focus on chronic immune system activation.

Whether it is through frequent infection, or the attempt of the body to accommodate toxic chemicals (for which defense is essentially lacking), or both, chronic immune system activation takes a toll on the body system. In the *New England Journal of Medicine* (March 8, 1990, Vol. 322, No. 10, pages 675–683), Mark Cullen indicates a potential relationship between multiple chemical sensitivity syndrome and chronic fatigue syndrome. This relationship has been anticipated by others[469a], including numbers of chronic fatigue and chemical sensitive people. An infectious agent is suspected as the cause of chronic fatigue syndrome. It is possible that chronic immune system activation is the key in both cases.

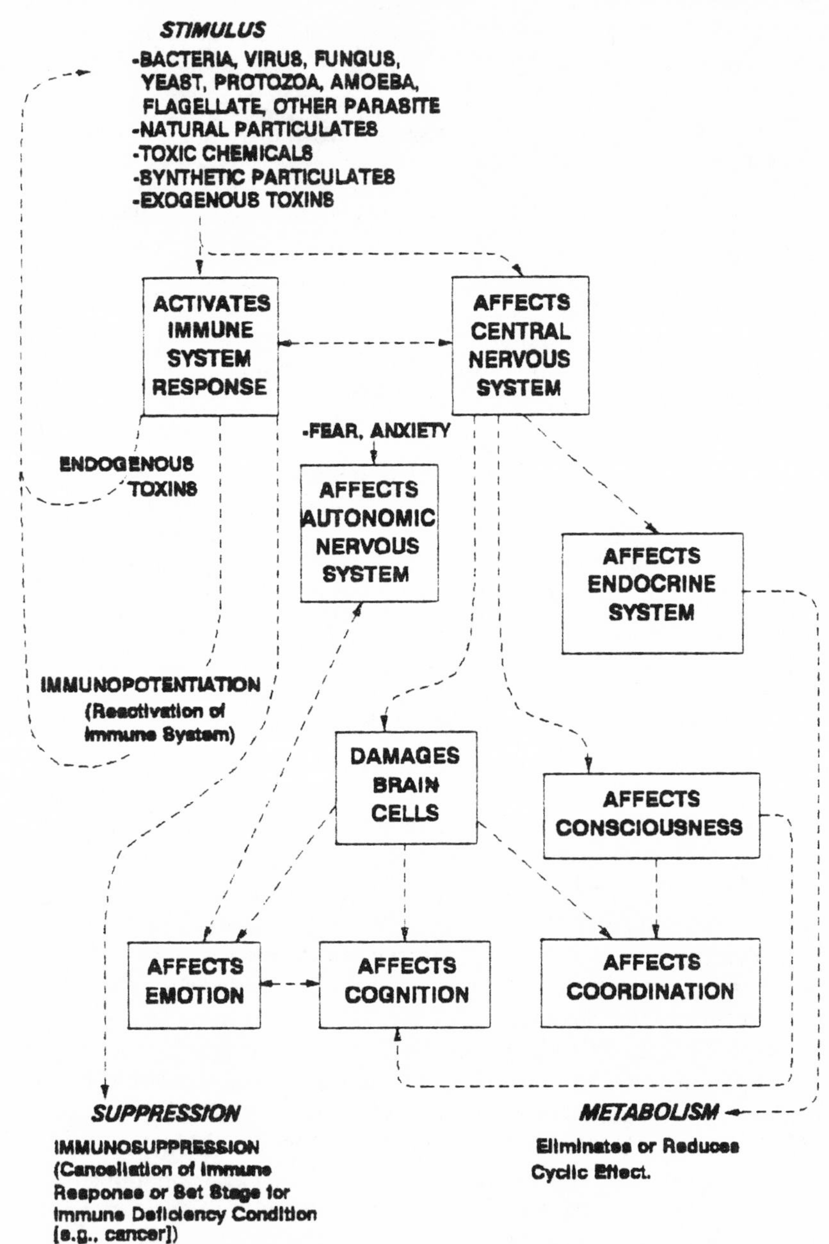

Basics of CS Self-Perpetuation.

Chemical sensitivity may result from an infectious chronic immune system activation, since the immune response involves endogenous toxic chemicals. It may also result from chronic low level exogenous toxic exposure (e.g. air pollution) which sets off a false but full blown immune response to attempt to repel the toxic. (See Basics of CS Self-Perpetuation chart, page 24.) Whether the immune system is involved in a full blown immune response to counter a viral, bacterial, or fungal infection or whether it is a full blown response to toxic exposure, the immune response on its own contributes to malaise and fatigue. Produce the full blown response on a repeated basis, and the cumulation effect may generate the critical pendulum swing—just sufficient to initiate self-perpetuation. The person whose immune system has been chronically activated may require less of a swing of the pendulum for self-perpetuation than one whose immune system is not chronically activated. Chronic immune system activation can be compared to a tilting of the framework which holds the pendulum suspended. If the framework is tilted (e.g., lower and lower levels of toxics can set it off or a breach in the blood-brain barrier has occurred), the effect is identical to adding swing to the pendulum. In self-quenching models, equilibrium is perceived when the pendulum returns to rest. In self-perpetuating models, equilibrium is perceived through the cyclic pendulum swing. One is passive; the other, active. By tilting the framework in the small-swing pendulum example, change occurs. Equilibrium becomes achieved through active, large swing, instead of returning to rest. Chronic immune system activation from chronic infection may weaken the body (tilt the framework) to the point where the disease becomes self-perpetuating. Tilting the framework, then, demonstrates a method of endogenous poisoning which contributes to self-perpetuating CS.

When dealing with the concept of toxics (poisons), it should be kept in mind that (1) the immune system actually produces toxic substances, and (2) poisoning means a breakdown or interference with normal physiological function. Poisoning can be either endogenous (caused by something inside the body) or exogenous (caused by something outside the body).

Understanding the concept of the cyclic, self-perpetuating nature of CS requires knowledge of the interaction of various systems and their cycles. Because of such interaction, one toxic may generate different symptoms in two identically exposed individuals; two individuals exposed to different toxics may exhibit identical symptoms.[600] Simple cause-effect is not the answer in dealing with dynamic systems. The major elements in the CS cycle are the stimulus, the nervous system, the endocrine system, and the immune system. Each component may have a role in the genesis and self-perpetuation of the CS cycle.[4] (See Appendix A.)

When a toxic is inhaled, absorbed, drunk, or eaten, it enters the circulating blood. Some toxics can actually damage capillaries or rupture blood vessels, causing swelling which damages brain cells, resulting in encephalopathy.[709] Blood may carry some toxics to the brain. Some neurotoxic chemicals—those which are small (low molecular weight) and fat-soluble—cross the blood-brain barrier with ease,[709] while other neurotoxics attach themselves to proteins which enable them to pass the blood-brain barrier. In the brain the hypothalamus responds to toxic exposure by initiating a certain firing pattern. Parts of the brain interact with other parts. In the response to the toxic, some parts may be destroyed. For example, a toxic which reaches the hippocampus and creates lesions or affects neurotransmitters at that site may have significant effects on behavior and cognitive function. The stimulated hypothalamus sends signals to the endocrine system, and in response the endocrine system sends signals to the immune system. This pattern is not totally directionally fixed. The immune system, for example, signals the hypothalamus when it detects antigen and when it produces antibody.[4] The presence of histamine stimulates the pituitary to release ACTH, setting off another series of signals.

The autonomic nervous system is the part of the body in which emotional reactions are translated to physical response. The sympathetic nervous system, a division of the autonomic nervous system, has the function of preparing the body for "fight or flight."

In the news coverage of the war in the Persian Gulf, a correspondent for CNN, Charles Jaco, provided the world with a clear picture of a false-alarm toxic event. During an air raid, the reporter caught a whiff of jet fuel and mistook the odor for nerve gas. His responses involved tremors and expressions of dizziness. War has a high potential for anxiety or panic responses. Thoughts of chemical warfare and a whiff of a strange odor are sufficient triggers for a strong sympathetic nervous system response.

At the same time the correspondent may have experienced along with the anxiety-panic reaction an acute (self-quenching) CS reaction. Petroleum products, whether in jet fuel or auto fuel or emissions, perfumes, plastics, dyes, solvents, fertilizers, and so on, are frequently identified as sources of neurological symptoms. Neurotoxics can affect any body system, but the nervous system is particularly vulnerable. Effects can be immediate following an exposure, or they may appear only after repeated exposures over weeks or years.[709] In 1990, Lisa A. Morrow, Thomas Callender, Stephen Lottenberg, Monte S. Buchsbaum, Michael J. Hodgson, and Nina Robin demonstrated in a *Journal of Neuropsychiatry* article, "PET and Neurobehavioral Evidence of Tetrabromoethane Encephalopathy,"[441] that organic solvents do produce brain dysfunction. It is worth mention that the patient on whom the study was performed had been misdiagnosed as having functional mental problems. How much of the CNN correspondent's reaction was illusion, producing a reaction of the autonomic nervous system, and how much might be attributed to

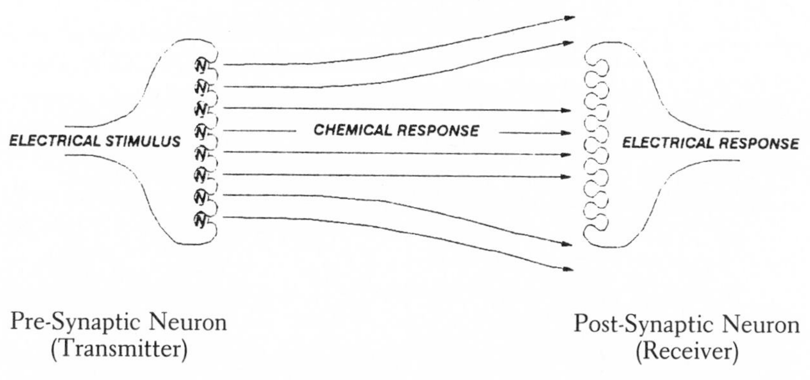

Neurotransmission

central nervous system response to the fuel is impossible to know. It is legitimate to question whether any exposure reaction qualifies as 100 percent illusory.

Considering the complexity of the relationship between the central nervous system, the endocrine system, and the immune system, the potential for a toxic to play havoc is staggering. It is comparable to the effect of a bug in a computer system. A computer system bug, however, is fixable. CS currently is not.

Neurotransmitters

A neurotransmitter is the chemical part of the electro-chemical nervous system communication function. In the chart above, there is an illustration of the fundamental neurotransmission process. On the left is the pre-synaptic neuron (the transmitter nerve). Each circle containing the letter N is a neurotransmitter. On the right is the post-synaptic neuron (the receiver nerve). Neurotransmission occurs in a four-step process:

(1) synthesis of the neurotransmitter (N) in the pre-synaptic neuron;
(2) release of the neurotransmitter;
(3) interaction between the neurotransmitter and the post-synaptic neuron receiver;
(4) end of the interaction by re-uptake of neurotransmitter into nerve terminals, destruction of neurotransmitter by enzymes, or diffusion.

• Synchronicity

The human has a need for what is called *synchronicity* in the brain. Synchronicity is non-random electrical firing. There are times when random firing is normal. An example of normal random firing occurs when

PHASE 1. NORMAL NEUROTRANSMISSION

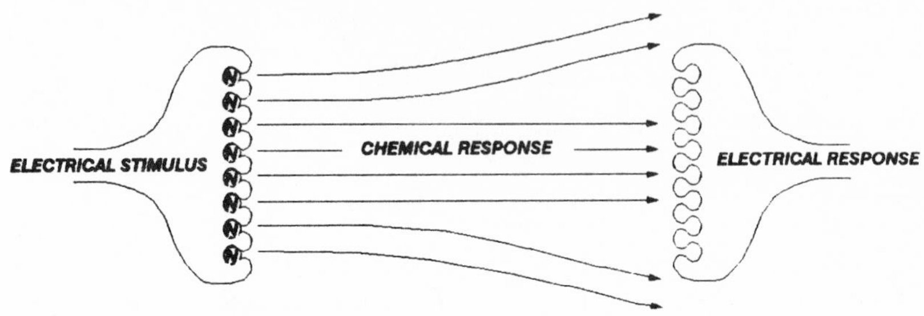

PHASE 2. REDUCED NEUROTRANSMISSION

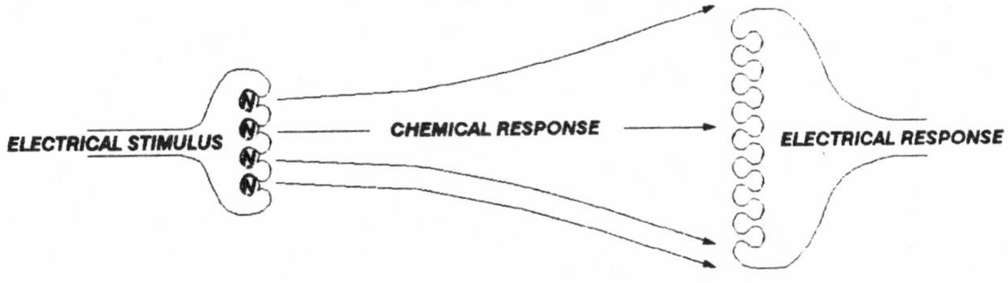

PHASE 3. ADAPTATION

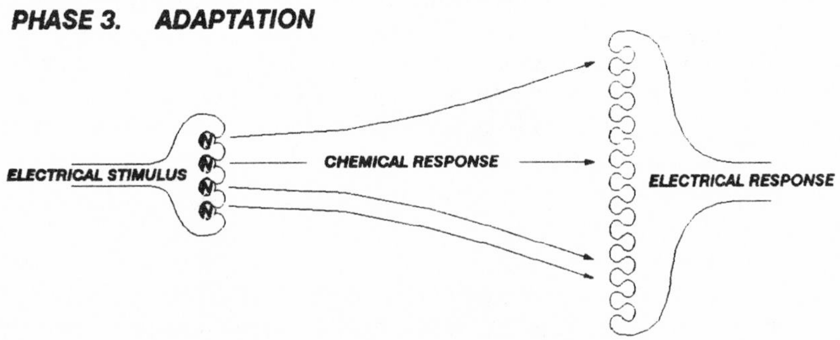

Neurologic Adaptation in Chemical Sensitivity.

the human is involved in new learning from a novel stimulus. Random firing results in increased vigilance (awareness) and dis-synchrony in the brain.

Physical systems adapt in incredible ways to achieve a sense of equilibrium. (See chart on page 28, Neurologic Adaptation in CS.) A relevant example occurs in the nerve depletion of neurotransmitter which takes place in the body in association with chronic immune system activation.[254] Normal function appears in the first block. A depletion of neurotransmitter is illustrated in the second block. The third block, showing an increased number of receptor sites, is the adaptation for equilibrium in the face of neurotransmitter depletion. Reception is enhanced by increased receptors.

Immunogenesis inhibits hypothalamic norepinephrine synthesis. Since norepinephrine inhibits firing rates of hypothalamic neurons, the decreased norepinephrine may explain increased firing rate during the immune response.[254] When neurotransmitters are decreased and receptors are increased and additional chemical exposure occurs, the CS patient experiences significant problems. The exogenous toxic may serve as a neurotransmitter, generating dis-synchrony. Dis-synchronicity causes cognitive hypervigilance (attention). This hypervigilance causes problems for the CS patient when the cause is pathologic. The CS patient becomes acutely aware of stimuli, both internal and external. Hypervigilance occurs, but with acute awareness of the multitude of stimuli, the CS patient becomes overwhelmed, and hypervigilance becomes distractibility. Multiple stimuli sent to the brain cannot be screened out, and the patient cannot attend to any specific stimulus. What occurs is "brain fog," a condition of intoxication. Thought processes are interrupted, mental ability deteriorates, and judgment is affected. The CS patient cannot take his mind off the stimuli, nor can he handle them.

Not only is cognition influenced, but also there can be an affective response. The National Institute of Environmental Health Sciences reports that increased numbers of receptors sensitive to the neurotransmitter acetylcholine are associated with depression.[713] In another example, a substance such as perfume may enter the bloodstream, find its way to the brain, and cause an emotional reaction such as intense rage. What effect variations in voltage may have on this pseudoneurotransmission remains to be investigated.

Neurologic communication goes both to and from the brain. The neurotransmission mix-ups from the brain produce symptoms such as tremors, difficulty walking, seizures, and loss of consciousness.

The nervous system and the immune system both need neurotransmitters. When equilibrium is off balance, a tug-of-war can occur between the nervous system and the immune system for neurotransmitters. Low neurotransmitter levels result in increased receptor sites and enhance pseudoneurotransmission. High neurotransmission levels, which occur when the mechanism for enzymatic destruction of neurotransmitter fails, can produce the same results. The patient can feel this pseudoneurotransmission as brain fog, paresthesias, electrical "short-circuiting," aberrant smell or taste, and so on.

• Systemic Implications

Neurotransmitter dysfunction cuts across physiologic systems. Not only is the nervous system affected, but also other systems sustain effect. For example, in the respiratory system when there is neuron failure to signal for the production of adrenalin (as would be the case in contact with a chemical such as trimellitic anhydride), asthma is the result. Another example is found in the effect on neurotransmission from nerve gas exposure such as occurs in chemical warfare, a massive and highly toxic acute poisoning. The toxics are colorless, generally odorless, tasteless, and they do not irritate the skin. Consequently, a lethal dose occurs without warning. Nerve gas prevents the enzyme destruction of acetylcholine neurotransmitter. The neurotransmitter builds up excessive amounts at the nerve ends, where only small amounts are needed. Excess acetylcholine can cause bronchoconstriction, abdominal cramping, heart palpitations, headache, anxiety, convulsions, coma, muscle twitching or cramping, and respiratory failure, to mention a few symptoms. It puts multi-system responses in chaos. Generally, standard treatment includes alkaline washing, clothing disposal, treatment with atropine to reverse the excess acetylcholine, and use of diazepam if convulsions occur. (For further information, see Munro NB et al.: "Treating Exposure to Chemical Warfare Agents: Implications for Health Care Providers and Community Emergency Planning." In: U.S. Health and Human Services, *Environmental Health Perspectives*, Vol. 89, pages 205–215.)

It would be convenient and certainly desirable to identify a sole mediator of CS. From our discussion of the immune system, it is clear that many mediators are involved. Mast cells release heparin, histamine, prostaglandins, and leukotrienes. T cells release interleukins and lymphokines, the latter of which set off cytotoxic T cells. B cells supply antibodies which can receive misinformation and begin cannibalistically to attack parts of the body. Add to all this activity the mental response(s) engendered by the CS patient who recognizes that he's been hit by something, and another set of internal mediators comes into play. An additional neurotoxic event, excitotoxicity, also contributes. In this case neurotransmitters flood adjacent cells, weakening their membranes and causing cell death.[709]

One investigated area that may be another factor is undiagnosed bowel syndrome. The intestine, composed of a significant amount of lymphocytes and covering 200 to 300 square meters of surface area, no doubt plays a role in CS, but the extent of that role is unknown. In some patients, bacterial, fungal, or viral agents, or protozoa, amebas, flagellates, or other parasites could factor into the etiology as a cause of immune system activation in chronic form. If CS in a patient is singularly tied to one of these, cure of the intestinal problem could cure the CS. If, on the other hand, CS resulted from another source, but undiagnosed bowel syndrome is involved, cure of the intestinal problem could improve patient condition. In reverse, CS caused by toxics could significantly affect or generate bowel problems.[562] The gastrointestinal tract is the largest endocrine gland. It affects and is affected by the brain and other glands. (Kerstin Uvnä-Moberg: "The Gastrointestinal Tract in Growth and Reproduction." *Scientific American*, July 1989, 261[1]: 78–83.)

Recently much information has focused on the effects of low levels of toxics as having very significant effect. It is possible that the damage they do initially is so slight that there is failure to trigger the cell repair function[712] and, therefore, the damage becomes permanent. Long-term exposure, then, could have a very significant cumulative effect.

Toxic contact can set off certain mental reactions: anger, depression, anxiety, and so on. Recognition by the CS patient that he has just encountered a toxic and a reaction is beginning can add a variety of mental states, depending on the individual. These include frustration, anger, depression, anxiety, panic, apathy, and so on. These mental states can add to the chemical soup already stirring within the CS person's body. Compromised integrity of the total system in CS is multifactored and modulated by multiple events. Neurological compromise examples are illustrated in the chart on page 32.

Toxic-induced, compromised systemic integrity can be viewed as: (1) an immune system that is hyperactive and cyclic; (2) toxic encephalopathy; or (3) a mixture of the two. Because the immune, endocrine, and neurologic systems each interact, it may be that there is no purely immune or purely neurologic compromise of systemic integrity, but in terms of presentation, there are cases in which one or the other appears to be significant while the other systems appear not to play a role. In other cases, it is clear that both the immune and neurologic systems are significantly compromised.

Intoxication and Addiction

Intoxication means an abnormal state resulting from poisoning by a drug or toxic substance, or overindulgence in alcohol. Intoxication can be voluntary (e.g. from consumption of alcohol, use of illegal drugs, or sniff-

Change	Level	Effects
Structural	**Cellular** (Often from oxygen deprivation, since neurons require large quantities of oxygen.)	• Contents swell; become more acidic. • Biochemical processes become inhibited (e.g., protein synthesis, neurotransmitter secretion)
	Morphological (Generally, prolonged intermittent exposure is required to produce effect.)	• Damages neuronal bodies. • Damages axons. • Damages myelin sheath.
Functional	**Sensory** (Effects result from destruction of myelin sheath, neurons, or damage to neurotransmitter system.)	Adverse effect on: -- sight -- hearing -- touch -- pain (numbness, tingling, hyperactivity, neuromuscular paralysis, weakness, vomiting, diarrhea, dizziness, coma, death.)
	Motor (Damage to sensory systems affects motor system.)	• Altered impulse velocity along nerve axons • Muscle weakness • Lack of control of muscular movements
Behavioral	**Emotional** Identified by neuropsychological assessment: can be exacerbation of existing problem or caused by toxic exposure.	Examples: Depression, irritation, anxiety, difficulty sleeping, agitation, loss of appetite, anger, rage, speech impairment.
	Intellectual Capabilities Learning, memory, integrative capability -- identified by neuropsychological assessment.	Examples: confusion, memory loss, reduced intellectual function, inability to organize information, difficulty learning new information, difficulty reading or writing or computing.

Effects of Neurotoxics.

ing glue) or involuntary (e.g. from taking a prescribed drug which generates unsuspected systemic reaction, or breathing polluted air). *Addiction* is dependence, either physical or psychological, upon a substance.

Where voluntary intoxication occurs, the action is initiated at a conscious level. It is quite possible that there occurs a quasi-voluntary use in which the action is initiated at an unconscious level. The initiator in this case is the workaholic. It is possible that workaholics are made in response to intoxication from low level toxic exposure. There is a legitimate reason for making this proposition, but *what follows in this section is hypothetical. No studies exist.*

According to anecdotal information of the group composing the Registry—Washington State Chemical Sensitives, the largest proportion of the group became chemically sensitive through workplace exposure. An interesting aspect of the stories of these individuals is the tenacity with which most clung to their jobs, despite the deleterious health effects obviously connected with the work setting. Most people surmise that the reason was economic and think no further. It is quite possible that other factors, perhaps far more significant factors, are involved.

Workaholism is not a medical term, but it is popular in the working world and in literature relating to individuals for whom work becomes the central focus to the exclusion of family and friends from non-work sources. The workaholic may accrue numbers of hours of overtime, or spend his time at home solving work problems or thinking about work situations. Vacations are worked through. The spouse of the workaholic may resent the intrusion of the workplace upon family life. Family relationships deteriorate. The compulsiveness of the drive to work is clear to everyone but the workaholic. The parallel to alcohol abuse or abuse of any intoxicant is evident to all but the abuser, whose likely reaction, if confronted, would be denial.

Office-setting poisonings are often very subtle. Beginning with the sick building syndrome symptoms, intoxication can appear to be nothing more than mild allergy or irritation, a cold or the flu. Over time, the worker may be performing quite well, accomplishing a noticeable amount of work in excess of what might be expected of the average worker. Then, suddenly and for no apparent reason, the super worker experiences major health problems that result in removal from the workplace.

With repeated exposure to toxics in the workplace setting, there is chronic immune system activation. That condition lowers neurotransmitter levels and increases receptors. Once the toxic (low molecular weight, fat soluble) enters the bloodstream, there is potential for the toxic to act as a neurotransmitter, causing damage and dysfunction.

It is known that intoxication alters mental states. The hypervigilance initiated by random electrical firing in the brain could initially contribute to enhanced thinking. By such means the super worker may be born. In cyclic self-perpetuation, enhanced thinking is pleasurable and rewarding. Workaholism follows. Hypothetically, workaholism can be viewed as addictive abuse of intoxicants to which the worker is unknowingly exposed at the worksite. Just as in alcohol abuse, the toxic-induced random electrical firing in the brain may be insidiously damaging the brain while enhancing the ability to think for a time.

That people who are becoming very sick on the job will fight desperately to retain that job may have more to do with addiction to intoxication[306] than any stated reason. The likelihood that any worker would recognize addiction to intoxication is virtually nonexistent. The perception tends to be, "I love my job." When a job disables a worker, whether the work is perceived as pleasurable (heightened ability to think, despite occurrence of undetected brain damage) or nonpleasurable (nausea), a fight to retain it may seem illogical; however, if one considers that the worker may have a literal dependency on the toxic in terms of neurotransmitter interaction, logic is restored.

When a CS patient is medically removed from the workplace, the experience can be as painful as removing someone from a drug dependency. Because the CS patient becomes sensitive to numbers of other chemicals, withdrawal from one may not change the condition, if others are able to provide the same or similar effect. A person who develops a type of hyperactivity from styrene in glued-down carpet in the workplace may discover that the same hyperactivity can be gained from other sources (e.g. gasoline fumes, laundry detergent), while being totally ignorant of the potential for more damage to occur from the new exposure. Unlike drug users who develop a tolerance to a drug and have to increase the dose to experience the effect, the CS patient learns fast that lower and lower levels are required to trigger the symptom set.

Once a person has become habituated to the effects of non-adaptive, destructive neurotransmission, whether at a conscious or unconscious level, or whether volitional (e.g. drinking alcohol) or avolitional (e.g. exposure to odorless toxic at low levels over time), the malfunctioning neurotransmission becomes *learned equilibrium.* Abuse of alcohol or drugs or environmental toxic exposure over time can result in the misperception that abnormal neurological states are normal. Thus in the absence of the abnormal neurotransmission, the affected person desires a return to the abnormal state, which for him represents equilibrium.

It is for this reason that the recovering alcoholic, though he abstains, is encouraged to continue to view himself as an alcoholic. It is more difficult to unlearn (perceive abnormal as abnormal) than to learn (perceive abnormal as normal) the behavior or attitude or perception initially. Once the toxic, whether alcohol or a chemical or set of chemicals, has done certain structural or functional damage, it may be that reestablishing equilibrium, let alone relearning it, is no longer possible. Brain damage may be a factor here. This is a possible explanation of the significant tendency of individuals who have attended substance abuse programs to return to their former pattern of abuse. It may be inevitable. Damage done by the toxic may prevent return to normal.

Of course there are fundamental differences between alcohol or drug abuse and CS. They include:

1. *Knowledge.* Alcohol and drug abuse begin with the knowledge that there is danger. CS occurs insidiously. The CS exposed individual rarely knows a risk exists.
2. *Control.* The alcohol or drug user/abuser can choose whether to use the substance and control the quantity. The person with CS is unwittingly exposed and has no control over quantity.
3. *Tolerance.* Use of alcohol or drugs typically leads to tolerance (more and more is required to achieve the desired effect). This tolerance may dissipate as the toxic effect becomes more pronounced. With CS, the amount required to produce symptoms declines.
4. *Avoidance.* Alcohol or a drug is uni-dimensional. Substances can be identified and avoided specifically. Avoidance is legitimate in social settings. CS is multi-dimensional, and it includes unknown and unidentifiable chemicals. Avoidance is not possible in social settings (in fact, when choosing to avoid, CS patients are viewed as antisocial). Even by group removal to isolated sites, avoidance may not be possible. One group in Texas found a "clean site" in which to build a community. Industrial pollution became a problem for those people.[50]
5. *Withdrawal.* Some alcoholics can relearn normal equilibrium, if not repair damage done by the toxic. The CS patient, unless he can find an isolated place free of any outdoor air pollution, rarely can reexperience it.

Is CS Psychosomatic?

There is a desire in our society to view CS as a psychosomatic disorder. That desire is strongly felt in medical, economic, and occasionally political quarters. The authoritarian voice of the medical community labels CS a *somatiform disorder*, one in which a mental condition finds expression in disturbed bodily functions. Essentially, the view is that mind and body are separate entities and that CS is caused by an illusion with a response perpetuated volitionally. The idea is that the person finds it easier to view his problem as physical than to face the emotional conflict from which escape is desired. Economic pressure to maintain the psychosomatic perspective is largely a result of concern over maintaining medical specialization status quo and liability; political pressure comes from special interest groups and concern over workers' compensation payments.

To label authoritatively any disorder as originating solely in the patient's emotional state is a demonstration of arrogance.[463, 745] Lack of evidence of a medical condition does not indicate that no disorder exists. The doctor may not know where or how to look for evidence, he may lack the tools to find it. Furthermore, any disease, especially any chronic disease, will have a mental component. For example, it was not until after 1982 that occupational asthma was recognized as reportable.[64] That did not mean that occupational asthma was illusory.

According to definition (*Taber's*, 16th edition) psychosomatic means "pertaining to the relationship of the mind and body." The text continues, "Partitioning of the human being is not possible; thus no disease is limited to only the mind or the body. A complex interaction is always present even though in specific instances a disease might on superficial examination appear to involve only the body or the mind." S. Michael Plaut and Stanford B. Friedman (in Ader: *Psychoneuroimmunology*, page 7) state that "the mechanism(s) by which psychological factors contribute to the etiology of any given disease is largely speculative."

Technically, it can be said that every human is psychosomatic; every disease is psychosomatic. However, the term has by now acquired a negative connotation. Popular belief is that psychosomatic means illusory illness caused by emotional factors. As long as that belief persists, the term will continue to present a picture of mind-body partitioning rather than integration, a picture that can have tremendous impact on the life of a CS patient. A statement such as "I suspect an emotional cause" can render a chemically poisoned individual financially destitute.

What is critical for anyone involved in CS issues to recognize is the concept of *integrity*. A functioning macro-systematic structure is classifiable into numbers and numbers of sub-systems, sub-sub-systems, to micro-systems and their subordinate systems. Integrity is the idealistic integration of all systems of the whole. A change in one part affects the whole. It is not a question of whether this occurs[745] but rather of whether it may be perceived and to what extent.

This being the case, one must also acknowledge that a view of unified mind and body integrated into the human whole does not imply that emotion does not serve as stimulus to response elsewhere in the human system. The question that one might pursue is, where does stimulus begin? Does irritability trigger high blood pressure, or vice versa? What other factors (e.g. environment, consumption of sodium, weight) are involved, if any? And, finally, it can be argued that even a precise answer fails to pass the "so-what?" test.

A patient who carefully avoids exposure to low level toxics and adamantly insists that certain places, people, or events are fraught with severe contaminants may, for example, be diagnosed as having obsessive-compulsive disorder (OCD). This is a severe, chronic psychiatric problem with biologic roots, though all too often society is unaware of any biologic aspects of OCD. In fact OCD has become popularized as an asset in some professional occupations (e.g., medicine). Ironically, PET scans of OCD patients show an OCD pattern.[518] That pattern is not congruent with PET scans of CS patients, which, if the patient can afford the test, can point to misdiagnosis. The problem of misdiagnosis can also be demonstrated by use of qEEGs. Patterns for schizophrenia, alcoholism, dementia, and so on are emerging.[19a] CS cannot be written off as casually as may be economically and politically desirable—an illusory stress-related transitory disorder.

Much has been written about stress and its role in CS, yet the term *stress* is so ill-defined as to be meaningless. As a consequence it is not helpful to identify "stress" as the cause of CS. Inhaling a toxic is stress, crowding too many rats in one cage is stress, bereavement is stress. Rather than focus on stress as a cause, it may be more beneficial to examine problem-solving ability as opposed to learned helplessness in the CS patient.

For example, a toxic poisons two patients who subsequently develop CS. One experiences severe depression as a CS symptom; the other does not. The one who experiences severe depression grew up in a home where child abuse was frequent; the other had a nurturing childhood. The one who experiences depression refers to the poisoning and subsequent development of CS as forms of victimization; the other does not. Exposure to detergent has a mood-depressing effect on both, though it is more evident in the one with severe depression.

It can be argued that the individual who grew up with child abuse in the home developed learned helplessness, which led to decreased perception of ability to solve problems. The intellectual problem of learned helplessness stimluated subsequent emotional response. The victimization perspective coupled with the effect of detergent vapor on the brain makes the patient's depression more evident to the observer. The depression in response to the detergent vapor is real. It's CS. However, the patient with such demonstrable depression will most likely be diagnosed as having an emotional disorder, and CS will be missed altogether (which will only reinforce the patient's learned helplessness).

In the case of the other patient, depending on the mind-body perspective of the examining physician, the diagnosis may be a "masked" psychiatric disorder or CS. Basically, the concept of masked psychiatric disorder is that the patient has a real psychiatric disorder of subconscious or intentionally hidden origin, and the psychiatrist or psychologist cannot find it.

Chemical sensitivity can develop when psychiatric problems exist and when they do not. Solving emotional or intellectual problems will not cure CS. However, it is known that learned helplessness has an immunosupressive effect, decreasing the number of T and B cells. Immunosuppression compounded by additional stressors (e.g. reinforcement of learned helplessness by mind-body separatists; loss of financial resources; harassment; and so on) can lead to immunoincompetence with enhancement of various pathological conditions. Because the mind and body form an integrated system, counseling to enhance coping skills will likely improve overall condition when CS is self-perpetuating.

Is CS psychosomatic? Certainly, in the sense that it involves integrated mind-body responses to stimuli. But then so do mumps and measles. When issues such as entitlement programs or litigation are involved, a "psychosomatic" diagnosis can cause problems for a CS patient. When a workplace toxic is clearly implicated, workers' compensation is appropriate, if the source of the toxic can be identified. When the toxic cannot be identified, the tendency may be to deny its presence. But because CS is not a single-cause, single-effect disease, and because so much remains unknown about the effects of chemicals in the environment, one should never assume that toxic exposure has not occurred simply because it cannot be proved.

With the expectation that some 37,306,481 people in the United States have heightened sensitivity to chemicals, this disease should be vigorously and ethically studied. In one view, 25 percent of those who develop CS eventually recover. If accurate, that leaves 75 percent who do not. Chemical sensitivity is a disease which society can ill afford to ignore. It is and will be expensive to recognize it, but that expense will be significantly increased if recognition is delayed.

2. What It's Like to Have Chemical Sensitivity

It is always easier to communicate facts than feelings. For example, it's easy to describe what a broken bone *is*, but to tell someone how it feels to have one is more difficult. It may help to use comparisons, that is, to draw on common experiences that are comparable to the ache of a bone, the stiffness of atrophied muscles, the weakness after removal from a cast. With CS, the symptoms are frequently so bizarre that finding comparisons in common experience is often very difficult.

Chemical sensitivity develops through a process with many stages. The individual may experience different complaints depending on the stage of the disease progression and how he relates to others during that particular stage.

Experience During Disease Development

Stage 1: Exposure

Only rarely during a chronic, low level toxic exposure does an individual recognize that anything is wrong. There are signs and symptoms, but almost everyone fails to recognize a problem because the buildup of poison is so gradual. Headaches, sinus problems, occasional hoarseness like laryngitis, sore throat, sneezing, watering or uncomfortable eyes, skin rashes, forgetfulness, and so on are characteristics of colds, allergies, and flu. An aspirin, antihistamine or anti-inflammatory cream will initially take care of symptoms the individual might consider an insignificant nuisance.

Initial symptoms generally are ignored until they become persistent or something significant occurs. Persistent symptoms will eventually result in a visit to a physician, who in most cases will diagnose flu. Persistent flu may be diagnosed as relapsing, or the person may be referred for an allergy workup. Treatment with some medicines may result in unexpected patient reaction. When a patient appears to have a psychological problem such as anxiety, a mild tranquilizer may be prescribed. In some cases instead of calming the patient, the drug may increase the anxiety. Immune system–related problems are frequently accompanied by inflammatory processes. Some CS patients will have serious reactions to anti-inflammatory drugs.

During the exposure period, the level of toxics builds up within the body and the person becomes sicker and sicker, but the overwhelming tendency is to deny that a serious problem exists. The patient denies it; doctors deny it; and so do friends, family, co-workers. Flu-like symptoms and fatigue are common feelings during this period.

Stage 2: Poisoning

With most chemical sensitives, there is a clear point even to the day when the toxic level became intolerable and recognizable poisoning occurred. Yet it is most unlikely that the patient with CS or his doctors or others will know *what* occurred, unless the event were an acute toxic exposure and symptoms were immediately and directly connected. Nevertheless, a time arrives when the individual can no longer deny that a serious problem exists.

Here are some examples of the event of poisoning: A person with no history of respiratory problems suddenly develops asthma, concurrently cannot think clearly, and begins to lose a lot of weight. A normal emotionally stable individual becomes extremely depressed, filled with anxiety, experiences systemic swelling and puts on a noticeable amount of weight, has "killer" headaches and a rash. Another has difficulty concentrating, feels confused, is extremely fatigued, has eye and sinus problems, and feels great pain in muscles and joints. Another who has never lost consciousness suddenly faints, lacks coordination, is mentally disoriented, has overwhelming nausea and vomiting, and keeps forgetting things. Another experiences depression, has an acute sense of smell, feels extreme fatigue, has nausea and diarrhea. Another experiences poor concentration, has difficulty sleeping, and experiences anxiety and vomiting. Yet another experiences sharp stomach pain, an upset stomach, intestinal cramps, muscle aches and pains, confusion, and loss of voice.

The poisoning event usually sends the individual to his doctor. At this point both the developing chemical sensitive and the physician recognize that something has happened. Unless the physician is trained to recognize low level or other than pharmaceutical poisoning, however, chances are that possibility will not be considered. The standard medical response is to consider psychological or psychiatric causes. Medical students are taught that when a person presents multi-system symptoms the problem is probably mental or emotional. Almost without exception, the patient will have already reached the same conclusion.

Both the doctor and the patient usually decide to wait to see what happens. Typically, the patient continues his activities. People who are employed return to work; those who are at home return home; those who attend school return to school. Life goes on as normal, and the illness progresses, while the developing chemical sensitive uses every bit of willpower to deny a serious problem, ignore the symptoms, and continue living as before the event. There arises a belief that continuing in familiar life pursuit, will cause the symptoms to disappear, because they are psychologically generated. By refusing to give in to the symptoms, the person continues to suffer increasing amounts of toxic exposure. Other substances begin to cause problems, and enormous energy has to be expended to perform simple functions. So it is that some of the strongest willed or most disciplined individuals become the sickest.

Stage 3: Chemical Sensitivity

While the person with CS is doing everything possible to conquer what he perceives to be a psychological problem, his immune system, if it is in a highly activated state, can cause him to feel increasingly worse. An absurd battle ensues in which the person fights to overcome the warnings his own body issues. The harder he fights, the louder the warnings become. Finally, at some point, the person knows that the problem is not a mental illusion. He recognizes that his behavior has changed, that he's fighting something he cannot see, but he does finally recognize that the cause is external to himself. If he is employed, he knows his performance is suffering. He knows his social relationships are deteriorating. He also knows that he does not want any of this to happen, and yet he's powerless to stop it.

Many chemical sensitives eventually discover their problem through trial and error. When the individual recognizes that there is a cause-and-effect pattern between road fumes and symptoms, detergent and symptoms, perfume and symptoms, understanding through trial and error begins. His feeling that he walks each day through an invisible mine field is accurate.

At the same time the undiagnosed chemical sensitive, his doctor, his family, friends, and coworkers have all reached the conclusion that he is really strange, if not crazy. To identify the problem, he has to convince himself first. Then comes the tremendous effort of convincing others.

Knowing the diagnosis is helpful, but hearing it the first time is a tremendous shock. The idea that your home or car or office or school has poisoned you takes some getting used to. Feelings of shock pass fairly soon, to be followed by anything from frustration to outright rage. At this point, the CS patient can be terribly sick. There may have been permanent brain damage. And he may be facing the toughest fight of his life at the time when he is least able to do so. He is likely to be exhausted.

What he faces may involve gaining entitlements (worker's compensation or disability retirement, if the exposure is work-related and he cannot safely work in other environments); recovery for personal injury (lawsuit, if the exposure is from a product); social security benefits or welfare (if he cannot work and there is no source liable for the injury). In numbers of cases, no benefits or entitlements are available and litigation is not possible.

Numbers of people with CS become so depressed, both from the illness and from the treatment they receive from others, that the only answer they find is suicide. In our society we like to think of ourselves as caring, enlightened peole, yet we allow such tragedies to happen.

Experience After Disease Development

The life of a chemical sensitive on a day-to-day basis is restrictive. Contact with chemicals to which the individual is sensitive brings on symptoms; careful avoidance decreases symptoms. Here are some of the things that create problems for people with CS.

A *Kitchen.* A chemical sensitive can easily become spooked in someone else's kitchen. As soon as he sees the sink, he wonders what lurks beneath it. Most homemakers keep all manner of products stored beneath the kitchen sink for handy use. Many typical ingredients in detergents, ammonia, chlorine, alcohols, glycol ethers, petroleum distillates, and so on can cause chemical intoxication. A gas stove can be the source of additional problems. Even the water that comes into the faucet can be a problem.

The Grocery Store. Most people would not be able to conceive of a grocery store as a source of minor hazards, let alone major ones. The chemical sensitive may put off going to the grocery store as long as possible. The detergent aisle can cause a person with CS to faint. The produce section can kick off the individual's symptoms, perhaps because of formaldehyde in particle board shelves or pesticides or fungicides used in growing or shipping the produce.

Hardware Stores. Many chemical sensitives will not enter a hardware store. The problem arises from plastic products which emit gasses, paint, solvents, adhesives, and who knows what else. These products confined indoors provide an environment that can exacerbate symptoms. They have a particularly severe effect on those with organic brain syndrome (toxic encephalopathy or false neurotransmission).

Service Stations. Petroleum products are potent. People sensitive to them can find a variety of their symptoms recurring quickly in the service station environment. Examples of these symptoms are respiratory difficulty, hoarseness, impaired consciousness, and nausea.

New Vehicles. The plasticizers (substances which make plastics bend) used in vinyl of new vehicles is frequently an initial sensitizer. For individuals who either are initially sensitized to plasticizers or become sensitized through the spreading phenomenon, new vehicles are extremely difficult to endure. The symptoms generated by this exposure are similar to those which occur in a service station, even though the chemicals are different.

Air Travel. Chemical sensitives usually are not eager to travel by plane. On the ground, if something is a problem, it is possible to exit. The same cannot be said for air travel. Once on board, you're there until the plane lands. There is no avoidance. Sealed up in a small space with other people wearing perfume,[454, 705] dry cleaned clothing, new leather, hairspray, or aftershave, or carrying newspapers or vinyl bags, the CS individual is surrounded by a wide variety of potential triggers which can set off the total array of symptoms. On takeoff the tail section may fill with jet fuel vapor, adding to the intoxicants.

Roadways. Chemical sensitives who haven't studied pollutants in outdoor air often complain about their difficulty with road fumes. The chemicals along the roadway from the vehicles using it can be extremely difficult for the chemical sensitive. To underscore the significance of this difficulty, it is helpful to examine a document from one's local air pollution control agency. These agencies have the responsibility of reporting to the EPA the quantity of certain pollutants from specific measuring points. An air quality data summary for a year is a very enlightening publication. Air quality limits often are exceeded during rush hour traffic in metropolitan areas. The levels at which a chemical sensitive has difficulty are much lower than what is anticipated by air quality limits. The worst offenders are diesel fuel users, anything emitting blue or black smoke, and vehicles using regular (leaded) gas, but vehicle emissions from any source may be a potential hazard.*

Aside from the vehicular emissions which compose road fumes there are additional sources of vapors and particles which contribute to the discomfort. These include hot macadam or tar, other road surfacing materials,

**See the following items in the Bibliography for more on vehicular emissions: 220, 260, 270, 296, 387, 412, 445.*

and wood or industrial smoke. A person with CS can easily recognize that road fumes are bothering him, but he may not be able to identify specifically what the chemicals are.

Aside from setting off physical symptoms, road fumes can be a sensitive subject to patients with chemical sensitivity. There are some physicians who are quite vocal in denying the existence of chemical sensitivity (more about this later in this chapter). One of the most frequent comments these doctors make about chemical sensitives is that "they keep talking about problems with road fumes." The remark is made in a disparaging manner. It's a real put-down. Chemical sensitives can be as emotionally sensitive to put-downs as they are physically sensitive to vehicular emissions.

Upholstery and New Carpet. New carpet is a well-recognized initial sensitizer. There are potent toxic substances in carpet, particularly in the glues and backings. Carpets give off gasses from dyes and substances added to the fibers. They also give off particulates, small particles which can be breathed into the lungs. New carpet and upholstery can be extremely difficult for the chemical sensitive, whether or not they were initial sensitizers. Some symptoms characteristic of contact with carpets and upholstery are respiratory distress (asthma), hoarseness, nausea, and impaired consciousness. (See Appendix D.)

Doctor's Offices and Hospitals. It is ironic that, of all places, doctor's offices and hospitals are typically located in tight buildings, that is, buildings where the windows cannot be opened for ventilation. These new buildings accumulate chemical substances inside the structure over time. The number of chemicals inside a hospital is frequently overwhelming for the CS patient.

Chemical sensitives often are required to report to hospitals for tests. For example, the gastrointestinal symptoms of a CS patient may require a colonoscopy, a procedure for examining the intestine. Prior testing has shown that the individual has been exposed to a chemical called trimellitic anhydride (TMA). The test proves negative for formaldehyde. On entering the hospital, the chemical sensitive has difficulty with indoor air without being able to identify the source. Disinfectants in one area are irritating. A refurbished waiting area wafts intolerable chemicals into the hallway. On finding and entering the room where the testing will be done, the person has to grab onto a wall for support. What's the problem? Medical instruments are soaking in a container of formaldehyde. There is no cover on the container. Is the colonoscopy a problem? Not at all. The patient was practially knocked out prior to administration of the mild anesthetic.

Parts of the United States have insect infestations. In those areas, medical offices and hospitals may be treated with insecticides. Insecticides are toxic, though some doctors will joke about pesticides as readily as about road fumes. Those who market pesticide products and services will often assure the public that they are safe. This is further evidence of the gradualistic deterioration of human reason. World War II wasn't all that long ago. Pesticides were used to murder countless individuals. Yet, in areas where insects abound, they are used routinely today. The substances may build through accumulation. People who encounter them and are sensitive to them find that their symptoms recur immediately and violently.

Other. For people with CS the sources of difficulty listed above are just examples, not a complete list. Trains and buses, which some people have to use, can set off an array of symptoms. Classrooms can be hazardous, particularly if the building is poorly ventilated. Magic markers may contain intoxicating solvents. Dissection in biology is difficult to impossible due to formaldehyde. Gas burners in chemistry are potent. Carpets in schools cause chemical sensitivity in our young people year after year. Gardening stores or nurseries are problematic due to chemicals for feeding and weeding plants and controlling pests. Clothing stores are difficult due to sizing in fabric. Printing and photocopy shops have significant toxic levels. Even the parks and forests, where clean air is expected, have their own set of problems. Parks and forests do use herbicides and insecticides. Wood smoke can be as significant a symptom generator as road fumes. The chemical sensitive knows there is no safe place.

There is probably no such thing as a "typical" chemical sensitive, but responses to a questionnaire sent out to one group of CS sufferers gives some idea of how the disease can strike and how it affects its victims. It should be noted that the results of surveys based on questionnaires illustrate characteristics of a group of participants willing to share experiences.

The data which follow illustrate experiences of one group of chemical sensitives. One cannot necessarily use these data to characterize other groups of those diagnosed with CS.

There are more than 500 chemical sensitives known to the Registry—Washington State Chemical Sensitives. The following data reflect a subset of just less than half that group. The participant group, for example, is 89 percent female and 11 percent male. The larger group is more evenly balanced according to gender. The group is 96 percent diagnosed by physicians, 4 percent self-diagnosed. Forty-two percent had organic brain syndrome diagnosed through neuropsychological assessment. Not all had been tested for organic brain syndrome, so the reported percentage may be an underestimate.

Of the chemical sensitives who had been wage earners, only 4 percent can continue to work.

Sources of poisoning:

64 percent occupational
16 percent home
10 percent school
2 percent product
6 percent outdoor environment
2 percent other

Major occupations involved in poisonings reported by the survey include: meatwrappers, manufacturers, office workers in "tight buildings," painters, construction workers (large or small projects), herbicide and pesticide applicators, medical personnel, chemists, printshop operators in "tight buildings," teachers, and people who work frequently with carbonless carbon paper.

Benefits available to the chemical sensitives are:

2 percent Federal Worker's Compensation
16 percent State Worker's Compensation
8 percent Disability Retirement
20 percent Social Security Disability Income
11 percent Self-Insured Employer Compensation
2 percent Welfare
2 percent Litigation
43 percent No Benefits

It should be noted that the percentages above are increased somewhat, because a few individuals had access to more than one type of compensation.

Prior to developing CS, 20 percent of the chemical sensitives smoked cigarettes regularly. Of that 20 percent, 55 percent quit smoking after developing CS.

Prior to developing CS, 27 percent of the group drank alcohol regularly. Of that group, 8 percent quit drinking alcohol after developing CS. It is interesting to note that 11 percent of the chemical sensitives, who did not drink alcohol regularly prior to developing CS, began to drink alcohol regularly after developing it.

Prior to developing CS 4 percent of the chemical sensitives used "recreational" drugs regularly. All of those who used "recreational" drugs prior to development of the disease have quit. Of those who did not use "recreational" drugs prior to developing CS, 5 percent have begun to use them regularly since developing CS.

Three individuals are known to have attempted suicide. One was successful.

Statements from chemical sensitives across the United States can also give some idea of how devastating CS can be:

What I really resent about chemical sensitivity is the restrictiveness. I am too sensitive for the metropolitan life, but I've been a professional all my life. Adjusting to life in the small town setting has some interesting dimensions, but I miss the life of the city more than I am really willing to admit very often. Every time the thoughts come creeping into my mind, I try to shove them down and do something productive.

When I tried to commit suicide, they put me in this room that didn't have anything in it. I was strapped down. Hospitals are just filled with stuff that bothers me. Why didn't they let me die?

My husband divorced me. He's got the kids. I miss my life. Even my parents won't listen when I try to explain this illness. They've written me off as crazy.

I've got three kids. The thing is so bad I can't drive. I black out. My oldest is 13. I have no income and I just can't think about taking handouts. I've been selling off all the things I've collected over a lifetime so we can eat. It makes me cry when I think I'll never see some of those things again. When the things run out, I don't know.

What am I going to do with my child? He can't go to school because of the stuff there. How's he going to get educated and how will he work? He keeps trying to do what the others do and then he's sick really bad for a week or so.

I thought attorneys were supposed to help. That's a laugh. Whenever I call I can't talk to him and he never returns my calls.

I feel guilty for not working. I start to feel better and I say to heck with it and go off and try working a different kind of job. Then it happens all over again. I feel like I failed my family. My wife knows about the problem, but when we can't do things or she can't buy what she thinks she should, I feel real bad. I think she'll leave. If I could get my benefits, we could make it. Looks like it'll take too long. It's not my fault, but that doesn't make it any easier.

Having this disease has taught me to hate. I mean really hate.

The Problem Patient with a Persistent Problem, Treated by Problem Physicians and Surrounded by Problem People

For many CS patients, the heading above is the most accurate and concise description of the CS sufferer. It would be understood immediately by most of those with the disease. The non-chemical sensitive may need an explanation. What follows may sometimes sound like the topsy-turvy world of Alice's wonderland, but to understand what it's like to have CS, it's critical to follow the CS patient on his journey down the rabbit hole.

The first thing most CS patients discover is that the rules by which they have so far successfully conducted their lives no longer apply. Doing what's right can be wrong; doing what's wrong is definitely wrong. For example, the chemical sensitive describing symptoms to physicians in open communication (doing what's right) can, by the very nature of the complaints described, lead the physician to the wrong diagnosis.

The following discussion is based on the assumption that the exposure prior to initial poisoning was chronic and low level and that the representative chemical sensitive developed organic brain syndrome.

The Problem Patient

A person with CS most often is a *regular patient*. He does not exhibit the signs and symptoms of severe illness. Appearing well groomed and having no visible signs of illness, the patient with CS is difficult to diagnose and treat. To appear disheveled is hardly an answer, since it will likely result in a diagnosis of psychological problems. Frequently, people are their own worst enemies, and chemical sensitives are no exception. By trying to do what is considered socially acceptable, they have a tendency, as the military puts it, to shoot themselves in the foot. Here are some ways it can happen.

First, chemical sensitives often fail to recognize initial symptoms of poisoning, or else ignore them or treat them as trivial. Ignorance is a large factor here. Because the public is uninformed, people have no cues that would cause them to raise questions about their symptoms. Second, when the palliatives (aspirin, antihistamine) cease to be effective or there is enough concern to visit a doctor, the tendency is to accept the diagnosis (flu, virus) without question. Unless there is an explosive event, the person with CS will continue to believe the continuing diagnosis (flu, virus, relapse). The tendency is to fail to analyze one's own symptoms, and to place too much confidence in the treating physician. Due to lack of public information, there may be no suspicion as to the cause.

When the event of poisoning occurs, it's obvious that something happened—but it's easy for the chemical sensitive to accept the diagnosis of stress. After all, who isn't affected by stress at one time or another? Chemical sensitivity can cause the feelings associated with stress. It's an easy answer to accept. It involves little analysis or critical thinking. It's socially acceptable. It continues confidence in the physician. And there may be no reason for anyone to suspect the real cause.

As CS develops, the chemical sensitive's symptoms make him more of a *problem patient*. For one thing, as the disease progresses, self-centeredness grows. It grows faster after the poisoning has produced recognizable physiologic dysfunction and the spreading phenomenon has begun to occur. The chemical sensitive may fail to recognize that self-centeredness, but others see it clearly. It is one of the aspects of personality characteristic of long-term illness, an aspect that tends to contribute in a negative way to the winning of friends and influencing people, particularly physicians.

Self-centeredness or any functional problem can be more obvious as the result of often bizarre multi-system symptoms which are fairly standard in CS. For example, an acute sense of smell is characteristic. A chemical sensitive may at times be able to detect odors so acutely that while walking down a cereal corridor in the supermarket, he can smell the entire garden of cereal odors, even though most cereals are double packaged. Unfortunately, this unasked-for sensory input is often not as pleasant as the garden of cereal odors. For example, a chemical sensitive who is experiencing acute sense of smell will be able to identify the level of personal hygiene of each person with whom he shares an elevator; recognize that a person waiting for a light to cross a street is sick (when it is not visually apparent); trail the path taken through a building by someone wearing perfume; and correctly list the contents of a metal lunch pail.

Yet the condition of acute sense of smell is not constant. In a single day, there may be a period of acute sense of smell, no ability to smell, and normal ability to smell. Some CS patients may have periods of months where ability to smell is nonexistent, and then briefly be unable to season soup because the ability to smell is overpowering.

Now imagine the CS patient trying to explain this to his doctor. He has no idea that the *Merck Manual* used by physicans has only one thing to say about the acute sense of smell: "Hyperosmia (increased sensitivity to odors) usually reflects a neurotic or histrionic personality" (15th edition, page 1357). Histrionic means theatrical or dramatic. It's attention-getting behavior. With multi-system symptoms and a super-sensitive nose, the patient will most probably be viewed as having a personality disorder, regardless of whether the physician communicates this view to the patient.

The trip through wonderland has only begun. Without communicating the symptoms, the patient cannot get a correct diagnosis. Yet, even if symptoms are accurately described, it is more likely than not that the diagnosis will be incorrect. The patient, expecting the physician to understand, shares information that may return to haunt him. Once there is written documentation of psychological or psychiatric problems (even when no such problems exist) successive doctors will rubber-stamp such a diagnosis.

Believing that open, honest communication is appropriate, the chemical sensitive referred for psychologic or psychiatric evaluation will continue to talk about his experiences and symptoms. It is characteristic to want to get to the bottom of the problem, and maybe he *is* stressed out. The tendency to self-diagnose a mental problem is almost universal in CS cases. If the problem is in his head, the patient wants to know, so he can get rid of it.

Psychological counseling involves intensive history-taking. The focus is not limited to the events leading up to the current problem. The psychologist or psychiatrist reaches back into the beginnings of memory and moves forward. It is not always the case, but many chemical sensitives have had some significant crises that turn up in such histories. Patients willingly share red herrings that prevent identification of the real problem, CS. Such red herrings include having had an alcoholic parent, having been sexually abused, having a significant amount of guilt about something, and so on. Even if the individual has resolved those conflicts, the diagnosis is usually based on their existence.

Ironically, once a CS patient does receive an accurate diagnosis, he may need psychological counseling for the rage resulting from prior inaccurate diagnoses, from having been poisoned, from chemical interference in the emotional center in the brain, from entitlements denied due to psychologic factors. The CS patient may need counseling through the grief that may follow chemical poisoning. He may need help to move from denial to acceptance; to develop coping skills; to set boundaries; to find releases from feelings of helplessness, victimization and hopelessness. But even where counseling would be helpful, it is likely to be rejected by the patient. A patient can overgeneralize his experience with psychologists and psychiatrists who have been unable to see beyond the functional, and thus fail to receive help from those who *can* sort out of the differences between functional and organic.

Aside from being his own worst enemy by communicating openly, honestly, and completely, the person with CS may also shoot himself in the foot by failing to communicate. Failing to communicate is a standard response to discovery that honest communication gets him in trouble. There is a distinct catch-22 operating against the CS patient.

It is important for the chemical sensitive to communiate what he knows to doctors, friends, family, and employers or school administrators. For example, with close friends and family (not children, unless done carefully and in a manner to protect their sense of security), there is nothing wrong and everything right with saying, "I know I haven't been easy to be around. Something is wrong, very wrong. Things are happening to me. Things I don't understand. I'm doing everything I know to find the right answer. I'm scared." Sharing feelings gives those who care a chance to provide support and show their caring. Some people who have never demonstrated strength can show amazing supportive capacity. Unfortunately, it is also true that some people either cannot or will not cope when the going is tough. Sharing reduces interpersonal tension and identifies those who cannot cope with another person's problem. It can also help to add perspective. Sometimes a friend or family member can see what is not obvious to the chemical sensitive, even suggesting that something in the environment may be a factor.

The chemical sensitive who withdraws into an impenetrable shell deprives himself of these potential benefits of sharing. Withdrawal also tends to confirm the diagnosis that it's simply a mental problem.

In addition to problems from use of normal communication skills, other problems may occur which make diagnosis difficult. With organic brain syndrome some patients experience communication problems such as aphasia (inability to express oneself or understand speech properly). Aphasia can result from the poisoning. Alexithymia can also cause the patient to be misunderstood. Alexithymia is inability to respond with proper emotional, psychological, or physical signals when expressing distress.[785a]

Problems with communication are only one obstacle the chemical sensitive faces as a patient. Another problem is that medications prescribed to alleviate one symptom may, because of certain ingredients, exacerbate other symptoms, or even worsen the problem the medication was intended to cure. For example, many CS patients develop asthma from toxic exposure. Those who do are likely to be given prescriptions for bronchodilators, aerosols which open restricted airways when inhaled. Normally bronchodilators provide initial relief, but the effectiveness tends to be short lived. The doctor increases the dosage, tries other products, and continues to hear complaints. It is not unusual for the chemical sensitive ultimately to refuse to use the products, because of the way they make him feel. He would rather have restricted airways than use medicine which makes him sick. The physician can easily become irritated with the patient and attach a label to him: "non-compliant." Neither the physician nor the patient recognizes that the propellants and in some cases the artificial sweeteners used in the aerosols are causing the problem that the medicine is designed to cure. (It should be noted that the Ventolin Rotahaler, recently introduced, has solved this problem of some patients, since only the bronchodilator is inhaled.)

The chart below illustrates three major propellants used in inhalers:

Propellant	Common Name	Inhaler Trade Name
dichlorodifluoromethane	Freon 12	Atrovent, Alupent, Azmacort, Intal, Proventil, Ventolin
dichlorotetrafluoroethane	Freon 114	Alupent, Atrovent, Intal
trichloromonofluoromethane	Freon 11	Alupent, Atrovent, Proventil, Ventolin

The general public is not unacquainted with the fact that chlorofluorocarbons deplete the ozone layer, or that chlorofluorocarbons in aerosol containers have a potential health risk, particularly for youthful and ignorant experimenters who separate the propellant from the product and breathe the propellant. What the general public has not addressed is the effect of chlorofluorocarbons on human health in common usage.

Propellants in the inhalers used by asthma sufferers are freons. Freons are chlorofluorocarbons. They are toxic. Freons are used as refrigerants and aerosol propellants. The toxic effects include confusion, pulmonary irritation, tremors, coma laryngeal spasm or edema, oxygen displacement, sensitization of the myocardium to endogenous catecholamines with subsequent ventricular fibrillation, cardiac arrest, respiratory paralysis, asphyxia, and death.[140]

Freon 12 causes lung irritation at high levels, and, if heated, it decomposes to HCL, CL_2, HF, F_2, and phosgene.[140] Freon 12 "if inhaled, will cause dizziness, difficult breathing," according to the Coast Guard CHRIS manual.[704] Freon 11 is not entirely inert, and had the most widespread use until it was banned for use as an aerosol propellant (i.e., 85 percent reduction in products such as aerosol hairspray). Freon 11 has the highest degree of cardiotoxicity in monkeys, and like Freon 114 it may cause central nervous depression.[140] These descriptions may be designed for large level, acute exposure, but it is clear from the literature that chronic, low level toxic exposures may do the greater damage.

Chronic, low level exposure is, of course, what inhalers provide. *Environmental Health Perspectives*, Vol. 11, pp. 215–220,[712] indicates that "halogenated hydrocarbons . . . would have to be suspected as potential health risks for the general population. . . . Though Freons are considered to be chemically inert in the environment, this may not be true in biological systems." Since there are alternatives (e.g. nebulizers, Ventolin Rotacaps), and since chlorofluorocarbons deplete the ozone layer, why they are used at all is an enigma.

Use of inhalers with freon propellants definitely can complicate the medical picture for the CS patient. Failure to recognize intermittent asthma when a breathing test demonstrates reverse results (breathing is worse after use of aerosol bronchodilator) indicates a lack of understanding, not necessarily a lack of asthma. Increasing dosage of inhalers for patients complaining of continuing problems, particularly when the patient points to the inhalers as a problem, may only make the asthma worse. The patient may have the answer and present it to a doctor, only to be written up as non-compliant, obsessive-compulsive, or histrionic.

The chemical sensitive may appear non-compliant or histrionic when standard pharmaceuticals generate significant and unpredicted side effects. Systemic reactions to drugs are common in the experience of the chemical sensitive, but that information is not standard medical knowledge. Those who have difficulty with formaldehyde may have difficulty with an array of pharmaceuticals having formaldehyde in the binding that holds the medicine together. Others may find that antibiotics, oral steroids, or other drugs are intolerable. Since chemical sensitives react to amounts at lower and lower levels, difficulty with medicine is routine. Doctors do learn quickly when a patient experiences anaphylactic shock from a standard dose of a prescribed medicine. One hopes that the doctor hearing the call of the chemical sensitive in shock will not write it off as histrionics of a "head case"—a potentially deadly and costly error.

Aside from appearing non-compliant, the patient may discover some side effects from exposures to certain substances and begin to use those discoveries to his own detriment. For example, exposures to gasoline vapors or the odors from the application of tar to roofs or roads produce in some people an initial reaction of hyperactivity and sleeplessness. A person who responds in that manner may use the effect to produce the energy he needs to counteract the extreme fatigue he feels. Finding that something (e.g. filling the car with gasoline or contacting some perfumes) provides a boost of energy, even though the patient may recognize that the energy is abnormal, can appear to be a great discovery. It can come as a big shock to learn from a physician who understands the mechanisms, that the "discovery" amounts to the voluntary destruction of one's own brain cells.

A problem patient may have other self-generated problems which contribute to the problem patient label, problems unrelated to CS. For example, some individuals are unprepared for medical professionals to be human. A doctor is no more immune to greed, no more incapable of lying, no more protected from error, no less susceptible to peer pressure, but no less admirable or deserving of respect than any other human. Once the chemical sensitive knows what the problem is, the pedestal upon which he may have set the doctor may crumble into an irreparable heap. It can be difficult for the patient with the stereotype to redefine his concept of doctors.

If the CS patient has had no problems with physicians in identifying the cause of the illness (rare, but it occurs), that picture may change once he begins to read adversarial medical reports (by "defense" doctors selected by benefits administrators or the opposition in a lawsuit). He may experience shock of another kind, one that can easily result in a functional problem.

The chemical sensitive may also be a problem patient by remaining loyal to a physician who does not have knowledge of CS or rejects it as a legitimate illness. When a physician is not successful in dealing with a medical problem, the patient should look elsewhere (e.g. the phone book for an occupational or environmental medicine doctor, if the cause is suspected).

Once diagnosis of CS is confirmed, the chemical sensitive should find out who's who in his area. He should know who recognizes the disease, who treats it and how, who serves as adversarial physicians, and so on. This information is available through support groups (see Chapter 4), physicians, other chemical sensitives, and attorneys; in some cases there are also clues in the yellow pages of the phone book. It is important to know how the primary care physician, who has provided the majority of the patient's care to the point of correct diagnosis, will deal with the diagnosis, if he did not suspect it himself. Patients may feel most peculiar educating physicians who treat them. Nevertheless, it is possible to work with many doctors, even if initially they vehemently reject the idea of CS. In these cases, the attitude of the patient is vital to a successful outcome. There is adequate information to provide these doctors, if they can entertain the possibility that CS may be the problem. The CS patient who works with these doctors helps not only himself but also other people who will develop the disease in the future.

The person with CS is a problem when he has an expectation that others should provide all his support and assistance. If there is a goal to reach, the person with CS must make the effort to reach it. Support groups are beneficial, but the member who expects the group leader to carry him is asking too much. Those who have CS are doing the best they can to carry themselves. If an advocate is needed, the answer is an attorney; but an attorney cannot begin to do the job unless the individual with CS does his. The chemical sensitive has to document his case (see Chapter 5). Nobody else can do it. If entitlements or litigation is the goal, it's either fight or eliminate the goal. Fighting involves considerable effort, especially since the chemical sensitive is often overwhelmed and exhausted. Essentially, the choice of whether to fight boils down to bloody battlefield experience. The enemy has shot the chemical sensitive in both legs. There's a choice: He can lie there and bleed to death, or he can crawl off the battlefield on his elbows (which may only set him up to be shot again). The chemical sensitive who successfully makes such a crawl will find a sense of satisfaction, a kind of joy, and respect from others. It is the crawlers who stand a chance of winning their wars.

Finally, there is a problem patient of a different kind, the one who permits himself to generate a poison from within: bitterness. Bitterness drives others away—avoidance of identifiable toxics is instinctive human behavior. A poisoned person who adds this additional poison to his system accomplishes nothing. Casting blame and hating others is self-destructive. Bitterness is one poison a person can eliminate by a conscious decision to change his way of thinking.

The Persistent Problem

Chemical sensitivity is a *persistent problem* for a multitude of reasons. There is a tremendous amount of information already available on the subject, but that information is not systematically organized and accessible. Much of the information is valuable and accurate; some of it is pointedly filled with bias and self-interest. It is difficult for the researcher to know which is which. There is a lot of money to be made at this time for those who will provide documentation that CS does not exist—even though, by the rules of logic, such proof is not possible. There is the medical principle, lack of evidence if not evidence of lack. There is the scientific principle, one cannot prove zero.

Part of the problem with CS is that medicine is structured in an over-specialized manner. A doctor sees patients in his field of specialization, even though the human is a composite of interworking systems. The primary care physician, who may be the only physician to see a patient in a generalized way, may lack the background necessary to recognize the possibility of or know how to treat a chronic, low level toxic exposure patient. Even those doctors who have spent years treating CS patients don't have all the answers. Not only does a chemical sensitive frequently end up with a patchwork of diagnoses—dermatitis, colitis, vasculitis, reactive airways, reproductive problems, fatigue, idiopathic edema, dehydration, hair loss, depression, to name a few—but the cause of the medical problem remains undetected. Consequently, it's a matter of treating the symptoms instead of searching for the root cause of the disease.

To further complicate the problem, those medical professionals who know the disease cannot agree. There is a battle in the medical world over who has authority to speak on the disease. The battle is well described in (1) *Chemical Sensitivity: A Report to the New Jersey State Department of Health* by Nicholas A. Ashford, of the Massachusetts Institute of Technology, and Claudia S. Miller of the University of Texas Health Service Center, December 1989 (copy available from National Center for Environmental Health Strategies, 1100 Rural Avenue, Voorhees, New Jersey 08043 at a cost of $17.00); and (2) *Chemical Hypersensitivity Syndrome Study* by Rebecca Bascom, University of Maryland School of Medicine, prepared for the State of Maryland, Department of the Environment. (The study and comments can be purchased for $27 from the National Center for Environmental Health Strategies at the address above.)

Mark Cullen, one of the pioneering researchers into CS developed in occupational settings, in the conclusion to his book *Workers with Multiple Chemical Sensitivities*[165] makes the following comment:

> The health problems of workers who react to low levels of environmental pollutants and chemicals, increasingly reported and recognized in recent years,

> has posed a serious dilemma for health providers from a wide array of disciplines, including generalists, internists, family practitioners, allergists, psychiatrists, social workers, and frequently occupational physicians and nurses. The inability of these professionals to provide satisfactory care from the patient's perspective has led to the emergency of new and alternative clinical theories and approaches, challenging traditional views. Unfortunately, the success of these alternative approaches has also not been demonstrated, fueling an ever widening and hostile debate in which the patient is held hostage and virtually all clinicians are rendered impotent because of widely known intraprofessional disagreements.

Aside from initial bias on the part of researchers, there are other significant problems. To perform the studies that are viewed as necessary, some scientists wish to use challenge tests with suspected triggers. At this point an ethical problem raises its head: The triggers can cause irreversible damage to subjects.

For example, the standard methacholine challenge test given to asthmatics whose asthma presents atypically can cause severe and unanticipated problems. A chemical sensitive with asthma can report for the challenge, demonstrate asthma, be given a bronchodilator to turn the reaction around, go home, and experience a massive delayed reconstriction which requires significant effort to restore opened airways. The effect may last for years, requiring the administration of drugs which the patient was able to do without until the challenge test. The Food and Drug Administration knows that this can occur, but getting the information out may take time because so few cases have been reported. Hospital data gives the impression that the drug is essentially safe for humans.

Meanwhile, researchers in some locations are gearing up for study by creating exotic inhalation chambers to study chemical sensitivity in human subjects. With the reactions people can have to a fairly standard challenge test, it is easy to imagine that inhalation chambers may create a much more significant problem than already exists. What is more, once the tests are conducted, there is no assurance that they will provide valuable information. It would be possible to interpret the results as psychogenic, even if they are not. People, doctors included, can interpret results any way they choose.

Considering the current lack of the sort of information that might lead patients and physicians to address some of these obstacles, chemical sensitivity is likely to remain a problem for quite some time.

The Problem Physician

Hippocrates, a physician of ancient Greece (est. 460–377 B.C.), is credited with generating one of the first principles of medicine, incorporated in the Hippocratic oath: *First, do no harm.* But sadly, where chemical sensitives are concerned, harm has been done. It occurs through lack of knowledge, misunderstanding, hasty decision-making, assumptions based on opinion rather than fact, and so on. Two major classes of *problem physicians* affect the chemical sensitive: (1) physicians unacquainted with CS, and (2) physicians acquainted with it. A third class might be reserved for physicians participating in independent medical exams (IMEs) or panels. Patients are required to participate in IMEs which are conducted by "defense doctors" and initiated by adversaries in litigation, benefits administration, or others contesting financial claims by CS patients.

• Physicians Unacquainted with CS

If the estimate by the National Academy of Sciences Institute of Medicine is correct,[710] this group comprises 98 percent of physicians who were practicing in the 1980s in the United States. A study of the effects of poisoning from chronic, low level toxic exposure with its resulting chemical sensitivity was not part of the curriculum when the majority of these physicians attended medical school. Very little literature about CS has been directed to the primary care physician. Even less emphasis is placed upon the relationship among the nervous, endocrine, and immune systems when toxic chemicals in the environment affect them.

Giving the medical profession its due, physicians are among the most educated people in the United States. To have medical authority requires great intelligence along with cognitive skills in analysis, synthesis, and evaluation; curiosity to stay current in the field; perseverance; stamina; a desire to heal; and so on.

Again to be fair, one must acknowledge that physicians are under great pressure, from their peers in medical and academic communities, to conform to standard practices. The medical professional who attempts a unique treatment may be labeled by his own profession as unorthodox, a term that sounds theological but is the rough equivalent of kook. Further, solid scientific methodological practice dictates that physicians not draw conclusions without proper proof.

Unfortunately, the very elements that are required in scientific research are the ones that hinder progress when dealing with a disorder such as chemical sensitivity.[241] Admission of recognition of the disorder may be enough to bias results. So is characterizing CS as an illusory mental problem. Most research is tied to universities. Universities have financial difficulties, and funding comes from sources where money is available for endowment. Most chemical sensitives, even collectively, don't fit that category. There are expectations tied to funding. Track down the sources of funds for CS research, and you will often find someone with a stake in the outcome. Certainly this can prevent effective research.

Also inhibiting the search for solutions are problems among some doctors that include inability to say, "I don't know"; inability to trust the patient; inability to see a problem from a different point of view; and lack of creativity. All of these problems stem from too great a focus on self and too little on the needs of the patient—that is, the all-too-human tendency to think more of oneself than one should. It may be difficult for a doctor who is proud of his medical knowledge to admit that a patient may know more about a particular disease than he.

Doctors are experts, but that does not make their observations 100 percent correct. It is unrealistic for a patient to believe that his doctor is always right. It is equally unrealistic for a physician to assume that his diagnosis is correct or complete when the patient fails to improve, or even gets worse, with the prescribed treatment. That physician needs to look further. A patient's failure to improve could be a result of non-compliance or a psychogenic problem, or it could be a misdiagnosis.

Individual patient responsibility exists. There is nothing wrong with asking a doctor to rethink a decision. There is everything wrong with continuing with one who will not. A doctor can think more of himself than he should, become locked into tunnel vision, have a bad day, fail to think, have mental confusion from chemical exposure from the tight medical buildings in which he works, and so on. Patients who run into these problems consistently with one doctor should not hesitate to go elsewhere.

• Physicians Acquainted with CS

In the few cases where CS is recognized, there is warfare among four groups. This display is intriguing to the outsider and extremely frustrating to the chemical sensitive. Essentially, here is a breakdown of the battle:

ORTHODOX MEDICAL PRACTITIONERS—MAJORITY VIEW

This view uses the term multiple chemical sensitivity syndrome (MCSS) to label the disease and concludes that it is characterized by (1) acquired multiple organ system symptoms and (2) symptoms precipitated by diverse environmental factors in the absence of a recognizable pathological process. According to this view, the psychological role, as cause or consequence, is unclear. Those holding to this majority view refuse to discuss the disease in terms of neuroendocrineimmune system dysfunction, because of the lack of double blind studies. (See Glossary for definition of double blind study.) Numbers of doctors who recognize MCSS will readily admit that they have significant ignorance of neurology, immunology, or endocrinology. They feel comfortable with a syndrome but not a disease. This perspective on CS is simple and aligns with all the other views—it is general enough to prevent scientific discredit.

Some medical researchers and practicioners go a bit further, forming subsets of the majority. One includes those who recognize central nervous system (CNS) involvement from toxic exposure which results in clinically recognizable organic brain syndrome. Muriel Lezak, an international authority on organic brain syndrome, deals with the subject in *Neuropsychological Assessment*,[369] in which she discusses organicity and the vagaries of damage to the brain from chemical exposure.

A second subset holds that MCSS is a function of psychologic vulnerability[629, 643] following environmental illness or injury with one of three mechanisms: (1) Pavlovian conditioning,[80] (2) "masked" psychiatric illness,[170] or (3) somatization[99]/hypochondriasis. Patients can be treated by behavioral deconditioning, relaxation training, and specific pharmacotherapy. (The source of this statement is course materials from "Recent Developments in Occuptional Medicine—MCSS," May 5, 1989, Northwest Center for Occupational Health and Safety, University of Washington, Seattle, Washington.)

Convenient though it may be—since it purports to narrow the cause of all CS to three mechanisms—there are four major problems with the disease model just described. First, in order to maintain this view, one must accept a double standard,[22] requiring double blind studies in order to accept toxic-induced chronic systemic disease while being willing to accept a psychological model requiring no double blind studies. Second, the recommendation for pharmacotherapy for chemical sensitives has some significant drawbacks: many CS patients have a poor response to drugs, and some drugs can mask the symptoms, so that the chemical buildup is overwhelming before it is recognized. If the problem is organic brain syndrome, extensive brain damage could result before the patient had any warning of danger. Third, the view is myopic. Fear or anxiety is but one disconnected stimulus in the cycle of CS self-perpetuation, but followers of this model see it as the sole cause. Fourth, this view requires a reversal of a standard medical principle that all avenues of medical investigation be thoroughly reviewed prior to assumption of psychologic or psychiatric causation. Ignorance or prejudice is a factor here. Quantitative EEGs with evoked potentials can easily document that exposure to a minute amount of a chemical can elicit a massive response as the brain perceives it. In the absence of such tests, doctors should remain silent.

To carry the concept of cure by behavioral deconditioning to conclusion, suppose a physician chose to treat a CS patient bothered by road fumes using this methodology. First, the physician and patient would have to accept the idea that road fumes are non-toxic. Road fumes, the lay term for vehicular emissions, contain significant toxic substances.[387, 412] According to the *Air Quality Data Summary*[7] published by the Puget Sound Air Pollution Control Agency, vehicular emissions contain:

carbon monoxide (reducing oxygen-carrying capacity of blood and weakening heart contractions)
particulate matter (injuring the respiratory tract by itself or in conjunction with gasses)
sulfur dioxide (constricting lung passages; associated with respiratory disease and increased mortality rates, and with particulates increasing the deleterious effects on health)
lead (affecting blood-forming systems, the nervous system and kidneys)
nitrogen dioxide (causing respiratory disease).

To treat a patient in this manner is illogical. If the patient has organic brain syndrome, such "treatment" is likely to destroy brain cells. There is no documented case of a chemical sensitive's ever having been cured through any treatment, including psychological or psychiatric channels. Part of the problem here may be a result of poor communication. Perception is altered when one's brain is compromised by toxic chemicals. A CS patient perceives a small level of toxic exposure as if it were enormous. That perception is correct. To one whose brain is not compromised it may be difficult to understand what the CS patient is expressing. Fortunately, medicine is not dependent on a doctor's having experienced every disease, disorder, illness, or syndrome they treat. Because a physician's assessment is so important to those chemical sensitives who attempt to pursue their entitlements or initiate a lawsuit, a further word is necessary here. Categorizing CS as a functional mental illness prevents people who are sick and cannot work from receiving their entitlements, if the injury is occupational but medical opinion considers it emotional. It bars them from legal recourse if there is an identifiable cause (product) linked to the illness. They get sicker; they are labeled crazy or lazy; they lose substantially from a financial angle. They wonder whatever happened to *first, do no harm.*

ORTHODOX MEDICAL PRACTITIONERS—MINORITY VIEW

Viewed from the perspective of this group, the disorder goes by the names chemical poisoning, chemical sensitivity, sick building syndrome, (occasionally) MCSS, and others. The progressive aspects of the disorder are recognized by immunologists and pathologists in California[692] and elsewhere, plus an increasing number of very quiet, strictly orthodox physicians. The sequence is as follows: toxic exposure; chemical poisoning (physiological dysfunction); development of an abnormal, activated immune system which leads to multi-system symptoms from the initial toxic and spreads to other substances at increasingly lower levels of exposure development of autoantibodies with potential for autoimmune disease; eventual suppression of the immune response; and frequent concomitant significant, documentable, organic brain syndrome (toxic encephalopathy) to varying degrees, uncommon for the general population.

An additional view of the spreading phenomenon taken by some immunologists is that CS may, in addition to being triggered by toxic substances, be triggered subsequent to poisoning by non-toxic irritants, which explode the already existing hypersensitive reactions. The psychiatric view of this group is unlike the model discussed in the previous section, which considers human "software" the problem and manipulation of it the cure. This group perceives the human computer "hardware" as the focus. Toxic substances have caused the computer (brain) to malfunction, and, no matter what one does to the software, it isn't going to work correctly. The issue is biochemical, not psychiatric.

There is increasing scientific data to demonstrate immunologic compromise and toxic encephalopathy resulting from toxic exposure. More attention is being given to the concept of compromised systemic integrity resulting from toxic exposure. The concept is not new. Over a decade ago work in this area was documented.[4] The concept is not a good fit in the current structured approach to medicine. When the structure and function of the nervous system is better understood, when PET scan metabolic evidence and brain topography electrical evidence becomes routine diagnostic technique tied with immune profiles and neuropsychological assessment, the current medical system may be forced to adapt. It is possible that it is this need to adapt that is the fundamental issue in the internal medical war. Established organizational structures are generally sites for strong rejection to change, or adaptation.

ALTERNATIVE MEDICAL PRACTITIONERS—MAJORITY VIEW

These practitioners characteristically use the terms environmental illness, twentieth century disease, and total allergy syndrome, and refer to patients as universal reactors. The major focus for this perspective, initiated decades ago,[504] is on finding and eliminating root causes of medical problems. Processes involve painstaking trials after removing the patient to a clean environment. Various substances are introduced to determine how the patient responds. Treatment associated with this view involves (1) identifying deficiency states that may contribute to the problem (e.g. vitamin, amino acid, and enzyme deficiencies) or any condition that may reduce ability to eliminate internal toxics; (2) detoxification (see Appendix B) to remove toxics from the body, reducing the load with which the body is burdened; (3) emphasizing feeling better; and (4) treating contributory infections or infestations such as Candida or internal parasites.

A very large number of patients, fed up with the obvious problems in the orthodox community of medical practitioners, have turned to these physicians because they find that the treatment makes a difference. The healthy lifestyle that some of these physicians practice and encourage is certainly advantageous to any human, though the approach can seem overly health conscious to some individuals, even those with chemical sensitivity. A distinct disadvantage is the expense involved in some of these programs, especially when reliance upon these doctors to the exclusion of orthodox practitioners is viewed negatively by benefits administrators in entitlement fights.

Orthodox doctors, too, frequently have a negative view of alternative practitioners. Such prejudice is sometimes demonstrated by subtle use of language in medical articles.* Total allergy syndrome, environmental illness, allergic to life, and so on are terms used by clincial ecologists, but when used by orthodox doctors they are twisted into arrogant put-downs of environmental medicine practitioners and their patients.

One of the orthodox attacks upon the environmental group is that their treatments are unproven, experimental. When one considers that less than half of medical treatment is "proven," such an argument loses some of its strength. Essentially the argument is designed more for the uninitiated than for the medical profession, despite the fact that the articles in which it appears seem to be targeted to the profession. It is important to recognize that "peer reviewed" articles are admissible in court as evidence. It is possible, then, that some articles may be written with at least a partial intent of having them available for testimony. With that in mind, and a knowledge of which doctors are serving a substantial amount of time as IME/defense doctors, objectivity in the literature may be called into question.

The major difference between orthodox-minority and alternative-majority doctors is the extent to which they are comfortable with risk management, that is, balancing the risks and potential benefits of new treatments and proceeding accordingly. Success may be achieved by unproven treatment. It happens all the time: antibiotics are given to prevent secondary infection when a patient has the flu; bone marrow transplants for those with leukemia; taking aspirin to reduce fever; and so on. These qualify as experimental or unproven. That does not in any way mean that patients may be experimented upon at the whim of a doctor. Successful risk management carefully identifies and weighs all the options. Consultation with the patient is critical. After evaluation and consultation, a management program is set in motion. Monitoring is an essential part. Ironically, it can be argued by the environmental medicine community that some of the most significant experimenting with CS patients is occurring at the

**Some examples of infighting through use of language in the literature are evident in the following references: 98, 128, 141, 251, 467, 573, 608, 629, 635, 674, 680. An excellent scientific review of some of these articles can be found in the following reference: 174a.*

hands of super-orthodox IME/defense doctors (more on this below) when they give challenge tests to CS patients. Taking risks is not the exclusive domain of the environmental medicine community or of any other group.

What CS patients should focus on is finding a doctor—regardless of category—who is knowledgeable in the field of toxic exposure cases; who will search for root causes; who has breadth to identify as many variables as possible; who informs the patient of treatment options; and who describes for the patient what he perceives to be the most likely means to achieve success and why. Last but not least, the doctor must be available to the patient when any treatment or change in treatment is instituted.

ALTERNATIVE MEDICINE PRACTITIONERS—MINORITY VIEW

A very few alternative medicine practitioners claim that they can cure CS. Some of these doctors may be doing harm to patients by use of colonics, by challenging extremely sensitive patients, or by using other questionable forms of treatment. Patients of these doctors will often claim cure. It is not unusual for the "cured" CS patient to insist that those who will not go to the miracle doctor just don't want to get well. In some cases, the relationship between patient and doctor seems to have developed into some form of personality cult.

Medical investigation into the practices of these doctors should begin without delay. If valid, they would alleviate the suffering of numbers of individuals. If not valid, patients should be warned about parting with financial resources for something of no value.

• Independent Medical Exam (IME)

Independent medical exam is a misnomer. The exam is not independent, but rather performed for the patient's adversary. The IME presents the chemical sensitive with another situation in which he may not only fail to find medical assistance but also be injured temporarily or permanently. The physician who takes part in an IME is legally protected if he misdiagnoses or injures a patient physically or psychologically. The IME, sometimes called a medical panel, has one purpose: diagnosis. The physicians are paid well and in a timely manner by interested parties. These physicians are given carte blanche to perform any tests, regardless of medical need, or to hospitalize a patient if they choose. Their diagnostic opinions are valued equally with those of the patient's physicians, if not more so, though the time spent with the patient may be less than an hour. In contrast it is noteworthy that some doctors who render positive reports on IMEs (positive to the patient) are frequently not paid. Doctors chosen by CS patients often are not paid. Eventually these physicians may deny access to CS patients.

Patients requesting, under the Freedom of Information Act, copies of reports written by IME physicians have had their requests denied. Even attorneys may have to resort to legal battles to gain access to these reports.[261] With non-federally ordered exams, such a practice may be legal. With federally ordered IMEs the practice is not legal.

Examination of reports written by IME physicians can be revealing. Some doctors perform these services on such a regular basis that when numbers of chemical sensitives manage to get the reports and compare them, they have discovered that the word processing system in the doctor's office evidently contains a standard report for an IME chemical sensitive patient. The doctor need only insert a word here, a phrase there to personalize the report.

Once the IME physician has seen the patient, contact between the two terminates. The patient is actually forbidden to contact the doctor. If, for example, additional medical data are generated after the IME and before the doctor writes his report, the patient cannot give those data to the IME physician. The new data could affect the report in some fairly significant ways. Consequently, in such cases, the written report at best is incomplete staff work. In workers' compensation cases, it is the taxpayer, both state and federal, who shoulders the burden of cost for a product which, if produced in the business world, would be rejected outright.

The Problem People

Aside from problem physicians, the person with CS encounters a variety of *problem people*. These people can have as much, if not more, impact on the life of the chemical sensitive as the physician.

Insurers

Health insurers are the single most baffling source of resistance to the recognition of CS and to the development of constructive risk management programs. The fact that chemical sensitives can see 15 to 30 or more doctors prior to diagnosis should send out a signal to insurers: namely, that the health insurance industry has a serious expenditure for tests and office visits where results demonstrate little, if anything. Recognition that CS occurs carries the potential to save cost. An informed and pro-active claims examiner could at the very least recognize the claims pattern and recommend consideration of toxic exposure as possible cause. Furthermore, acknowledging that the longer the person is exposed, the worse the disorder becomes, should generate cost-saving practices. Finally, group insurers often carry the heavy costs of initial testing, when, in workplace poisoning, workers' compensation should be paying the medical expenses. Subrogation (retrieving funds from the responsible party) for initial diagnostics often costs more than taking the loss.

Resistance from insurers other than those involved with health claims is easier to understand. Whether a person is chemically poisoned at work, at home or elsewhere, frequently the only recourse is litigation. Insurers who provide liability protection to employers, or to manufacturers and retailers of toxics, stand to lose when CS has extensive recognition.

Instead of meeting the problem head-on by training insurance loss control representatives in air pollution detection, adequately researching or contributing to research on new chemicals and their potential effects, reviewing product packaging for clear communications, and requiring organizations to fix problems or lose coverage, insurance companies tend to shrug the problem off. If workplace toxics are evident, the typical attitude is "Workplaces are like that," or, "If people can't work there, they can go work somewhere else." When consumers use products indoors that are labeled for outdoor use only, the liability issue ends not with the manufacturer of the product but rather with the user. But what if the user is dyslexic, illiterate, or a recent immigrant unfamiliar with the language? What if the package says to use the product outdoors and the pictures show indoor use? What if the product instructions state that a mask is required, but one is not included in the product package and the pictures show the product in use without the safety device?

With increasingly sophisticated methods of identifying the occurrence of chemical poisoning, increasing evidence of the problem, and no alternative for the injured party but to seek relief legally, insurers should be managing the problem now. So far, the only evidence that insurers recognize the devastating effects of CS is the fact that a person with organic brain syndrome, regardless of type, will not be able to purchase health or life insurance at any price except through conversion on a group policy if that applies.

• Employers

It is not difficult to understand why employers might wish to ignore the problem of chemical poisoning. Consider our analogy to the canaries in the coal mine. When profit is the motive, it's easy to adopt a policy of burying dead canaries and purchasing new ones.

Putting the ethics of such a policy aside, ignoring the problem may well be suicidal for businesses. Toxic exposures exist. In June 1987, the Environmental Protection Agency published *The Total Exposure Assessment Methodology (TEAM) Study: Summary and Analysis: Volume 1.*[741]

Much has been learned since the study was published, but it is significant as a first legitimate documentation of cause and effect in chemical sensitivity. In addition to documenting exposures and identifying possible sources, the report briefly addresses health effects. Essentially the concern was carcinogenicity (potential for cancer), but the cogent points made include the following from page 107 of the report:

> *Under the section dealing with chronic effects:* A second chronic effect of interest is chemical sensitivity. This is an ill-defined condition marked by progressively more debilitating severe reactions to various consumer products such as perfumes, soaps, tobacco, smoke, plastics, etc. The incidence of this syndrome is unknown; however, anecdotal accounts indicate that it may be increasing sharply. The effects on productivity of affected persons can be severe.
>
> *Under the section dealing with acute effects:* A second ill-defined group of symptoms, sometimes known as Sick Building Syndrome, affects numbers of office workers. The symptoms include sleepiness, nausea, eye irritation, irritability, forgetfulness, and a number of other respiratory and central nervous system disorders. One experiment has determined that the symptoms are unlikely to be related to mass psychology or otherwise psychosomatic. A second experiment has shown that mixtures of common organic pollutants (mostly xylenes) at levels similar to those in new buildings can cause both subjective and objective symptoms in a group of sensitive individuals.

Where employers are concerned, the significant word in the first quoted paragraph is *productivity*. Low productivity affects profits. Whether exposures are chronic or acute or both, simply having toxic substances (identified or unidentified) and irritants in the building can affect productivity.

Beyond the effects on productivity, another issue is turnover. The path of least resistance when an employee is confronted with illness from substances within the workplace is to leave willingly. Perhaps he may have to leave unwillingly, through termination from excessive absence or poor performance. Frequently the chemical sensitive has no idea what is wrong and may actually come to believe, "I'm just a poor performer—worthless." Once the poor-performer label is attached, nobody challenges with, "Are you sure?" Failure to meet performance standards is the obvious problem, but the poor performance may be a symptom of toxic exposure, a compensable workplace illness.

In other words, an employer can unwittingly create an environment which poisons an employee and then remove the employee for performance problems which are a direct result of the environment. For the former employee who cannot find another job or is too sick to work, financial disaster follows.

It is worth noting that not all workers who are chemically poisoned will exhibit performance problems severe enough to remove them from the workplace. Chemical poisoning can also cause mental impairment to those who remain on the job, thus draining an organization of critical brain power.

In all fairness, employers are not out looking for ways to poison employees. Most employers are simply not aware that workplace poisoning can occur. If there were a campaign to educate employers, CS might be reduced through their intervention, rather than perpetuated by their ignorance.

Some employers may fear that if one employee is diagnosed with CS, other workers would suddenly come down with psychologically generated CS symptoms. Fear of this effect, known as the Hawthorne effect, need not stand in an employer's way, for there are tests which actually show immune system activation in response to toxics. People cannot fake their blood tests. Neuropsychologic assessment and tests measuring brain metabolic and electrical activity are other indicators. Toxicological studies are available, and the results cannot be manipulated. Doctors who routinely deal with numbers of individuals from a single workplace estimate the number of somatizers to be at about 2 percent. That is hardly a ripple characteristic of the Hawthorne effect.

When the highest management levels recognize a toxic problem, they can choose to address it or to create deception. Deception is unethical. It stems from placing greater value on immediate profit than on human life. It is also illogical, for profit depends on the good condition of the workers who produce. Failure to act in the long run costs even more.

Deception can also be motivated by an emotional reaction to the very concept that poisoning can exist in the work environment. Poisoning is a very strong word. There is an element of horror associated with the subject. Workers—including managers—who hear of poisoning will recognize that they too are at risk. That is hard to deal with. Fear can surface.

To use an analogy, there are numbers of intelligent people who develop potentially malignant growths. They know that the growths should be examined. They put off going to a doctor, hoping that the thing will go away, if they ignore it. Then, when they finally go for examination, it's too late. People react in a similar way to the possiblity of poisoning. One emotional reaction to horror is to shut down the thinking process. Playing ostrich-with-its-head-in-the-sand is unworthy behavior for those who would aspire to management. So is crisis-reactive, defensive behavior. The appropriate response is pro-active behavior. It starts with listening to the canary. The canary can tell management more about the working environment than anyone would guess.

Chemical sensitives are diagnosed through medical tests. What do these tests reveal about the environment? What places in the environment do they pinpoint as sources of the problems? In most cases the location of the source can be identified. What does an unbiased chemical laboratory identify as the actual exposures (regardless of "safe" levels) in the working environment? What can be done to eliminate the hazards or reduce the risk of exposing more employees? Do other employees have the problem and not know it? Would running an annual health analysis profile be helpful? Generating such questions, pursuing them to the end, and acting in a mature manner free of deception is appropriate, pro-active management responsibility. It is behavior worthy of respect.

• Environmentalists, Industrialists, and Government Officials

Environmentalists have a penchant for scolding manufacturers of toxic substances, whether the substances are designed for commercial or domestic use. They also point fingers at industrial manufacturers who pollute, knowingly or unknowingly, as a result of the processes they use. They are right, but perhaps their methods are self-defeating. Doom-and-gloom perspectives have a tendency to retard progress in reaching desired goals. Use of fear as a motivator is self-defeating. A normal response to the doom and gloom is to close the mind. On the other hand, continuing to pollute the environment with poisons and irritants is nothing to conceal. Somewhere in between lies government with regulatory and enforcement responsibility at federal, state, and local levels, trying to effect a balance between what is safe and what is economical.

Concerns of safety and economy create a hotbed of issues. Environmentalists blame government officials for poor regulation and enforcement. Industrialists and the workers who earn their living in the industry complain of the economic impact of shutdowns. "Safe levels" of toxics become an issue. Ingredients and processes are shrouded in secrecy. Injured workers or people in the area who attempt to issue health warnings may be called "radical environmentalists" or "chemophobics." Put issues from environmentalists, industrialists, those who have been chemically poisoned, and government officials into a large pot and you have a witch's brew out of which can surface civil disobedience, violence, political games, and corruption.

The United States as a whole has an acceptance mentality where pollution is concerned, while giving lip service to avoidance. For example, Puget Sound, located in Washington State, is vigorously defended from pollution by environmentalists and Native American groups. Before dredged material is disposed of in the Sound, tests have to prove that the substance is safe for mud worms. Mud worms tunnel through the sediment. Their value in the ecosystem is unknown, but because they exist, they are protected. With water column analysis, taking readings at various depths is not enough for this environmentally sensitive area. Analysis is also performed at the bottom. Mud from the bottom is brought up and tested for its effects on actual living organisms (e.g. sand fleas).

When dealing with indoor and outdoor pollution, we consider ourselves less than mud worms. Our own immediate environments are subject to no such rigorous testing. Further, our thinking is provincial. A source of pollution 20 miles away is not perceived as an immediate danger, let alone one in a state 800 miles away. Yet toxics can be carried by wind from Texas to New York. It is time to restructure our thinking. Remember the coal mine? What happens if, when it's time to get out of the mine, there is no place to go?

• Friends, Family, and Co-Workers

Family and friends may be the first to recognize that the chemically sensitive person has a problem. They may suggest a visit to the doctor, and be rebuffed. Comments they may make in an attempt to be helpful—"You surely do seem to need a lot of sleep these days," or, "You really have been testy lately. Too much stress?"—might be perceived as criticism. A kind of alienation may begin which tends to grow as the symptoms escalate.

Because the person being poisoned may look and sometimes act normal, family and friends may begin to make assumptions about motivators—assumptions which are dead wrong. Some characteristic assumptions are: so-and-so must be having a mid-life crisis; so-and-so just doesn't want to be included; so-and-so lives for work and really doesn't care about anything else. In this way they tend to seek emotional or mental causes for the problem.

Eventually those assumptions appear to be verified as the chemical sensitive becomes more and more self-centered. Resentment can easily build up, particularly when the well friends and family begin to carry some of the load that the chemical sensitive used to carry. Parents can feel frustration regarding their undiagnosed children, who appear lazy at one time, hyperactive at another, or sickly and not responding to medical treatment. Bitterness may develop, and the already poisoned person may absorb that bitterness which can cut quite deeply into a person who is already struggling.

Consider the mother whose daughter was poisoned in a school setting. The child was diagnosed as having an aversion to attending school so the mother insisted, day after day, that the child continue in the environment. Finally, after seeing the child come home early, unable to walk, nauseated, and obviously quite ill, yet trying with everything she had to comply with her mother's wishes, the mother sought and found the answer. When she finally discovered that her child was poisoned and had difficulty with CS, the mother developed and carried a tremendous burden of guilt. The child has learned to go to school regardless, and resents the idea of a different school or, perish the thought, homebound teaching. This case demonstrates how problems of guilt and unlearning may be added to the burden of life with CS.

If the chemical sensitive works, there are co-workers. The essential difference between friends or family and co-workers is that, generally, co-workers are less likely to be understanding. Already overworked employees can resent another's absence or lowered productivity. As a result, they tend to react more readily in a negative manner. This is not a rule, just a generalization.

Co-workers can participate in gossip about the person, diagnosing the problem and arriving at cures as if they had the tools to do so. This is the same process by which friends and family draw assumptions about the cause of the behavior. However, friends and family are unlikely to carry their assumptions into the territory of harassment; sadly, co-workers are often less restrained. Examples of harassment actually experienced by chemical sensitives include refusing to recognize the presence of the chemical sensitive; placing more work on him than he can accomplish; moving the person's worksite to a more deadly location; refusing to give him enough work to do; excluding him from work-social activities; letting him know he is the butt of office jokes; surreptitiously placing announcements of jobs in Saudi Arabia or Afghanistan in his in-basket; bringing a substance into his presence when that substance is known to cause problems; and a number of other mean and less printable ideas.

If co-workers hope that by such behavior they can change the behavior of the chemical sensitive—get him to act more "normal"—they are wasting their energy, for the sick person is likely already straining to appear as normal as possible. On the other hand, if co-workers, family and friends choose to spend some energy in a positive fashion—namely, in striving to understand chemical sensitivity—the result may be a better environment for all.

3. Coping with Chemical Sensitivity

Chemical sensitives are first poisoned and then confronted with a sea of other chemicals which can cause significant problems, sometimes quite literally repoisoning an individual. How do they cope? The range of responses runs anywhere between two extremes: becoming a virtual hermit or denying the problem and attempting to continue life as it was before the initial poisoning. It would be unjust at this point to conclude that either extreme is an inappropriate response or that the solution lies in some program falling somewhere in between. Because too little is known about this disease at present, any program of treatment other than avoidance of offending chemicals is experimental.

The word *experimental* carries different connotations depending on its application. It is fair to estimate that far less than 50 percent of current standard medical practice is proven. The rest is experimental—it is known to work, but *why* it works may not be fully understood. This type of experimental (unproven) treatment is normally acceptable. In other applications, "experimental" is associated with unacceptable practice. According to the norm, anything which is untested or which has potential harmful effects is clearly unacceptable for use on humans.

In the case of the CS patient, the norm is inappropriate. What may be experimentally acceptable for the standard population may be unacceptably experimental for the CS patient, and vice versa. For a chemical sensitive patient to try different coping methods or vary medical treatment with the concurrence of his physician is legitimate. Each CS sufferer has to learn through trial and error what is a problem and what is helpful. What bothers or helps one may not do the same for another, and a medical solution for all is far in the distance. It could be helpful for the medical community to monitor the various methods chosen for coping and identify commonalities which prove beneficial to the CS subgroup.

The "experimental" label often results in denial of medical benefits to people who may have a real need. It is more a health care funding issue than a real dispute over efficacy of treatment. For example, some states will not cover any allergy treatment for welfare recipients despite the fact that a child suffers terribly with hay fever and desensitization shots could control the problem and prevent chronic immune system activation. CS patients who might improve with detoxification may be denied the treatment because it is considered experimental. Toxic encephalopathy sufferers who need oxygen are being told that the use of oxygen for their condition is unproven and not covered. The cost is frequently beyond the reach of CS patients. Those who cannot work, have no financial resources, and must depend on welfare often are excluded from access to the doctors who could help. The reason is not refusal to accept the patients but rather the bureaucratic perception that the disease is one which is not covered or that treatment is experimental. Patients who are insured may discover that some patients using the same carrier may be given access to expensive diagnostic tests (e.g., PET scans, qEEG with evoked potentials) while others are refused pre-authorization.

Health care costs are skyrocketing. One way to decrease the costs to insurers would be for all insurance coverage to exclude medical payments for experimental (unproven) treatment. If, let's say, 35 percent of standard medical treatment were proven and coverage for the remaining 65 percent were excluded, health insurance companies would find their costs reduced to almost nothing—while AIDS patients would die more rapidly; heart patients would have shorter life spans; infants needing liver transplants would not see their school years.... In short, the public simply would not stand for it. Yet today the poor and the sick are being denied treatment that is acceptable, appropriate, and necessary because some of the medical community is willing to make sweeping statements regarding what is experimental, statements which those with responsibility to pay medical expenses willingly believe. It is vital that those who can make a difference in this distressing situation hear and accept two facts: (1) that some CS patients are subjected to harmful "acceptable" experimentation by medical practitioners uneducated in the effects of chemicals in the compromise of systemic integrity; and (2) that some CS patients are denied beneficial "experimental" treatment which only a few practitioners have studied carefully and trained to provide.

Physician and Patient Decisions Regarding Exposure

Because people with CS vary in their levels of sensitivity and the triggers which set off reactions, it is very difficult for the physician to offer advice or to establish a management program. Even more difficult for the physician is to express an opinion as to whether the patient can work or attend school, an opinion that may be required even when the poisoning occurred in a location other than the work site or school. Much hangs on this opinion, not all of it connected with the patient.

Physicians have reputations to establish and uphold. Those involved in claims or litigation usually attempt to establish a reputation for fairness, generally interpreted as that which reflects a balance. Judgments which tend to fall heavily on one side or the other may lead to a reputation for bias often without any knowledge of specific cases.

A physician who sees numbers of CS patients may recognize that many of them are (1) not equipped safely to contact vehicular emission in venturing to and from the workplace or school, and (2) once there, unlikely to be able to tolerate the chemicals on the site. For that physician continually to offer the opinion that these people should not work is a difficult choice. It skews his judgments in the eyes of others, and can result in quite vocal "peer jeers." However, those who consider these judgments unbalanced should consider that a physician who sees significant numbers of chemical sensitives is not seeing a representative group of the population, or even a representative group of sick people.

Physicians who make decisions on returning a CS patient to the workplace or school must do so based on a very thorough examination of the data available. It is not possible for a physician to follow patients to various places to determine to what degree their symptoms flare. Some patients react immediately; others, up to three or more days following an exposure; still others have both immediate and delayed reactions. The physician must trust the patient's reports—which may complicate the situation because individual tolerance to pain varies, and what is severe discomfort to one may be hardly noticeable to another. Even the immunological data which physicians use is not necessarily standard. For example, data studied at the time of poisoning will show an abnormal, highly activated immune sytem. For the patient who has been avoiding exposure to intolerable chemicals for several years, the blood work may show nothing, because the immune system has become suppressed. The signs of CS may be apparent without supporting blood test corrobation.

Essentially, the physician's opinion regarding return of the patient to the workplace or school boils down to what can be evidenced through tests and the physician's trust in the accuracy of the patient's reporting. The physician who sees a substantial number of CS patients can make his determinations with some degree of confidence. For those not familiar with the patient or the disease, a decision can be quite difficult.

The standard decision is that the patient may continue in any situation where he is unaffected by chemicals. Initially, this decision is safe for both physician and patient. It provides time for both to take a hard look at the situation. When time passes and the patient continues to experience great difficulty with exposures common to many environments, particularly when organic brain syndrome is an issue, there should come a point where the physician is comfortable with recommending removal from workplace or school. Such a resolution is ultimately necessary for all involved. Without it, the CS patient who has a strong desire to return to work will hold out hope and alternate between denial and acceptance; without it, a chemical sensitive who is pursuing entitlements or litigation may be blocked from income of any kind; without it, friends and family may waver in support, unable to accept once and for all that the individual is sick; without it, all the players remain in limbo. For the patient, learning to cope with CS is a problem; doing so in limbo adds to the difficulty.

A final decision is particularly critical in workers' compensation cases. Legally, doctors are prohibited from making decisions regarding disability. In the case of CS, the physician is requested for information on "impairment." Whether the word disability or impairment is used, it is the physician who determines whether a CS patient may return to the workplace. When facing workplace issues, the physician and the patient must communicate openly, even if the discussion becomes heated. A statement such as "This patient may work in any situation where he is unaffected by chemicals which bother him" must eventually become more specific. Either the patient can work or he cannot. To drag the matter over years and years leaves the CS patient in a state of stress. There is constant haggling, while the workers' compensation claims examiner sends the patient to one IME after another, waiting for the return-to-work flag. The chemical sensitive wonders whether his payments will be cut arbitrarily, and, if so, how will he survive. In an attempt to solve the problem on his own, he may decide to work just to see whether there will be damage. This can make present disabilities worse, add to the number of symptoms that already exist, or create additional permanent disabilities.

Without medical guidance for the physician, the difficulty in decision-making will continue. Given the variety of toxic chemicals and the endless array of combinations and the divergent physical manifestations of poisoning, a standardized approach is impractical, at least at present except for the position expressed by Gunnar Heuser[453a] in terms of diagnostic markers. That said, it should be noted that the dilemma will certainly remain as long as the medical community chooses not to address it. One solution for the present might be to decide that the existence of recurring disabling symptoms for a given period of time constitutes disability.

Patient Education

Patient education is the foundation upon which specific coping mechanisms are built. One way or another, a person who develops CS must become educated. Some preparation through physician counseling, support groups, or psychologic or psychiatric counseling can be of immense value to the new chemical sensitive. Basically, this is what the new CS patient needs to know:

1. The medical profession knows little about the disease. Only a few practicing physicians have any concept of compromised systemic integrity. Little is known about the neuroendocrineimmune systems interaction. Most doctors have no knowledge of CS.

2. Among doctors who have heard of the disease, an internal war rages regarding CS. The war developed because the orthodox medical machine has difficulty responding to the new in an efficient manner. The alternative medical practice has reacted to this inefficiency by using unorthodox procedures for diagnosis and treatment. The orthodox establishment complains that such procedures are inadequately tested. Little orthodox research has been done on the subject, and the projects begin with bias. The war is really over who has authority and power, not whether CS exists.

3. Political and economic pressures can and do affect the behavior of medical professionals. The patient who expects all physicians to be all-knowing, altruistic, and truthful is in for a heavy dose of reality therapy.

4. Medical practice is specialized, and few doctors are able to see systemic (whole body) disease. Reports will reflect this tunnel vision, and that complicates the picture for the CS patient who must deal with litigation or entitlements when the condition is systemic.

5. Significant changes in relationship with friends, family, and others should be expected.

6. Those whom the person with CS trusts initially (e.g. employers, administrators, vendors, friends, doctors) may lie, if entitlements to compensation or lawsuits are at issue.

7. Entitlements designed to be no-fault in nature (worker's compensation, disability retirement, social security) are very difficult for the person with CS to obtain.

8. The chemical sensitive must thoroughly document his case.

9. Attorneys are almost invariably necessary if action is to occur (entitlements, lawsuits).

10. Information is available from many sources, and the chemical sensitive should know and use the resources.

11. Life for a CS patient is not easy, but even with severe restrictions, life is not over and can still be fulfilling.

12. Many chemical sensitives have enjoyed excellent health prior to their poisoning and CS development. Consequently, many have little or no idea how to deal with doctors (e.g. stand in awe of them or lack trust in them) or react with something akin to horror at some of the procedures frequently used in CS diagnostics (e.g. MRI, colonoscopy). The new CS patient should prepare himself for these experiences.

13. If the CS patient is female the problems will be compounded. Sex discrimination in diagnosis is a fact of life. Men stand a far easier chance of receiving better psychological/psychiatric evaluation than women. As far as the literature is concerned, most studies are focused on men.

Perhaps the most difficult aspect of early patient education, but perhaps the most important, is to establish whether organic brain syndrome (toxic encephalopathy or false neurotransmission) is a factor. Because there is pride connected to intellectual function, the suggestion that damage may have occurred is often resisted. The idea is frightening, and when the individual has compensated well through unconscious mechanisms, he may honestly believe—along with family, friends, and doctors—that no brain damage has occurred. It may show only in very subtle ways, until a task is required which demonstrates the problem, and then poor performance may be attributed to stress.

Compared to skin problems, gastrointestinal reactions, or mild asthma, organic brain syndrome requires increased patient care to avoid triggers. Those other problems, tough as they are, can be treated. The cells in those structures can regenerate. Brain cells, once killed, are gone, though some brain function may be regained through different pathways. The general public recognizes the criticality of brain involvement. Entitlements or lawsuits may be decided in favor of the chemical sensitive because of brain damage. On the unfavorable side, a pivotal determination in insurance underwriting is the appearance of organic brain syndrome. Once a patient is diagnosed as having the problem, new coverage for life and health insurance will be denied.

Unlike the toxic encephalopathy sufferer, a CS patient who develops asthma and gastrointestinal problems from the workplace may be a given a return-to-work order by the treating physicians. Remember, those physicians will be seeing only lungs and the GI tract. The compromised systemic integrity (immune system) which is a probable mediator of the respiratory and GI problems is not an issue, generally speaking, with pulmonary specialists or gastroenterologists. They will be, in effect, treating a symptom, rather than a disease. If the person with CS shares his immune test data with these doctors, they may respond quite truthfully that they have no idea what the tests mean. If, however, these physicians are presented with a well-written, well-documented report illustrating organic brain syndrome and the level of brain damage, they will generally stop and think. Suddenly the specialized symptoms are part of something bigger, perhaps not understood, but definitely something to consider.

All of this points to the need for patient education—the chemical sensitive must learn, and, having learned, he must educate some of his doctors. That is an intimidating task, to put it mildly.

Essentially, the chemical sensitive must undertake a multi-disciplined education. A college major (business, education, math) is a discipline. The information a chemical sensitive needs to know beyond the basics involves aspects of the following disciplines: medicine, chemistry, engineering, safety, weather, architecture. He also must have a firm grasp of problem-solving techniques. In addition, knowledge of the political process is helpful. To achieve any progress toward any goals, a solid understanding of human behavior is essential. Sales skills are beneficial. A logical mind is an asset. Developing such a set of knowledge, skills, and abilities would be mind-boggling for a healthy person at the graduate level in a university. Imagine trying to accomplish any part of the task when fatigued, sick, and brain damaged.

Part of the value of early patient education is that it provides the person with CS something to do, particularly if he is accustomed to working and cannot. By hard, constructive effort, tasks get accomplished. There is no time for pity-parties. Effort focuses on a beneficial goal, even if the chemical sensitive has to write out that goal and stick it on a wall so he won't forget. All of this will be easier for the chemical sensitive who does not have brain damage, but hard effort expended by those with organic brain syndrome can have compensatory value in re-establishing some ability to function. At any rate, using time profitably to work toward a goal contributes to a healthy attitude.

General Coping Strategies

As the CS patient becomes educated, he begins to make decisions regarding exposure. The wilderness hermit and the person with CS who denies it are rare. The majority of chemical sensitives make decisions regarding their environments somewhere between these extremes.

The Extremes

Regardless of symptoms, the person with CS, like other humans, has physical, mental, emotional, spiritual, and social needs. The hermit has eliminated social needs to cater to physical needs. The chemical sensitive in total denial has eliminated physical needs to cater to social or emotional needs. Because there are degrees of sensitivity, each may be coping at maximum effectivenesss for the moment. Individual values play an important role in overall health. Our society teaches us that balance in things is best. It's easy to turn that concept into a rule or law. In doing so, we may have some knowledge, but we lack wisdom.

The wilderness hermit may be an individual at the highest level of the sensitivity continuum. Environmental exposure of even a small mountain town may be greater than that person's physical needs can bear. On the other hand, the chemical sensitive denier may have a sensitivity at the lower end of the scale. Being able to function, even with persistent symptoms, may frequently be possible.

Concern arises rightly when the wilderness hermit chooses his lifestyle because of the pain generated by thoughtless others, especially those who persist in slapping the label of "crazy" or "lazy" on him. Running away from a problem of that nature is not a good solution. Concern arises for the denier when he either cannot accept the diagnosis or is pressured by others to deny it. Continuing life-as-usual under those conditions asks for trouble, even tends toward the suicidal, but it may be the only way the person has to give himself permission not to work or attend school. He may be attempting to provide proof to himself, to family members, or to his physician. If continuing life-as-usual generates significantly disabling reactions, that will provide the proof, costly as it may be.

The Balancers

Most people with CS balance the risk of exposure with the value they expect to derive from an experience. There are times when the value of doing some particular thing outweighs the result of three to ten days of rough recuperation. There are some things a chemical sensitive will want to do enough to risk even more significant brain damage. The rules and guidelines for CS patient behavior are unwritten. Each person has to make the choices and live with the consequences.

• Journal Keeping

One of the least pleasant activities that some physicians will require and that some CS patients will do on their own is keeping fairly extensive records of daily exposures and symptoms (some will also include their emotional level). The purpose of this activity is to identify places and activities which cause certain symptoms. Such a record can be extremely helpful to physicians who have to determine whether to return a patient to work or school; to attorneys who are demonstrating the severity of injury to a client; and to the patient himself. The down side of journal keeping is that it keeps the patient's focus on CS. A sample journal checklist is included in Chapter 5. Using a pre-set format helps to maintain focus, reduces time spent, and keeps the writing required to a minimum.

• Work

For chemical sensitives who are employed, the choice of whether to continue working is very difficult. Some chemical sensitives will continue working even after having been medically removed. The reason given in most of these cases is financial. It can take months or years for some CS individuals to receive compensation, and some people will continue working, despite health risks or poor performance, because of perceived economic necessity. Sadly, sometimes that perception is incorrect.

Sam, for example, employed in accounting, was poisoned by a painting activity which took place on the ground level of the building in which he worked on the second floor. He became quite ill. He asked to have his location moved, and after several months his request was granted. The employer moved him into a small office in another building nearby which was used as a storage shed. He continued working, knowing that he was developing cancer. Sam knew that he had one year remaining to work before he would qualify for disability retirement. He had been assured that worker's compensation did not apply in his case. As Sam worked alone in the storage shed, the employer decided to spray pesticide in the shed. The timing was during Sam's work shift. Sam remained at his desk while the pesticide was sprayed. He became quite ill and had to leave a number of times to vomit. Yet he continued working to make his final year.

Sam's case is not at all unique. His story is repeated day after day somewhere. If he lives to qualify for his disability. retirement, his quality of life will be less than it would had he followed the medical advice and left the environment. In Sam's case, he had been misinformed about workers' compensation. He was entitled. It might have taken a battle, and he might have been without compensation for up to a year, and he might have lost financially in the meantime, but he might have had less of a physical problem to deal with in the long run. Sam needed a smart attorney along with his physician.

Being uninformed, Sam (1) lost money (workers' comp is not taxable, and it includes complete medical expenses; disability retirement is taxable, and out of it the person pays insurance premiums and part of the medical expense); (2) lost health (continuing in the environment compounded a serious medical problem); (3) lost quality of life (by becoming more ill, some of the things he might have been able to do may no longer be options).

Not all chemical sensitives have to stop working. Some people with CS have no significant difficulty with transportation to and from the workplace. They may respond with significant reactions to a limited number of chemical substances. In those cases, finding the proper environment is the right answer.

In those cases where the CS patient is returned to the workplace because a doctor reports that the degree of illness (impairment) does not warrant permanent removal, the chemical sensitive must return even if he disagrees, unless he is independently wealthy. A fine line exists in some cases. To cope with the effects of decisions which are counter to what the CS patient feels is right, the chemical sensitive ordered to return to work should at the very least secure a copy of the return-to-work slip from the physician, and he should remain under the care of the physician. The reason for this is potential litigation. By following orders of a physician (and keeping a copy safe in the possession of the chemical sensitive and his attorney), the CS client has coped with the situation to the best of his ability. If his condition becomes worse, the treating physician has the ability to remedy the situation. If he doesn't, and the chemical sensitive can prove that his condition became worse by following the medical treatment, the chemical sensitive can initiate a suit and be fairly sure of a favorable outcome.

One option that is being investigated by some employers of CS patients injured on the job is to provide a work-at-home opportunity. This concept reduces the financial burden of workers' compensation payments, because there is a return (product) for the compensation. The employee is provided a safe means of earning income, and usually the CS patient responds very positively to the chance to continue working.

For those who cannot work, finding some productive activity is very helpful. What the person does will depend on interest, motivation, availability, and so on. This may require creativity on the part of the CS patient or help from others. The chemical sensitive may have to redefine work, but there are always some things that need to be done which the individual who is determined to make some contribution can do.

• School

Many students and teachers are developing CS in schools (from preschool through college). Some of them will be disabled for a lifetime, unless some cure is found. Adults follow the standard employee profile. As for children, the decisions made for them by their parents and their doctors will be critical as they develop into adults. Decisions will have to be made with respect to whether they can continue in the same or different school, or whether they cannot tolerate such environments and may require homebound teaching. At the elementary level, the classroom is less likely to contain some of the toxics (perfume, hairspray, chemicals) that abound in the higher school levels.

What has occurred with disastrous results is to misdiagnose a child's CS as a desire not to attend school. Severe damage can be done to a child who is misdiagnosed.

Essentially, the manner of coping with the school environment is similar to that described for the work environment.

• Where to Live

Numbers of chemical sensitives report an inability to cope with the outdoor air in metropolitan areas. If the chemical sensitive lives in or near one of these areas, he may be faced with having to select another place to live. Such a selection may be very difficult, particularly if family members are tied to a particular place. Moving may require a change of occupation for the chemical sensitive or a family member. Such decisions are not simple and cannot be made in haste. Yet it may not be possible to remain long in the dangerous location. There are some physicians who will not continue to treat a CS patient unless that person moves out of the area, simply because the threat to that patient is too great if he remains.

In some situations, a family may go to great expense too fast, possibly due to physical urgency. Being required to move from the metropolitan area, Susan, for example, chose a location on the coast. She sold her home and purchased a home that gave her no physical problems. The ocean air was clean, and her health began to improve. Finally, she felt well enough to attend to the crop of weeds growing in the yard. Her family discovered her collapsed in the yard. What had seemed like the answer actually created another problem. The yard had been treated with pesticide which the CS patient could not tolerate and to which she responded violently.

In another case, a CS patient fleeing a metropolitan area moved to a secluded wooded area in the mountains. He thrived on the outdoor life, until winter arrived. Then, to his dismay, he discovered that his neighbors heated their homes with wood-burning stoves and fireplaces. The wood smoke was intolerable.

In these cases, haste may have been necessary, but the move did not solve the problem. Continuous moves trying to find the right place can be very expensive. Any opportunity to try out an area prior to making a purchase is worth pursuing. It should be kept in mind that numbers of CS patients who move away from metropolitan areas find that their health does improve, along with their quality of life.

For some CS people, the isolation of a small town is not acceptable. They may find that by removing toxics from their homes, and then spending most of their time there, they can remain in the large city they prefer. Others choose to move to an established colony of chemical sensitives, much as an elderly person may move to a retirement community. There are advantages and disadvantages. The advantages include the sense of community and the ability to control a given space. The disadvantages include the fact that such environments reduce social variety. Individual growth can be inhibited, and there is potential for pity-parties. Residents may also find that they are less willing to push themselves to reach goals.

• Cleaning House

It is likely that the chemical sensitive will spend significant amounts of time at home. If the home is the problem, as in the case of mobile homes with high levels of formaldehyde, another living space will have to be chosen. Finding one that is not built with toxic materials may require looking for an older home, built prior to the mid-1960s. The chemical sensitive can usually walk into a building and determine whether it will create problems. For individuals who develop immediate reactions it is a simple task. For those who develop delayed reactions, the person should be away from exposure for several days, taken to the new place for testing, and returned to a "clean" environment. He should remain there for four days to a week. In that length of time, a delayed reaction, if there is one, will occur.

A non-toxic structure is important. What goes inside the house is also important. Painting walls, installing carpet, using glues, even using aerosol products can be hazardous to the health of chemical sensitives. These are the hazards that come instantly to mind. Others are more subtle: soap, detergent, fabric softeners, hairspray, nail polish and remover, shoe polish, new leather, upholstery, floor wax, carbonless carbon paper, parts of computers, how the home is heated, the flooring and sub-flooring, the material that composes the mattress, newspapers, books, ink, disinfectant, insecticide, room fresheners, deodorizers, candles, animal flea collars, cleansers, glass cleaner, felt-tipped pens, scented or colored toilet paper and tissues, polyester fabric, and so on. All of these things and a long list of others can cause a CS person a lot of difficulty. The home should be cleared of any products which generate CS symptoms. If some items are precious enough to keep but offensive enough to cause problems, they can be removed to a garage or storage area outside the living area where they cannot contribute to the indoor air through ducting.

Because the home is the place most CS patients spend the majority of their time, the following checklist may be helpful. It is used with the kind permission of William J. Rea of the Environmental Health Center, Dallas, Texas. It should not be seen as a complete list, but the information is a helpful beginning.

HOW TO ACHIEVE CLEANER INDOOR AIR BY REDUCING CHEMICAL CONTAMINATION

Eliminate as many as possible to reduce and eliminate your chemical sensitivity symptoms:

1. **FUELS:** Use electric heat and cooking. Avoid hydrocarbons, i.e., kerosene, coal, oil, gas, wood.
    1. These should not be in house or garage if attached.
    2. Gas appliances must be removed. Won't help if only disconnected.
    3. If heating is electric, remove motor driven fans. These utilize oil. Use cool electric heat in form of radiator or heat pump installation—two stage controls of baseboard.
    4. Be sure there are no plastics in heating ducts.
    5. Be sure filters are not oiled.
    6. Electronic filters dry dust and can give out dangerous gasses.
    7. Use activated carbon filters.
    8. Be sure refrigerator has no leaks.

2. **PAINT:** Avoid fresh paint and varnish and wood stain. Paint must be non-odorous. Casein paint is best. Use no rubber base paint.

3. **CEMENTS, ADHESIVES:** Avoid the following:
    1. Fingernail polish.
    2. Nail polish remover.
    3. Paint remover.
    4. Hinge looseners.
    5. Adhesives used in model airplane and other types.
    6. Adhesives containing tars for floors.

4. **CLEANING, LIGHTER FLUIDS**
    1. Be absent for several days if rugs are cleaned.
    2. Clothes should be aerated in the sun after being sent to the dry cleaners.
    3. No lighter fluid in the house.

5. **NEWSPRINT:** Newspapers and magazines should be opened and read by someone else first.

6. **ALCOHOL:**
    1. No rubbing alcohol.
    2. No shellac, brush cleaning preparations.
    3. Flavoring extracts have alcohol in them.

7. **REFRIGERANTS, SPRAY CONTAINERS:**
    1. Slow escape of gas from air conditioners or refrigerators or freezers can cause trouble.

2. Same type gas is commonly used propellant in spray containers of insecticide, hair sprays, and other cosmetics.

8. **INSECTICIDES:**
   1. DDT and related compounds are usually dispensed.
   2. Avoid lindane, methoxyclor, DDT, chlordane, malathion, or thyocyanates.
   3. Rugs are often moth proofed with fluids containing DDT while in storage. Rug shampoos can contain DDT.
   4. Exterminators use dieldrin, chlordane, pentachlorophenol.
   5. Blankets are often moth proofed similarly.
   6. Moth balls, cakes, crystals containing naphthalene para-dichlorobenzene can cause symptoms.

9. **SPONGE RUBBER:**
   1. Odors can come from rubber pillows, mattresses, upholstery, rug pads, seat cushions, typewriter pads, rubber backing of rugs and various noise reducing installations.
   2. Look out if one has restlessness, insomnia, night sweats, etc.

10. **PLASTICS:** The more flexible and odorous a plastic the more frequently it contributes to indoor chemical air pollution. Hard plastics like vinyl, formica, bakelite, cellulose acetate—are rarely incriminated.
   1. Vinyl and radiant floor heating fumes should be avoided.
   2. Plastic pillows, combs, powder cases, shoes can give symptoms.
   3. Avoid plastic air conditioning ducts.

11. **MECHANICAL DEVICES:**
   1. Evaporating oil from any motor.
   2. Air filters of glass wool or fiberglass usually have oiled filters, but one can get them without.
   3. Fans and motors in hot water units.
   4. Small kitchens may have too many motors.
   5. Cars in garages or near elevator shafts can volatize gasses.

12. **MISCELLANEOUS:**
   1. Toxic fumes and odors can come from detergents, naphtha containing soaps, ammonia, clorox, cleansing powders containing bleaches, some silver and brass polishing materials.
   2. Storage of bleach-containing cleansers.
   3. Highly scented soaps, toilet deodorants, disinfectants, especially pine scented air improver.
   4. Phenol and other chemicals are sometimes placed in wallpaper paste.
   5. Pine Christmas trees, pine in woodburning fireplaces, creosote odors.
   6. Odors from prolonged use of TV sets.

CHEMICAL CONTAMINATION OF INGESTANTS

A food additive is any chemical substance that makes its way into food. Susceptibility to chemical additives and contaminants of the diet has long been confused with specific susceptibility of foods. One may be sensitive to the food or the additive—or both. If one eats a food at one time and has no reaction, and then eats it another time and has a reaction, he probably is sensitive to the chemical and not the food.

1. **FOODS COMMONLY CONTAMINATED BY CHEMICALS:** Foods often containing spray residues: *fruits* (apples, apricots, berries [cranberry, blueberries, boysenberries, raspberries, strawberries], currants, grapes, grapefruit, lemon, orange, nectarine, peach, pear, pineapple, plum, cherry, rhubarb, olive, persimmon); *vegetables* (brussels sprouts, broccoli, cauliflower, cabbage, head lettuce, celery, asparagus, spinach, beet greens, tomato, chard, mustard greens, endive, escarole, leaf lettuce, romaine lettuce, chinese cabbage, artichoke)
   1. Most commonly used sprays permeate the food to which they are applied.
   2. They are not removed by washing, peeling, soaking in water or vinegar, or cooking.
   3. Root vegetables are apt to be free of spray residues unless contaminated in transit or in market.

Meats: Lamb, beef, pork, fowl may be contaminated by the animals having eaten sprayed forage and concentrating such oil-soluble insecticides, herbicides, or their vehicles in their fats. Chicken and turkey often contain residues of stilbestrol, a synthetic hormone.

2. **FOODS OFTEN CONTAINING FUMIGANT RESIDUES:** Dates, figs, shelled nuts, raisins, prunes and other dried fruits, wheat, corn, barley, rice, dried peas, lentils.

3. **FOODS OFTEN CONTAINING BLEACHES:** White flour (unbleached flour is usually available). Freshly stone-ground whole wheat is much safer.

4. **FOODS OFTEN TREATED WITH SULFUR:**
   1. Often dusted with sulfur: peaches, apricots, nectarines.
   2. May be treated with sulfur dioxide as an anti-browning agent: commercially prepared fresh apples, peaches, apricots, and french fries.
   3. May be bleached with sulfur dioxide: molasses, dried fruit, melon, citrus candied peel, fruit marmalade.
   4. Usually treated with sulfur dioxide in the process of manufacture: dried apple, dried pear, dried peach, dried apricot, raisin, prune, corn syrup (glucose), corn sugar (dextrose), cornstarch, corn oil.

5. **FOODS ARTIFICIALLY COLORED:**
   1. Oranges, sweet potatoes, Irish potatoes, maraschino cherries (and other colored fruits).
   2. Ice cream, creme de menthe, candy, cake, frostings, and fillings.
   3. Butter, oleomargarine, cheese, bologna, wieners, etc.
   4. Root beer, cola drinks, and other soft drinks (not all) usually contain coal-tar dyes.

6. **FOODS ARTIFICIALLY SWEETENED:** with saccharine or sodium cyclamate

7. **FOODS EXPOSED TO GAS:**
   1. Ethylene gas: bananas, apples, pears.
   2. Open gas flame: Coffee is often roasted this way and absorbs products of combustion.
   3. Filtered through bone char (the filters usually reactivated periodically in gas-fired kilns and the absorbed products of combustion apparently are imparted to the next batch of syrup filtered through them): Cane and beet sugars.
   4. Have usually been fumigated in shiphold: chocolate, arrowroot, tapioca, carob, and sassafras tea.

8. **FOODS CONTAMINATED BY CONTAINERS:**
   1. Dispensed in odorous plastic bags: carrot, parsnip, turnip, tomatoes, mixed shredded greens.
   2. Other plastic containers may contaminate certain other foods transported, stored, or frozen in them.
   3. Cellophane wrapped foods are usually tolerated by chemically sensitive people.
   4. Plastic refrigerator dishes: commonly incriminated.
   5. Fungicide-treated containers: citrus fruit.
   6. Golden brown lining of metal cans: This is a phenolic resin which prevents the metal from bleaching the contents but it also contaminates their food contents chemically. Only such foods that the manufacturer desires to bleach, such as asparagus, grapefruit, pineapple, artichoke, and some citrus juices are apt to be packed in unlined cans.

9. **FOODS OFTEN WAXED WITH PARAFFIN:**
   1. Waxed and lightly polished: cucumber, eggplants, green pepper, parsnip, rutabaga, turnip.
   2. Waxed and/or polished: apples, oranges, grapefruit, tangerine, lemon.

FOODS THAT ARE LESS CHEMICALLY CONTAMINATED:

1. Fish and meat: Fresh or frozen seafood: fresh or frozen fish in large pieces and not packaged.
2. Vegetables: Fresh if undyed, home peeled, not waxed, frozen or canned in glass, only the tops sprayed.
3. Nuts: In shell only: brazil nut, coconut, walnut, hickory nut, pecan, filbert, hazelnut.
4. Sweetening agents: honey, sorghum, pure maple syrup or sugar.
5. Fats and oils: olive, cottonseed, peanut, soy, coconut, sunflower, sesame, safflower, preferably cold-pressed.
6. Uncontaminated food sources: Foods from approved local sources should be secured for canning in glass and freezing in glass during the season of availability. Membership in state or local Natural Food Association groups or Organic Gardening Clubs is helpful in finding sources of supply.

• Clothing

Over time, particularly if a chemical sensitive has difficulty with petroleum products, polyester fabric may cause problems.

In addition to fabric, a clothing problem that a significant number of chemical sensitives face is substantial weight loss or gain. Why this happens is not clear, but it is seen quite often. A change of some 30 pounds in adults is not uncommon. Depending on the size of the individual prior to poisoning, that can mean that an entire wardrobe change is required. A woman, for example, whose pre-poisoning weight was 146 may lose weight to 110 pounds, going from a clothing size 12 to a 4–6.

People whose clothing is geared to an office environment may need to make changes in their wardrobe if they can no longer work. Clothing that requires dry cleaning may be unwearable because dry cleaning uses chemicals many CS patients cannot tolerate. Most chemical sensitives prefer cotton clothing.

• Going Out

Most people with CS will balance where they are willing to go with the expected value of the trip. For example, quality of life is definitely enhanced by social events. Even if it would be wise from a physical point of view, few chemical sensitives wish to be housebound for the rest of their lives. Consequently, a CS person may choose to attend a social event, even knowing that the event will mean exposure to a mass of intolerable chemicals, recuperation may take a couple of weeks, and for some damage (brain damage) there will be no recuperation. The price is justified by the long-term value of being able to interact with people, even if symptoms require having to leave early. The memories of the social event will linger.

Other trips, such as to the grocery store, pharmacy, doctor's office, post office, or department store, carry fewer social rewards and may cause problems each and every time. To cope with these trips, which are necessary unless someone else takes the major responsibility for running errands, it may be beneficial to do some planning for consolidation. Running several errands at the same time can be helpful in reducing exposure. Using the telephone in advance of trips can also help. For example, the CS person who needs something from a hardware store can call the store, explain the problem, tell the clerk what he needs, and have the item waiting and payment prepared when he arrives at the store. People can be very accommodating, especially when aware of the problem. Nobody in a store is eager to have to call 911 because someone has a severe reaction to a substance in their store. Planning helps prevent drawn-out shopping—the person can get what is needed and leave.

Automobile travel can be difficult because of the car, its interior, and the emissions from other vehicles.[709] Use of effective filtering devices and ionizers and limiting vehicle travel to older cars can help. Some states provide disabled parking privilege to CS-disabled individuals, reducing the need for walking great distances through traffic and cooling vehicles. For people who cannot tolerate metropolitan air and must go to a city for medical purposes, the best choice is either for someone else to drive or for the person to take a taxi. Mass transportation such as the bus or subway not only provides exposure to the more intolerable forms of fuel, but also means coming into contact with numbers of other individuals, who may be wearing intolerable cosmetics. It's bad enough to deal with road fumes without adding a multitude of other intolerables for synergistic effect.

It is important for people with CS to drive with their windows closed—the air recycled internally if possible—and to keep their vehicles well maintained. States which provide disabled parking privilege usually provide for service to the disabled at the self-serve pumps of service stations which also provide full service. That permits the CS patient to have gas pumped at the self-serve price. However, regular use of this service will not include checking the levels of fluids, a task which can be a problem for chemical sensitives. Occasional full service is wise. When maintenance is necessary, it's helpful to have someone follow the chemical sensitive to the service center and take him away while the service is done, returning him when the work is completed. In some cases a service center will pick up the vehicle and return it. This service is a tremendous help, even if there is a small charge. It is of particular benefit when changing oil or maintaining radiators, since it means that someone else will drive the car immediately after service. Frequently fluids spill on the surfaces, which heat up when operating the vehicle. The resulting fumes can be a very unpleasant surprise, if the CS patient happens to be the driver while the spill is burning off. Good car maintenance will keep the car available and postpone having to find another safe one, which can be a tremendous chore in itself (many chemical sensitives cannot purchase new vehicles due to the off-gassing of plasticizers, matting, upholstery, rubber, and so on).

Travel in automobiles may not be a person's only contact with roadways. For the chemical sensitive who enjoys walking or jogging, some modifications may be required. When exercising, more air is taken into the lungs. When exercise is performed along a roadway, the vehicular emissions can be devastating to the chemical sensitive. Finding exercise pathways in parks or protected areas is important. For those who choose other forms of exercise, some care is necessary. Membership in an indoor swim club may seem just the thing, but the chlorine in the water can be a real problem for some. It is helpful to check to determine whether alternative exercise areas are safe prior to signing up. Another option is to equip one's home for an exercise program.

• Safety Equipment

One way to cope with unavoidable exposures is to use a safety device for breathing. Some chemical sensitives have tossed aside their pride (which is a definite requirement) and purchased a silicon mask, available at safety equipment stores for industrial use. The device fits over the head and hooks behind the neck. Two canisters are screwed onto the mask. Canisters are available for many industrial uses. Some of the canisters themselves can be a problem. It takes a trial-and-error period to find what is suitable for each person. To provide protection, most people begin with canisters designed to screen out VOCs (volatile organic compounds) and acid gases. Canisters have to be replaced from time to time, and when not in use the device has to be stored in an airtight container. The cost is about $30. Canister replacement usually is less than $10. The other cost is looking like a giant mosquito and having strangers stare. Another option is the 3M Dust and Mist Respirator (#9913). It is lightweight and easier to carry. This means of protection has other drawbacks. Masks reduce oxygen intake. They should be worn for no longer than 45 minutes at a time. Reduced oxygen is even more of a problem for the CS patient who habitually practices shallow breathing. Consequently, to use the protection for running short errands is helpful. To use it to make trips downtown for medical tests may be impractical. If the CS patient has organic brain syndrome, the mask may protect the brain while making the trip to town; once there, however, he is going to have to remove it. Trying to communicate with a mask on is virtually impossible. If the CS patient encounters toxics while the mask is removed, driving back home even with the mask is not safe.

Safety equipment doesn't have to come from a safety equipment store. Some of the coping means CS patients find are creative. For example, for those who love to read, books may be a real problem. New paperbacks can be taken outside the home, clipped with clothespins to hold them open, and aired. Some people find that the cellophane type of page protectors available at office supply stores can be opened to serve as a barrier between the ink on paper and the reader. Some people build airtight boxes and read through glass.

• Planning Ahead for Illness or Emergency

Some CS people have had the disease long enough to recognize what others may need to know in the event of an emergency. Some chemical sensitives wear medical identification to prepare for such an event. These identifiers may contain medical alert insignia, the person's name, the medical condition, some do's and don'ts, names and numbers of treating physicians, and the medical coverage name and charge number.

It is a good idea for the CS patient to explain his problem to other caregivers, such as dentists. Some chemicals used in dentistry can create real problems for the chemical sensitive. One material for making impressions may be better than another; an aluminum temporary cap may cause GI symptoms; amalgam fillings may cause symptoms; cosmetics used by people in the office may be intolerable. No one will know unless the CS patient communicates. With prior warning some dentists may take CS patients to the dental chair and start oxygen rather than expose the patient to waiting room environments and dental chemicals. Some CS patients will notify their local fire department and police, in advance of potential need, to prepare the individuals who might respond in an emergency. To some this might appear over "symptom focused" behavior, but it could be important to the chemical sensitive. For example, a CS person who is having severe difficulty breathing needs help, but attaching a plastic face mask fresh out of its airtight container may be met with resistance—the off-gassing plasticizers may cause additional bronchospasm and bronchoconstriction or damage the brain.

Hospitalization

Facing a stay in a hospital can be traumatic for a CS patient. There are some considerations which should be dealt with up front. Some general precautions can be taken. For example, oxygen can be useful with some patients to reduce effects of exposure. Those with nervous system compromise or metabolic hyperactivity may be aware that during and following toxic exposure a significant amount of oxygen may be required by the body. Some patients use oxygen at about 2.5 liters per minute for 20 minutes three times a day, and find that it makes a real difference after a symptom-producing exposure. Plasticizers in face masks and tubing can be a problem. If so, a cannula can be used. If that is ineffective, Tygon tubing can be soaked for two weeks in one-half cup of baking soda for every two quarts of water, rinsing daily. Otherwise, stainless steel tubing and porcelain masks may be necessary. The patient should be encouraged to bring his own bedding, pillows, and clothing. Rooms should be prewashed with vinegar and water or borax (no Lysol). Avoid plastic mattress covers, foam pillows, bed pads, synthetic products. The room should be in a location that has not been recently renovated, without residue of pesticides, and with a window that opens (not toward heavily trafficked streets, parking lot, incinerator, truck delivery area).

If blood transfusions may be required, the patient should donate his own, preferably to be stored in glass containers, three weeks prior to surgery. Pre-test patients for tolerance to surgical scrub, tape, suture material, metals, acrylics.

Anyone present in surgery should refrain from wearing hair tonic or spray, pre-shave, aftershave, cologne, perfume, fragrant deodorant, or residue of scented soap. As for anesthetics, regional is preferable. Avoid products with preservatives. Avoid carbocaine and halogenated hydrocarbons. Pentothal appears to be generally tolerated.

Problems may occur with IVs. The bags in which these products are packaged contain PVCs. Those chemical leach out of the packaging and can be toxic to the CS patient whose threshold level of sensitivity to PVCs is very low. For that reason, any way to avoid plastic packaging will be beneficial. Glass is the safest packaging material.

Staff and visitors should be barred from entering the patient's room if they are wearing perfume, cologne, aftershave, scented deodorant, hair tonic spray, scented cosmetics, fresh shoe polish, dry cleaned clothing, new leather; if their clothes have been washed or dried with fabric softeners; or if they carry tobacco odors.

• What to Do Following Chemical Exposure

On February 6, 1991, a local Seattle television news program aired pictures from a school where a teacher and some children wore respirators due to poor indoor air quality. Numbers of schools across the nation have experienced problems with indoor air quality. It isn't a new problem. Wearing respirators while in the building isn't a satisfactory answer. First, respirators reduce oxygen intake. Second, canisters for respirators require some knowledge of what the pollutant is. A respirator that screens out volatile organic compounds (VOCs) and acid gases, for example, will not protect against formaldehyde. Third, respirators are effective only for screening out breathable vapors and particles. Vapors and particles with which skin comes in contact make another route of exposure likely. That route is absorption.

Absorption as a means of exposure is often overlooked. Imagine the potential for such exposure in a tight building where the walls are painted, new foam-backed, heavy indoor-outdoor type of carpet is installed (attached to the floor with adhesive), new furniture in vinyl with new upholstery and foam padding of ergonomic design is purchased. All of this brightens up the office. Office workers at their desks rest their bare arms on the arms of the chairs, touch the upholstery, and remove their shoes to rest weary feet on the carpet. When the temperature drops, space heaters keep unshod feet warm. If toxics are present in the carpet, its backing, or the adhesive, human skin can absorb the vapors. Heaters enhance off-gassing, so unshod feet can absorb a significant quantity. Arms, hands, or feet in direct contact are not the only means of skin absorption. Vapors can penetrate clothing. For people with CS, setting off symptoms requires only a minute amount of toxic, and toxics can come from a wide array of sources. It is virtually impossible to live free of exposure. So what can be done to reduce the effect?

Immediately following a reaction-causing exposure (e.g. appointment in physicians's office in tight building or trip to the grocery store), removing clothing to a remote location until it can be washed and taking a hot shower and shampooing can remove substances with which skin has come in contact. Shampooing is important. Because the surface area of hair is large, chemical accumulation in hair can occur in unexpected quantity. Other helpful measures include:

Use of Alka-Seltzer Gold (in gold package): After toxic encounter, a CS patient frequently becomes dehydrated, as if he might have participated in some form of athletic event. The dehydration occurs not as a direct symptom but rather as a secondary response to the coping with various symptoms generated by the exposure to toxics. In water, Alka-Seltzer Gold contains principally sodium citrate and potassium citrate. It reverses the metabolic acidosis that occurs with some toxic exposures. Reasons for using this product are largely hypothetical: (1) to reduce neurological symptoms from the imbalance of electrolytes occurring during the dehydration process; (2) to add water to the system; and (3) to settle upset stomach. Hypothetical or not, numbers of CS patients rely on the product, because it works. An alternative is Emergen-C. It is a powdered electrolyte product containing vitamin C and fructose, though buffered vitamin C may be more effective.

Anti-inflammatories: If inflammation is a problem, an anti-inflammatory product such as aspirin or Tylenol may be beneficial. Warning: For those who have problems with the nightshade family plants, products such as Nuprin or Advil may provide immediate relief only to provoke later exacerbation of symptoms.

Use of oxygen: Oxygen reverses metabolic acidosis felt by the CS patient as if he were a sprinter who gets cramps in his legs due to acidosis. Oxygen is used in great quantity when a toxic exposure affects the neurological system. Neurons are known to consume large quantities following a toxic event; therefore, oxygen treatment for toxic encephalopathy is intended to replace oxygen used to prevent additional brain damage from lack of oxygen. For other CS patients, oxygen can reduce severity of symptoms because it assists in the detoxification process. Detoxification mechanisms are urine, feces, sweat, and respiration.

In the absence of oxygen it is important for the CS patient to be where air is as clean as possible and focus on deep breathing. The patient may require some medical help to learn proper breathing, as it is not uncommon for CS sufferers to develop shallow breathing as a coping measure of sorts. Shallow breathing is not inappropriate for the CS patient undergoing exposure to intolerable substances; it reduces the respiration of harmful materials. However, the effect of continual shallow breathing is to reduce the already depleted level of available oxygen in a person's system. Deep breathing assists in detoxification through respiration, increases oxygen availability, and is psychologically relaxing.

A CS patient can be taught to breathe properly by having him lie on his back and place his hand on his abdomen. His hand should rise when he breathes in and fall when he breathes out. The patient should be observed while initial practice occurs and on office visits afterward. The patient should be encouraged to use the hand-to-abdomen technique after exposures.

Rest: Following exposure, physical and mental rest is beneficial. In some cases the exposure generates what feels like great energy. Some patients describe this feeling as hyperactivity, recognizing that it is not normal energy. Part of the reaction to the feeling is a strong drive to accomplish something, to do something, with the idea that activity will reduce the discomfort of the exaggerated energy. Some may express the feeling as being "wired" and their activity as seeking to "get un-wired." When physicians prescribe tranquilizers for patients experiencing this symptom, the reaction may be (1) to appropriately balance the patient's energy level; (2) to increase the level of energy; or (3) to decrease the level of energy to the extent that the patient "crashes" for days.

If the feeling of need for activity interferes with rest, attending to chores which require little analytical effort is a good outlet. Trying to solve problems just after chemical exposure symptoms appear is usually not a good idea, for often thinking is affected. For those who have organic brain syndrome, judgment may be sorely lacking. In addition, expenditure of large amounts of abnormal energy can lead to an exaggeration of the inevitable crash which follows.

Disciplining one's self to rest despite an urge toward activity can reduce aggravation of fouled neurotransmisson and reduce recovery time. Ironically, at the time when self-discipline may be most needed, it may not be easily accessible. The CS patient needs reminding, following symptom-generating chemical exposure, that he has been exposed to chemicals which are affecting him. People who have the organic brain syndrome effects of rage, depression or feelings of excessive energy may also experience memory lapses and forgetfulness, and thus fail to tie the feelings to the toxic rather than to something else. How a person reminds himself is individual. A red string tied to a watch band is a possibility. For those who live with others, reminders from them may be helpful, even if not readily accepted or appreciated. In that way, a person who feels his life is falling apart may remember that the impression will pass; a person frantically pursuing a task may remember that the crash will be greater if the activity pulls out too much real energy. Toxic exposure can color perception and cause a transference from the real to the imagined. For example, a person exposed to a perfume may arrive home feeling angry. As a result of the road tar he passed acting on the brain he may view his life as bad or unendurable. At home someone may make a casual remark which is interpreted as injurious by the toxic-exposed individual. Then, illogically, the person who made the remark is perceived as the cause of the anger or depression. Remembering the real cause of the feeling—perfume or road tar—can keep the feeling in perspective.

Sunshine: Provided that the outside air is clean, going outside and getting some sunshine[319] on the skin can be very beneficial to the recently exposed patient. However, the person who feels sleepy should sunbathe only cautiously, since a sunburn will add to the difficulty. Walking in the sun may be the only way to remain awake. The individual who is consumed with the drive to do must take extra precautions. Working frantically to weed a garden may seem like a great idea, but if the activity continues unabated for four hours, exhaustion and dehydration may be harmful effects. And remember, the sky does not have to be clear of clouds to provide the benefits—and risks—of sunshine.

Using Survival Mechanisms: The CS patient may develop certain survival mechanisms. These include hypervigilance, hyperosmia, and shallow breathing. Hypervigilance in the early stage may warn of the presence of neurotoxics. Hyperosmia can serve the same function. Both can alert the CS patient to vacate an area. Shallow breathing can buy time for the individual to get away from toxic exposure.

Staying "Up"

Like it or not, a chemical sensitive has to think constantly about his environment and how it affects him. It is a self-centered focus, but it does not have to consume that person and those with whom he shares life. Some doctors will maintain that every chemical sensitive experiences depression or anxiety, but in one group of chemical sensitives, 3 people out of 500 did not experience either. In each of these three cases, the patient cited religious faith as the reason for his lack of depression. Each of these patients is the type who expects life changes and looks at them as containing some form of blessing. That pattern was established prior to exposure and did not change with poisoning. Part of the explanation for the lack of depression or anxiety may rest in the expectation of life change and the fact that hunting for the blessing is a time-consuming exercise. The posture is active, not passive, and the expectation is that some good will result from the person's having the disease. It may also be of some significance that these three people report no fear of death.

For most people with CS, getting "up" and staying there generally is very difficult. Finding a psychologist or psychiatrist who understands CS may be helpful to those who have functional depression or experience anxiety. (It should be recognized that a chemical depression can occur in people who have organic brain syndrome. This is not the standard functional depression. It can be remedied by identifying what chemicals are causing the problem and being extremely careful to avoid those exposures.) Some chemical sensitives find that involvement with a support group helps them raise their spirits and gives them something to do. This is particularly true if the group actively pursues education or some constructive project. It can have the reverse effect if the focus is on complaint and continues to emphasize the problem.

Activity is a great help, and those with CS who insist on getting up in the morning, getting dressed, and accomplishing some meaningful tasks each day tend to keep up better than those who give in quickly to complaints. The person who presents himself well, appears cheerful, and has interest beyond himself is someone others like to be around.

It is important to develop daily routines and to stay in synchrony with the hours of others (particularly spouse and children). Otherwise, those non-chemically sensitive individuals may feel left out, deserted, and their support and caring can change to rejection or disgust.

• Planning for the Future

There are ways to get out of the pits. One asset that chemical sensitives have in abundance, if they cannot work or go places as much as they would like, is time. After the initial shock wears off, time can be very valuable. The chemical sensitive can take the time to take stock of his life and plan for the future, to examine wants and don't wants. It is often helpful to list them:

I Want	I Don't Want
1.	1.
2.	2.
3.	3.

After making his list, the chemical sensitive can perform his own reality check. With the situation as it currently exists, which of the wants is realistic? Which of the don't wants is realistic?

After eliminating the unrealistic items, the CS person can reevaluate the list. Another dimension can be added by asking a spouse, mature children or a close friend to write similar lists as if they were the CS person. All lists should be written down and kept; having things written makes them easier for the person with organic brain syndrome to remember.

Once the realistic list is written, it is a very enlightening experience to explore the "why" behind each item: Why does item one fit in the I-want list? What does the list show about the things valued? What about the don't-want list? What values are tied to the statements? It is helpful to write a list of things the CS patient values:

What I Value:

1.
2.
3.

Listing one's values and why those things are valued can result in a bit of a shock. It can lead a person with CS to identify some apsects of his own nature which are quite nice and some which are not so nice. He should remember, however, that a lot of time to think provides a great chance to grow, and the opportunity to grow is enhanced if one's values are always available for study. Another step toward growth is to perform another reality check. How realistic are the values? For example, if financial security is the highest value, how realistic is that? To what extent does any human have control over financial security? By doing some thinking about values and determining whether those values are realistic, the chemical sensitive has accomplished a task that many non–chemical sensitives never accomplish in a lifetime.

The CS patient can take that list of wants/don't wants, realistically valued and assigned priority, and set some goals. It is helpful, again, to write down those goals:

My Goals:

1.
2.
3.

Goals can be small (I'll do this by the end of the month) or large (I intend to do this before I die). Once goals are identified, the CS person has the time to identify any barriers to overcome before accomplishing each goal. The barriers have to be assessed. Can they be overcome by the CS person himself? Will he need assistance? If assistance is needed, how can it be obtained? Or, is the goal just too hard? By setting goals and working a piece at a time to accomplish them, the CS person can get out of himself and become involved in living. One very common cry of the CS patient is, "Oh, God, I just want to live." Life is setting goals and working toward them. It is identifying and solving problems. These things are true whether one is healthy or has a disabling disease. Here are some little examples of problem-solving or coping mechanisms that worked for some people:

1. Carol, who values tidiness, found that her tremors caused her to spill coffee on the drainboard when she fixed coffee. She solved the problem by purchasing a syrup container and storing the coffee in the container. When she fixes coffee, she pours it from the container, recognizing visually the proper amount. No longer does she have to keep cleaning the drainboard just to fix a cup of coffee.

2. Mike was determined to overcome brain damage which made it impossible for him to subtract a two-digit number from another two-digit number. He spent three months working to find another part of his brain to pick up the task. Mike discovered that no matter how hard he worked, the function would not return. He readjusted the value he had placed on being able to perform the mental calculation, and now he carries a small pad and pencil or calculator.

3. Andrea wanted to write an article. Writing had become very difficult, and she could not seem to organize her thoughts. Because she had something to say, Andrea did not give up. She took a tape recorder and tried to speak into it, but found that she needed a person to spur her ability to communicate. A friend came by. The friend suggested that Andrea tell her what she wanted to say while they tape-recorded the conversation. Afterwards, Andrea transcribed the taped conversation. From that transcription, she was able to write out the material well enough that with editing, it was quite effective and was published in a local paper.

4. Tyler was up to his ears in an entitlement battle. Between the information he kept getting from doctors and the calls from his attorney, he couldn't keep it all straight. By purchasing a spiral notebook he solved his problem. Each day, he wrote the date in the margin. Every call that came in he recorded in the notebook. The notebook was his "brain" and a great resource, he discovered later, for remembering things that were important—things that in the past, without the notebook, he'd overlooked. It kept a history for him, which was helpful many times during his battle.

5. Gail and her husband, Tom, both retired, enjoyed eating out. They discovered that they could continue this pleasure by careful choice of places to go. For example, restaurants with divided sections for each eating area, those with high-backed booths, and those that had neither new paint nor newly reupholstered furniture were tolerable. To avoid the contaminants brought into places by customers, they chose the less

frequented hours for their dinner (between 2 and 3 p.m.), which often carried the additional benefit of reduced prices.

6. Sara was devastated when she experienced severe hair loss. To add body to her hair, she went to a beauty salon and got a permanent. The salon was filled with intolerable chemicals, and the permanent was a disaster for her remaining hair (as well as making her very sick). Discontented with her appearance, Sara decided to try a wig. She explained to the salesperson what the problem was and found a helpful, interested salesperson. With the additional weight she had gained, her former hairstyle did not really enhance her best features. The salesperson helped her find a style that was becoming and did not require spraying to maintain. (A scarf protected the style on windy days.) Sara was delighted with the effect.

Warning

Because CS is a chronic disease developed insidiously and has some of the characteristics of intoxication and addiction, there are some patients who adopt patterns of behavior similar to that of alcoholics or drug abusers. Others experience significant anger, depression, or anxiety. Some of these behaviors are chemically driven while others are psychogenic. Unless trained, the people who interact with CS patients are not equipped to help the chemical sensitive cope with chronic disease. The necessary tools are in the hands of the psychologists, neuropsychologists, or psychiatrists *who recognize* CS.

The CS patient who demonstrates fear, panic, depression, or anger needs to find help from those equipped to provide it. A spouse, relatives, friends, and support group leaders are not appropriate sources of help. To keep him from establishing a destructive pattern, those upon whom a CS patient begins to lean too heavily must insist that the patient seek help in appropriate channels. Most people hesitate to push another away, particularly when that person has a disabling disease, but such reluctance to hurt the CS patient may contribute to the problem, ultimately hurting the person more.

There is nothing wrong with explaining the situation calmly to a CS patient, saying something like, "You are leaning too heavily I care a lot. I feel you may need some tools to cope with chronic disease. Let's try to learn where those tools can be found." This prevents buildup of anger, resentment, and hostility in the caregiver and helps the CS patient begin to get perspective.

It is important to determine whether the CS patient does lean too heavily. For example, a patient with brain damage may not be able to drive.

It is normal for the caregiver, family or friends to offer to transport the CS patient. If, however, the patient will drive with only one person, demands transportation when it is inconvenient to the caregiver, or refuses to use the alternative of a taxi, the CS patient is leaning too heavily. Characteristic attitudes of the too-dependent CS patient are demanding, manipulating, withdrawing, fearing, clinging.

The normal needs of CS patients may be somewhat burdensome to family members. For example, the CS patient who stays at home and cannot use cleaning products requires assistance from others, either family or a cleaning service. The CS patient in such a case may feel guilt and the busy others may feel burdened. This is normal. If these feelings persist, a psychologist or treating physician can help the involved individuals gain appropriate perspective. If the CS patient refuses to permit anyone to clean, the problem may need extensive intervention.

Guilt and blame have never been effective in fostering human interaction. If a problem needs solving, those involved should try to identify reasonable accommodations. Options require discussion to find the most mutually satisfying.

4. Resources for the Chemical Sensitive

For the CS patient who becomes too disabled to work or attend school, knowledge of financial resources may be critical. Because the illness is newly recognized and many physicians are not prepared to diagnose or treat it, medical resource identification is likewise very important. Information on support groups; answers to questions about chemicals; data on regional air quality—all these can be of vital importance to the person with CS. Knowing the resources can be the key to surviving physically, emotionally, and financially. There is as yet no state-by-state directory of resources, but certain information can put the CS patient on the right track. That is the purpose of this chapter.

There is one rule for people with CS. It's a no-risk rule and applies to filing claims, securing service of an attorney, asking for information and so on. The rule is: Ask. If the answer is "no," nothing is lost. The answer may be "yes."

Legal Counsel

Probably the single most valuable resource available to the CS patient is legal counsel. Having a personal injury attorney who knows the chemical poisoning/chemical sensitivity legal picture merits all the time required to locate one. But bear in mind that a personal injury (PI) attorney generally cannot help the CS client who hasn't done his homework. (That "homework" is the subject of Chapter 5.) For the client who has done his homework, the PI attorney can do everything legally and administratively to assure that the CS client secures all that is available in terms of assistance.

The book *Your Medical Rights* by Charles B. Inlander and Eugene I. Pavalon (Little, Brown and Company, 1990) is an excellent guide to understanding medical rights.

Financial Resources

Financial resources fit into an entitlement perspective. The claims examiner's job is to assure that eligible individuals get their entitlements. Many CS patients will comment, "I've put all this into Social Security for years, it's time for them to take care of me." This viewpoint is unrealistic. The CS patient has to demonstrate that entitlements are due. Chapter 5 addresses the documentation necessary for such demonstration.

SSI

For adults and children who have never worked, there are various programs, which can work hand-in-hand. One of these programs is Supplemental Security Income, otherwise known as SSI. It is administered by the Social Security Administration of the U.S. Department of Health and Human Services. To apply for SSI, the person with CS either visits his local Social Security office or calls 1-800-772-1213.

In the article "When Life Is Toxic" (The *New York Times Magazine*, September 16, 1990, Section 6, Page 70), Robert Reinhold writes that in 1988, the Social Security Administration indicated that environmental illness is to be evaluated by claims examiners on a case-by-case basis. Though not specifically identified as a disabling condition, such as blindness, it can be a covered disability through the Social Security Administration. Numbers of CS patients are covered by Social Security programs.

SSI pays monthly checks to people who are aged, disabled or blind, and who don't own much or have a lot of income. It's not limited to adults. Monthly checks can go to disabled and blind children. People who get SSI usually receive food stamps and Medicaid also. Medicaid helps pay doctor and hospital bills.

The 1992 basic federal SSI check for one person is $422 a month; for a couple, $633 a month. The precise amount depends on the state of residence and the calendar year since amounts change. A recipient can get more if he lives in a state that adds money to the federal check. The amount may be reduced if other income is available.

Basic eligibility for SSI is the disabled category, which means that the claimant has a physical or mental problem which prevents working. To qualify, the condition has to be expected to last at least one year or to result in death. Children, as well as adults, can qualify. Eligibility for SSI depends on income (including non-cash items received such as food, clothing and shelter) and financial resources available and it varies by state and sometimes by area within a state. The income and resources of the spouse of a married claimant or the parents of a child under 18 are considered.

In addition to income, SSI has a resources qualification for eligibility. A single person may qualify with resources up to $2,000. For a couple the amount is $3,000. There are some resources that do not count: the home the claimant lives in and the land it occupies; personal and household goods and life insurance policies, depending on value; the claimant's car (usually); burial plots; and up to $1,500 in burial funds may not count.

In addition to income and resource limitations, there are other qualifications. The claimant must (1) live in the United States or Northern Mariana Islands, (2) be a United States citizen or in the United States legally, (3) have applied for Social Security or other benefits if eligible; and (4) accept vocational rehabilitaton service, if offered.

To apply for SSI, the claimant will need: (1) a Social Security card or record of Social Security number; (2) birth certificate or other proof of age; (3) information about home, such as mortgage or lease and landlord's name; (4) information about income and resources (payroll slips, bank books, insurance policies, car registration, burial fund records); (5) names and addresses of doctors, hospitals and clinics where claimant has been seen and names and addresses of social workers or institution superintendents.

Local Social Services and Public Welfare

People with CS who receive SSI may also be able to obtain additional assistance from the state or county. It isn't necessary to receive SSI to qualify for local assistance, but the CS claimant who can get benefits from both programs will find life a little easier.

Frequently, the major difficulty in applying for local social service programs appears to be overcoming pride. It is very difficult for some individuals even to consider going on welfare. Others may have heard that many programs won't pay their medical expenses because the expenses are categorized as experimental. That may be true, but there may be other financial benefits available. For the CS claimant with dependents, medical and dental costs of those dependents may be covered. Even this one benefit may prevent some irreplaceable family possessions being sold just to provide basic food, shelter, and clothing needs.

In general, there are income and financial resource eligibility requirements. Because benefits usually are not retroactive, the claimant should inquire when the need is felt. The telephone book is the place to look for the nearest social service, public welfare, or public assistance office.

SSA

Social Security (SSA) is a program administered by the U.S. Department of Health and Human Services, Social Security Administration. It provides retirement, survivors protection and disability protection to covered workers. Disabled workers or the widowed spouse of a covered worker, who is either disabled or caring for children under 16, may qualify for benefits of the deceased spouse.

This program differs markedly from SSI and public assistance benefits. Instead of focusing on income and resources, SSA eligibility depends on the number of credits earned. For example, if a claimant becomes disabled before age 24, he needs six credits out of the three-year period ending when disability began. If disability occurs at age 24 to 30, the claimant needs credits for half the time between age 21 and the time of disability. If disability occurs at age 31 or older, the claimant needs the same number of credits required for retirement benefits, and 20 of the credits must have been earned in the 10 years prior to disability.

Under SSA, the disabled claimant may be eligible for Medicare hospital insurance. A monthly premium is required for Medicare coverage.

If it appears that SSA due to disability is an available benefit, the CS claimant should file as soon as possible. Payment cannot begin before the sixth full month of disability. If the claim is filed after that time, the first payment may include some back benefits.

Social Security may be affected by workers compensation, public disability payments, or pensions based on work not covered by SSA. Payments are adjusted annually in January to rise in relation to the cost of living.

For the claimant whose SSA disability is approved, the Social Security Administration will issue a Certificate of Award, which indicates the amount of award and when payment begins. It also identifies the time the claimant can expect the first disability review.

Disability reviews may occur as frequently as every six months or as infrequently as every seven years. First, a Social Security representative will contact the CS–disabled person. That representative explains the review process and appeal rights. The person disabled by CS will be expected to provide information about medical treatment, any work activity and how CS affects him. Second, the updated folder is sent to the state agency which makes decisions on disability on behalf of Social Security. If the information is not considered complete or sufficiently current, a special examination or test may be required. If so, a written notice is sent to the claimant. The claimant also receives written notice of the decision of the state agency's disability decision. A negative decision can be appealed. If the decision is that the claimant is no longer disabled and no appeal is filed, the claimant receives a benefit for the last month of disability and two additional months.

Two special rights accompany a negative decision if requested during the first ten days of receiving notice of end of disability: (1) *Disability hearing*—the claimant can meet face-to-face with the decision maker and explain why he feels he is still disabled, submit new evidence or information or bring someone who knows about his impairment. (2) *Continuation of benefits*—he can have his disability benefits and Medicare coverage (if he has it) continue through a decision by an administrative law judge. If the appeal is not successful, the claimant may have to repay the benefits unless a waiver of overpayment is granted. The claimant has 60 days after receipt of notice that he is no longer disabled to file a written appeal at any Social Security office. The first step in the appeal process is reconsideration. The case will be reviewed independently by people who were not involved with the decision to stop benefits. The second step is a hearing before an administrative law judge; the third, a review by the Appeals Council; the fourth, a civil action in a federal court.

It should be kept in mind that sometimes SSA is taxable. When the claimant receives his Form SSA-1099, he will have to determine whether the amount qualifies, along with other income, as taxable income for that year. If so, he must file a tax return.

After receiving disability benefits for 24 months, the SSA–disabled claimant is eligible for Medicare to help pay hospital, doctor, and other medical bills.

Social Security disability payments continue as long as the medical condition has not improved and the claimant cannot work. If still disabled at age 65, disability benefits convert automatically to retirement benefits, generally in the same amount.

From time to time SSA disability recipients may be contacted by phone or in person. If someone appears at the door and the disabled person has questions about him, the disabled person should call the Social Security office and verify that they sent the representative.

Representatives from state vocational rehabilitation services may contact the SSA disability recipient about possible services to help him regain his ability to work. If offered services are refused without good reason, monthly benefits may be terminated.

Disability Retirement

For the worker whose CS disability did not occur from or cannot be proved to have been caused by the work environment, disability retirement may be available. This benefit is available to those employees having disability retirement provisions through employment programs or an insurance plan. Qualification depends on being disabled and unable to work, though some programs will continue payment until the disabled worker earns a certain percent (e.g. 80 percent) of the income of his former job.

Some plans provide coverage for only a brief period of time for disabilties viewed as psychogenic. A CS patient with a somatiform label may lose benefits if an accurate diagnosis does not occur quickly.

In addition to a monthly payment, disability retirement programs generally provide life and health insurance through conversion policies. It should be noted that disability retirement is taxable income and the life and health insurance premiums have to be paid by the disabled person. It is easy for the CS patient with organic brain syndrome to overlook what is vital. When filing for disability retirement, the CS–disabled person who has organic brain syndrome should ask about insurance coverage under a group plan or conversion and write reminders to himself to assure that the conversion opportunity is not missed by oversight. The significance of this point is that certain diagnoses (e.g. organic brain syndrome, occupational asthma, reactive airway disease, chemical sensitivity) are bases for denying insurance coverage. Conversion policies may be the only medical or life insurance the person with CS is able to purchase.

Generally, disability retirement programs have reporting requirements of continuing impairment. Usually, the treating physician is asked to report the continuing impairment and that opinion stands. Some programs may require annual exams. These programs tend not to carry the adversarial appearance that workers' compensation tends to have.

Because of the lack of adversarial appearance of these programs, some individuals who may be entitled to either disability retirement or workers' compensation may choose the disability retirement program to avoid what they perceive to be harassment. One should make such choices with care. In most cases, disability retirement is lower income, and it's taxable. Insurance premiums must be paid in full, and deductibles and copayments apply. However, some people may feel that the disadvantages are offset by the relatively uncomplicated nature of the program. It is a personal decision.

Workers' Compensation

Workers' compensation programs, whether state administered or approved or federally administered or self-insured by the employer, are designed to provide compensation for wage loss and medical expense coverage for injury or illness which resulted from employment. The programs were designed as a no-fault form of employee protection that would prevent employees from taking legal action against an employer. If an employee falls and breaks his hip, a workers' compensation program can work with efficiency. The efficiency and no-fault perspective are considerably weakened when dealing with an illness such as CS.

Some state programs will provide coverage when the individual with CS submits a claim and the proper documentation accompanies it. Payment begins with the provision that it will have to be repaid if the claim is denied, unless the claimant successfully claims a hardship waiver of overpayment. Other programs may initiate no payment whatever unless and until the claim has been accepted. In some cases this can take more than a year. Some plans cover stress-related workplace injury for limited periods. For CS-injured workers a clear diagnosis is important early on.

The eligibility requirements for workers' compensation are (1) that the medical impairment prevents the worker from working; (2) that the individual must have been employed; and (3) that the injury or illness resulted from or was exacerbated by that employment. The burden of proof rests on the disabled employee. The employee who became ill from work-related toxic exposure has to prove that toxic exposure existed in the workplace, that those toxics are the cause of his illness, and that his illness prevents him from working. That proof is available only from medical professionals and medical tests, all of which can be time-consuming and very expensive. In cases where workers' compensation approval will take a long time, the worker with CS may be able to take disability retirement until the workers' compensation is approved. This can help financially while the disabled employee works to establish the proof needed for workers' compensation. Once workers' compensation is approved, the employee can opt for that program.

Litigation

If a product or service performed is responsible for the individual's developing CS, the person with CS may file a lawsuit. In some cases a CS-disabled employee, disabled through on-the-job toxic exposure, may also file a suit in court. There is little legal precedent for products, service or employer suits. The tendency is to offer settlement when it appears that the plaintiff may be successful in court.

Medical Resources

Finding orthodox physicians who can diagnose CS is extremely difficult. In Washington State in 1990, for example, there were only two recognized points for CS diagnosis. One of these was an occupational medicine program. The other was a practicing allergist-immunologist. The occupational medicine program physicians were available only to patients with work-related CS.

Some alternative physicians can diagnose CS. These physicians can be located in the telephone directory under "environmental medicine" or "clinical ecology." When searching for a diagnostician for CS, it is advisable to call to be sure that the doctor has an M.D., is board-certified, and takes CS or potentially CS patients.

If benefits programs or litigation is the patient's goal, at least one diagnostician should be an orthodox practitioner, regardless of whom the patient chooses for treatment. Right or wrong, the diagnosis of an orthodox physician carries more weight.

In addition to selecting a physician, the CS patient should keep in mind that, if he is pursuing benefits or litigation, psychological or psychiatric diagnosis will almost always be required. Diagnosing physicians should be able to refer the patient, who should obtain diagnosis from a psychologist, neuropsychologist or psychiatrist who understands the effect of toxic chemicals on the function of the brain.

Advocacy and Support Groups

There are several national-level advocacy and support groups that focus on chemical sensitivity issues and events. People with CS can contact the groups to identify their specific goals, objectives, and services:

Susan Molloy, Editor
Reactor Newsletter for the Environmentally Sensitive
2 Park Circle, #202
Marin City, California 94965

Mary Lamielle, President
National Center for Environmental Health Strategies
"The Delicate Balance" Newsletter
1100 Rural Avenue
Voorhees, New Jersey 08043

Natural Resources Defense Council
(The Amicus Journal)
40 West 20th Street
New York, New York 10011

Human Ecology Action League
P.O. Box 66637
Chicago, Illinois 60666

Environmental Defense Fund
National Headquarters
257 Park Avenue South
New York, New York 10010

Chemical Injury Information Network
Attn.: Cynthia Wilson
P.O. Box 301
White Sulphur Springs, Montana 59645

Organization for the Advancement of Environmental Health (OAEH)
"Environmental Health News" newsletter
3865 E. Delhi Rd.
Ann Arbor, Michigan 48103

Sick School Syndrome
Irene Wilkenfeld
52145 Farmington Square Road
Granger, Indiana 46530

Well Mind Association
4649 Sunnyside Ave. North
Seattle, Washington 98103

In addition, the person with CS may find local advocacy or support groups. Group meetings frequently draw interested people who are not well-informed in terms of what substances cannot be tolerated by extremely sensitive individuals with CS.

Other groups that may relate in some manner to CS issues are environmental, ecological, and toxic control action groups.

Useful information is often available from groups that study the relative safety of commercially available products. The Washington Toxics Coalition, listed below, is the pioneer in this field.

Washington Toxics Coalition
4516 University Way NE
Seattle, Washington 98105
(206) 632-1545

Green Seal
1733 Connecticut AV NW
Washington, D.C. 20009
(202) 328-8095

Green Cross: 1 (800) 829-1415

Another CS advocate that may be helpful indirectly to the person with CS is:

Earon S. Davis, J.D., M.P.H.
643 Hibbard Road
Wilmette, Illinois 60091

Earon Davis consults with other attorneys regarding chemical sensitivity cases. He is recognized as a national expert in this legal field.

Information on Chemicals

Industrial hygienists can provide beneficial assistance to people with CS. Industrial hygienists can be found in university environmental health units or in federal, state, or local government labor or environmental units. To identify industrial hygienists who are willing to assist those with CS, contact them by phone. It takes little time to find out their opinions on CS. Even those with negative views can be helpful, if the CS individual is searching for toxicological information on a specific chemical.

Some groups in some states have formed for the sole purpose of examining materials in commonly used products to determine comparative levels of safety or toxicity. The people in these groups may develop newsletters or pamphlets with their findings. These can be helpful, if the studies relate to substances which the person with CS cannot tolerate.

There are some books which are excellent resources for people with CS. *Dangerous Properties of Industrial Chemicals* by Irving Sax and the Kirk-Othmer *Encyclopedia of Chemical Technology* are two of them. They are available in libraries, or industrial hygienists can provide data from them. The U.S. Government Printing Office Bookstores occasionally have valuable material. An example is the little CHRIS manual (Chemical Hazards Response Information System) used by the Coast Guard. The manual briefly identifies the chemical, its form, color identifiers, odor, what it does in water, hazard information, what the chemical does in fire, what happens to people exposed to the chemical, what the chemical does in terms of water pollution. The Environmental Protection Agency (EPA) has publications available in U.S. Government Bookstores and available through EPA. Its toxic release inventories can provide a general picture of state outdoor air quality.

For a more precise local view of the quality of outdoor air, the person with CS can contact his local air quality control agency and request an annual data summary. These agencies provide feeder information to the EPA. Their collection points may be near enough to explain some reactions to outdoor air. To read the data summary, one must understand chemicals and weather patterns to some extent. One should also keep in mind that only a very few more than 65,000 chemicals available are monitored. For example, one data summary tracks the following: carbon monoxide, ozone, sulfur dioxide, lead, nitrogen dioxide, and in some cases arsenic, along with particulate matter (particles of dust, soot, organic matter and compounds containing sulfur, nitrogen, and metals).

A chemical sensitive can use such a resource as a tool to identify the quality of air that surrounds his home, workplace, and the general driving area. The person who develops asthma symptoms or "brain fog" when driving in traffic may discover that heavy concentrations of sulfur dioxide, nitrogen dioxide, and particulate matter either trigger or exacerbate the asthma symptoms or generate the "brain fog."

The outdoor air and its pollutants enter homes and workplaces, where weatherization efforts, particularly in the winter, tend to keep the pollutants indoors, adding to the effect of the indoor pollutants.

The air quality data summaries can be helpful when people with CS are searching for a place to live where air is less polluted. The prevailing wind flow and a drive to locate business or industrial activity upwind from potential home sites can give some expectations of air quality for the area.

Information on specific chemicals is available from Chemical Injury Information Network or Washington Toxics Coalition (see page 109).

Material Safety Data Sheets (Indoor Air)

Material Safety Data Sheets (MSDS) are available from the workplace (to identify hazards of commonly used substances which contain some hazardous chemicals) or from the local fire department. You may be able to obtain them by phoning or writing the manufacturer.

The MSDS format consists of ten sections: (1) product identification, (2) emergency and first aid, (3) toxicology and health information, (4) physical data, (5) fire and explosion data, (6) reactivity data, (7) special protection information, (8) special precautions, (9) spill, leak, and disposal procedures, and (10) transportation information. The sheets provide the name and address of the manufacturer and telephone numbers for information. The information focus is acute exposure.

For the known chemical sensitive, an MSDS is of limited value. Consider the information offered in an MSDS for a computer toner. Ingredients are identified as styrene/acrylate copolymer (55–60 percent), magnetite (35–40 percent), polyolefin (5–10 percent), metal complex azo dye (less than 5 percent), amorphous silica (less than 1 percent) and metal oxide (less than 1 percent). First aid for inhalation exposure is removal from exposure. Toxicology data indicate that the toner is "practically non-toxic" when ingested, absorbed, or inhaled. Data conclude that the toner is not an irritant, sensitizer, mutagen or carcinogen. Physical data identify the toner as a black powder with a faint odor. Special protection information reveals none is required when in use as computer toner. According to the sheet, no special precautions are necessary.

These data would lead the user to conclude that the product is safe for human use. This conclusion for some chemical sensitives is a dangerous and uninformed one. Some CS users develop itching eyes, serious respiratory problems and central nervous system symptoms from using the "safe" product. It should be kept in mind that the CS-compromised individual may have difficulty at increasingly lower levels of chemical exposure. A re-examination of the data is required.

The ingredients should be evaluated. The CHRIS manual provides the following information on styrene: (1) it produces an irritating vapor; (2) vapor is irritating to eyes, nose, and throat; (3) if inhaled, it will cause dizziness or loss of consciousness; (4) it can cause respiration to stop; (5) the liquid will burn skin and eyes; (6) spills into water must be reported.

The toxicological data indicate that the toner is "practically nontoxic"; this is an unfortunate and unclear choice of words. Further comment—"This material has been tested and evaluated. When used as intended, it does not represent a health or safety hazard"—is untrue for some chemical sensitives. The assumption that the product is safe for humans is based on low level substance testing on rats and rabbits. The evaluation group neglected to account for the numbers of CS-compromised individuals who experience symptoms when reading material printed with use of this product, even after it had been permitted to lose its vapor for weeks. No comment is made regarding potential effects of inhaling particulates (black powder).

Finally, MSDS data do not address exposure to combinations of chemicals. Many printers, for example, give off ozone when operating. What is the effect of ozone and toner in combination? The problem with Material Safety Data Sheets is that our society really asks the wrong question. We ask, "What's wrong with a chemical?" instead of, "What's safe about a chemical?" The first question narrows scope; the second one widens it.

Government Agencies

Government agencies often have information available to the public, either free or for a fee. Examples previously identified are the U.S. Government Printing Office Bookstores, the Environmental Protection Agency and local air quality control agencies. Other relevant agencies include:

Consumer Product Safety Commission
5401 Westbard AV
Bethesda, Maryland 20207
(301) 492-6580

Department of Health and Human Services

1. National Institute of Environmental Health Sciences
   P.O. Box 12233
   Research Triangle Park, North Carolina 27709
   (Publishes *Environmental Health Perspectives*)
   (919) 541-3212

2. Social Security Administration
   1-800-772-1213 or local Social Security office

3. National Institute for Occupational Safety and Health (NIOSH)
   (404) 639-3286

4. Food and Drug Administration
   5600 Fishers Lane
   Rockville, Maryland 20857
   (301) 443-1544

5. National Institutes of Health
   9000 Rockville Pike
   Bethesda, Maryland 20892
   (301) 496-4000

Department of Labor

Occupational Safety and Health Administration (OSHA)
200 Constitution AV NW
Washington, D.C. 20210
(202) 523-8017

Environmental Protection Agency

401 M Street SW
Washington, D.C. 20460
(202) 382-2090

Legislators

Whether they are at the state or federal level, legislators (senators or representatives) can be a valuable resource to the chemical sensitive. They can be called upon for assistance in dealing with bureaucratic tangles affecting financial entitlement or benefits. They can also provide information, when they are directly involved in environmental legislation or investigations of adverse health effects from air pollution.

The U.S. Congress, for example, has had some information published which is interesting to people involved with CS. Sample publications are:

Neurotoxins [sic]: *At Home and the Workplace,* 99th Congress, 2nd Session, Report 99-827, Sept. 16, 1986, U.S. Government Printing Office, Washington, D.C.: 1986 (71-006 O).

Health Effects of Indoor Air Pollution, 100th Congress, 1st Session, Senate Hearing 100-70, April 24, 1987, printed for the use of the Committee on Environment and Public Works, U.S. Government Printing Office, Washington, D.C.: 1987 (73-934).

Issues Related to the Use of, and Exposure to, Various Chemicals, 101st Congress, 1st Session, Senate Hearing 101-112, March 6, 1989, printed for the use of the Committee on Environment and Public Works, U.S. Government Printing Office, Washington, D.C.: 1989 (96-831).

Indoor Air Quality Act of 1990, 101st Congress, 2nd Session, Report No. 101-304, May 24, 1990.

H.R. 1530—The Indoor Air Quality Act of 1989, 101st Congress, 1st Session, No. 89, Congressional Hearing, July 20 and Sept. 27, 1989, printed for the use of the Committee on Science, Space and Technology, U.S. Government Printing Office, Washington, D.C.: 1990 (26-090).

Neurotoxicity: Identifying and Controlling Poisons of the Nervous System (352 pages), GPO Stock Number 052-003-01184-1, price $15. Superintendent of Documents, Government Printing Office, Washington, D.C. 20402-9325. Call (202) 783-3238 to verify prices.

5. Documenting the Chemical Sensitive's Case

Whatever the cause of chemical sensitivity, some level of documentation is necessary, if only for members of the medical profession who provide future treatment. People are poisoned in a variety of ways, and they have different means of pursuing financial resources to cover medical expense and wage loss, if they were working. In this chapter we will focus on just one case as an example of how documentation might proceed. For the purpose of affording the most in-depth approach to this topic, the assumptions in this case are:

1. The employee has developed CS.

2. The CS was developed through chronic, low level toxic exposure on the job.

3. The injured worker must deal with entitlements through a workers' compensation program.

4. What the employee knows at the beginning of documenting is that he is sick and there is reason to suspect that the sickness is connected with something in the environment, probably at work.

Documentation required for other purposes (e.g. litigation or other entitlement programs) can be adapted from this example. Documentation is also necessary for children and adults who are not working, even in cases where litigation does not apply.

Note: Copies of actual personal documents are used in this chapter. Blotches are intentional and protect the identity of the individuals. If the document is desired only as an example by the reader, it will not be necessary to strain to read. If the reader wishes to read specific documents and has some difficulty, a magnifying glass will help.

As each kind of documentation is discussed, the reasons why such documentation might be necessary will be explained. These reasons may seem far-fetched to those unfamiliar with the war in which most CS patients find themselves embroiled. Nevertheless, it *is* a war, and without awareness of the battle, a purpose, a plan, a lot of effort, and persistence, the person with CS has no chance of surviving.

Initial Phase

Case documentation begins with a medical record. Something occurred to make the CS patient aware that a physical or mental problem exists. On the job, the sick employee must notify his supervisor. That should be done in writing, and the employee should keep a dated, signed copy of that communication.

Recognition of illness requires pursuit of medical answers, so the chemical sensitive begins the search for diagnosis. If the individual can make the link with toxic exposure, the potential for rapid diagnosis is enhanced. During the problem identification stage, it is very important for the employee to remain on the job. Sick leave may be required. If so, the employee should obtain a physician's letter or prepared form stating the nature of illness and need for removal from the workplace for whatever time the doctor deems necessary. The employee should give the original to the supervisor and keep a copy. Written medical excuses may not be required by the employer and may be perceived as superfluous by the physician, but having them will establish the important paper trail for the future.

Sample

The employee in our case study obtained from his physician a signed, handwritten note reading as follows:

Medical leave of absence for 2 weeks starting Monday 1/9/XX. He is bothered severely by air quality at work and should be observed away from the building.

There is great temptation at some point during the diagnostic period for the chemically sensitive employee to quit his job. What may appear to be a flu-and-relapse cycle can be annoying to any employer. People in the workplace may be outright nasty. Regardless of the situation, it is important that the employee weather the storm. To quit prior to medical removal complicates the case. It could easily remove access to entitlements. At this point, the war has not even begun. Weathering the storm is good preparation for the future conflict. The CS patient may not be prepared for unkind treatment, and the easiest answer may appear to be to leave and seek employment elsewhere. Depending on the degree of damage, this decision may be counterproductive. The right answer is to remain employed where the problem appears to be occurring, so it can be identified.

During this initial phase, doctors who suspect that there may be a workplace-related problem (even if they know nothing about CS) may put the employee through workplace removal-return trials repeatedly, while they observe. If the employee suspects the symptoms are occurring from some substance at work, documentation should begin immediately, and findings should be provided to the physician. During this phase there are a number of things the employee should do.

1. The employee should *remain in his job*. (Reasons: Until it is medically determined that the illness is work-related, the potentially heavy medical cost just to diagnose CS can be covered by group policies through the workplace. If the illness is CS, the sickness remains. Another job may be extremely difficult to find, and, if found, may not provide a better environment. It is unlikely that a group policy provided in another place of employment would cover a pre-existing condition, such as the individual is experiencing. In addition, quitting may cause the employee to lose entitlements from the employer where the toxic exposure occurred by metabolizing evidence from the body before tests can be run to detect its presence.)

2. The employee should *keep a daily journal* of symptoms; what appears to make symptoms worse and what is suspect; when symptoms are worse (day of the week and time). The employee keeps a copy and gives one to the physician. (Reason: This provides the physician with essential information for diagnosis.)

3. The employee must *follow physician advice*. Removal/return-to-work trials and medical requests for change of location in the workspace can be difficult for both employee and employer, but they may be essential. Most employers are aware of the need to provide "reasonable accommodation" for physical or mental impairment. (Reason: An employee, even in the medical world, is not equipped to be his own doctor. By not following the doctor's advice, the employee could compromise entitlements. Moving to another workspace may solve the problem or demonstrate its severity.)

4. The employee should *communicate with the physician*, especially if there are problems with the physician's advice. (Reason: Doctors are not

mind readers. The information that a certain prescription or certain advice is increasing the level of difficulty can be the single piece of critical information to steer the diagnosis in the right direction.)

5. The employee should *keep copies of every relevant piece of correspondence* from doctors and employer—sick leave request slips and so on. (Reason: The paper trail is critical if the employee eventually must pursue entitlements. Trying to get these documents after the fact may be very difficult, if not impossible.)

6. The employee should begin to *develop the history of the illness*, going back in time to identify when he first began to feel sick. The history should begin with the time when the employee last felt well. It is important to trace the illness and any other symptoms which may or may not appear to be relevant, dating each as accurately as possible. (Reason: If the employee has CS, this information is required to pursue entitlements. To gather it as quickly and as accurately as possible will strengthen the case.)

Sample

Below are some excerpts from the documented history of illness in our case study.

Date	Occurrence	Doctor	Diagnosis
Summer 19XX	Reaction to antibiotic — never had a systemic reaction to anything previously	(Doctor's name) came to my home and administered adrenalin	Systemic reaction
19XX	"Something" in the air in the room in which I worked bothered me (sinus congestion)—while substance falls from ceiling.		
19XX	Voice began to become "strained." Use of antihistamines at night helped.		

8/XX	Increasing "laryngitis"		
. . .	. . .	. . .	. . .
8/22/XX to 10/10/XX	out from work for convalescence (from surgery)—no "laryngitis" during this period		
10/11/XX	"Laryngitis" returned . . .		

This employee's history went on through the end of 1988, documenting increased problems with "laryngitis," a feeling of "sandpaper" in the lungs, fainting, weight loss, and other symptoms, plus the diagnosis of asthma, which he had never had previously.

7. The employee should go back in time and *try to recall any changes in the workplace* that occurred which might relate to the illness (e.g. installation of new carpet, painting, a new business located nearby, renovation, new furniture, any problems with plants growing in the area, any other people often sick or exhibiting signs of allergy, and so on). (Reason: This information can help to pinpoint the source(s) of the cause of CS; tie it to a real event; and provide strength to the case, if entitlements must be pursued.)

8. The employee should *identify locations or processes which, when he passes them, make him feel worse.* (Reason: This information can identify sources of the cause of CS and or the extent of the illness.)

9. The employee should begin to *document his past health history* briefly. If he has never had a history of medical conditions relating to the symptoms he has developed, he should get a letter from his physician stating that information. (Reason: Filing for entitlements will require this to rule out pre-existing conditions.)

10. It is important for the employee to *identify the products which are in the work area.* (Reason: Numbers of commonly used substances are toxic. Items in offices such as carbonless carbon paper, cleaners, photocopy machines, toners for computers and copy machines, and so on can cause problems in certain situations. It isn't necessary to work with what are generally perceived as extremely hazardous chemicals to develop CS.) Note: This should be done during the lunch hour or prior to or after work.

This is not work for which the employee is paid, and it should never be done "on the clock."

11. The employee should *discuss the problem with his supervisor* and ask whether he may have the freedom to look around the office and see whether he might identify substances which could be causing his problem. It is important to identify problem substances and eliminate them or reduce the exposure, if possible, in order to perform work. If approached in a polite manner, many employers will be willing to permit this activity, assuming it isn't too time-consuming. It is also important to ask the employer for copies of any Material Safety Data Sheets applicable to processes within the building space occupied by the employing organization. (Reason: The employee will have a better idea what products are daily exposures. Also, it should be kept in mind that ventilation systems can carry toxic substances from one place to another within the building.)

12. If the employing organization shares a building with other organizations, the employee should *identify the function of those other businesses.* This can easily be done before or after work. In addition, it is important to identify what other businesses are located in the vicinity. (Reason: Shared office space usually involves shared ventilation systems. What is in the air in another organization can be transported into the workplace where the sick employee works. The identification of other businesses in the area can pinpoint or rule out sources of toxic substances which can contribute to indoor air pollution.)

13. The employee should *identify whether the building in which he works is a tight building.* Tight buildings have windows which cannot be opened. (Reason: Anything in the air of a tight building remains there. Toxics can accumulate. Ventilation systems do not have the capacity to provide the kind of air exchange necessary, without great expense, which many organizations are simply not willing or able to provide.)

14. The employee should *note the ventilation provided into and out of his workspace.* Many office-injured employees work in rooms where the ventilation is a function of seepage of air around unvented fluorescent lighting fixtures. (Reason: Part of the war is a function of ventilation. Air studies to disprove work-related CS claims will point to good ventilation when there is either ventilation around light fixtures or inadequate frequency of air exchange. If an air study is requested by either the sick employee or the employer, ventilation can be increased for the study and lowered afterward. Air studies will be performed using guidelines that the Environmental Protection Agency provides, even while EPA recognizes

that the standards are set too high for safety for the entire population. Lower levels than those assumed safe are making significant numbers of people sick.)

During this phase, there are also some things an employee should not do. The temptation may be great, but there are legal issues involved:

1. The employee, unless he has written permission from a person with the authority to grant it, *should not carry into the workplace any device to test the air.* (Reason: In terms of law, the air in the workplace may be viewed as belonging to the employer. The question would involve whether the employee was authorized to test it. An employee who may be suffering from CS definitely does not need to find himself sued by an employer.)

2. The employee, unless he has written permission from a person with authority to grant it, *cannot carry off materials for independent testing of toxicity.* (Reason: These materials belong to the employer. Taking them is theft.)

3. The employee *should not believe everything he is told by medical personnel.* If an employee is convinced that workplace toxic exposure exists, and the treating physician continues to diagnose flu, the employee can get a second opinion. Unless aware of a physician who is trained to recognize CS, the employee could choose one or both of two routes: occupational medicine specialists or environmental medical specialists. (Sources can be identified through CS support groups, national organizations which recognize CS, or referral from the treating physician. Resources identified in this book may be helpful.) If the employee suspects toxic exposure, he *should not wait.* He should seek out three diagnostic tools: (1) an immune system profile, (2) a toxicological survey (blood and fat), and (3) a neuropsychological assessment. (Reason: These sources can reduce the time required to identify the problem and find the substances which may be causing the problem while those substances can be found. Because the body does rid itself of toxics and because the immune system eventually becomes suppressed, failure to get these tests during exposure can demonstrate lack of evidence of the problem.)

4. The employee *should not believe everything he is told by the employer.* The worker injured on the job is entitled to workers' compensation of one variety or another. Many employers will perceive CS injury as being solved through disability retirement. The employee should beware. If it appears that the injury is work-related, the wise employee will find a good personal injury attorney. (Reason: CS is as new to the people who

work in a personnel office as to the medical community. Not all people in personnel offices have a thorough grasp of workers' compensation. To the CS-injured employee, there is a big difference in workers' compensation and disability retirement programs. Workers' compensation is nontaxable; disability retirement is taxable. Workers' compensation fully covers, or is supposed to cover, medical expense; disability retirement deducts for premiums and the coverage is like group insurance—the sick person pays part of the medical expense.)

Filing the Initial Claim

Cause and Effect

In order to solve problems, it is necessary to establish the link between cause and effect. Toxic environmental exposure is a problem, when it makes an employee sick. The first place to look for the potential cause is the place where the symptoms appear to worsen. If removal/return-to-work trials reveal a worsening of the symptoms in the workplace, that is the point where the documentation begins. To demonstrate cause and effect for work-related toxic exposure and poisoning, here is what the employee must establish:

1. That toxic chemicals exist in the workplace and that the employee has been exposed to those chemicals either through a massive single exposure or through chronic, low level exposure.

2. That damage consistent with chemical poisoning exists. A full blown immune response in the absence of other identifiable disease is an indicator. Toxicological data can point to some exposures, but there is no screen for all potential chemicals. Neuropsychological testing can initially demonstrate CNS involvement.

3. That there is a probable (or in some cases more probable than not) link between the toxic exposure(s) in the workplace and the employee's symptoms.

It sounds simple. It is incredibly difficult.

• Workplace Mapping

One of the first tasks is to illustrate the environment of the workplace. Not everyone is an artist. The point is not to prepare a perfect architectural drawing but rather to communicate aspects of the employee's working environment as completely as possible. The charts on pages 124–126 are samples from our case study. Along with these charts, the employee kept information from an Air Quality Data Summary relating to the chemicals found on his worksite.

The Medical Tests

While establishing the potential for toxic exposure at the worksite, the medical process continues. In our case study, it was obvious that neurotoxic exposure could exist in the workplace, since over half the identified chemicals are known neurotoxics. It is critical when one suspects that a patient has had a toxic exposure to test for evidence. Tests which identify a full blown immune response in the absence of identifiable disease are important. Tests which identify toxic exposure are critical. The employee in our case study had both kinds of tests, with results that pinpointed exposure to trimellitic anhydride (TMA), producing a full blown immune response. He also had the same tests a year later, following scrupulous avoidance of known TMA sources. They showed that immunosuppression had occurred.

Key to the interpretation of immunological testing is the presence of IgE, IgM and IgG (see Chapter 1 for discussion of these substances). It is important to recognize that IgE shows only during exposure and for about two weeks following the exposure. Its half-life is a day and a half. On the other hand, IgM may be found in blood for a year following exposure, and IgG may last for many years. Some doctors, through either ignorance or deception, will test for IgE a year after exposure and state that the patient is no longer having problems with the chemical. Whether the doctor is aware of the half-life of IgE is not something which can be established, but the CS patient must be aware of it for his own protection. In the case of a chemical such as TMA on which there have been no neurotoxicity studies, sending the person into an environment where contact with it is likely could do substantial additional damage. If damage were neurological a case could be made that such an occurrence is human experimentation with a known toxic. That particular chemical, TMA, is low molecular weight, fat soluble. In a compromised neurological system that chemical could do significant damage by acting as a neurotransmitter or simply by directly or indirectly causing brain cells to die.

It is worth noting—in order to acquaint the CS patient with possible objections to immunological data—that there have been claims and counter-claims regarding the value of immunoglobulin data with respect to various toxic substances. It has been asked whether the production of IgM, IgG, or IgE in response to exposure to TMA or other chemicals actually proves anything. As the bibliographic entries make clear, much research

Workplace of *name of claimant* from Month, Year to Present

F C S
12345 N West Street
P. O. Box 9876
Pacific, State 99999-9999

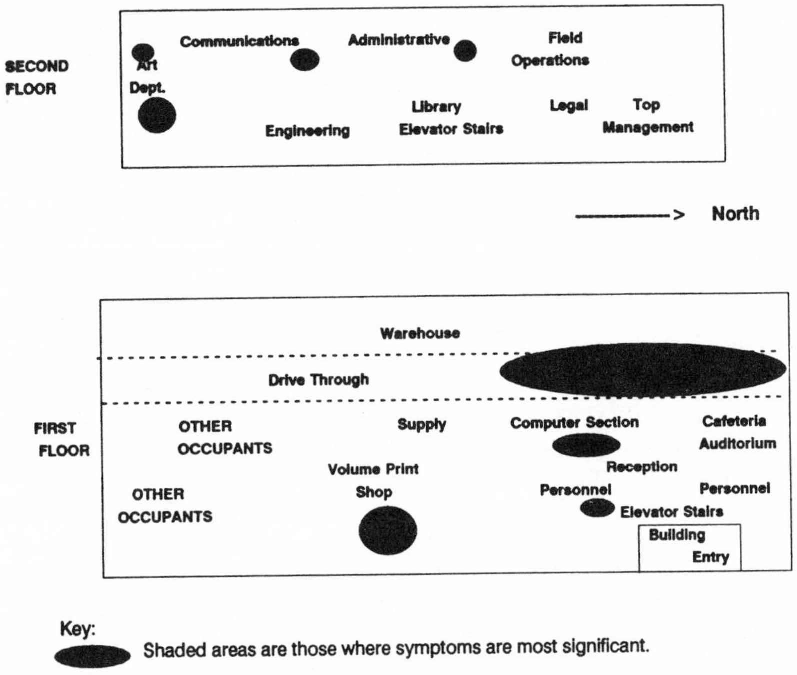

SECOND FLOOR
Art Dept.
Communications
Administrative
Field Operations
Engineering
Library
Elevator Stairs
Legal
Top Management

------------> North

Warehouse
Drive Through
FIRST FLOOR
OTHER OCCUPANTS
Supply
Computer Section
Cafeteria Auditorium
Volume Print Shop
Reception
OTHER OCCUPANTS
Personnel
Personnel
Elevator Stairs
Building Entry

Key:
Shaded areas are those where symptoms are most significant.

Workplace Location: Industrial Area

The building faces a 6 lane, heavily traveled highway
A train track, used on a daily basis, lies between the highway and the building
To the south is a paper manufacturer
To the north and south are cement production sources
There are metals manufacturing operations in the area

Former Uses of Building

Automobile manufacturing plant
Aircraft manufacturing plant

Workplace map showing exposure sites.

Substances Known to Exist in the F C S Building:

Substance	Source
Acetone	Cements
Acids/Alkalis	Cleaners
Ammonia	Cleaners/Blue Prints
Art Media (wide range) [inks, lacquers, thinners, retarders, developer bath chemicals, fixers/stabilizers, paints, etc.]	Graphics Section
Benzene	Cleaners
Carbon Monoxide	Vehicle Exhaust
Carbon Tetrachloride	Cleaners
Detergents	Car Washing Operation
Dry Cleaner Fluid	Garments Worn
Ethanol	Photocopiers
Formaldehyde	Building Materials, Carbonless Carbonpaper
Gardening Chemicals	Outside/Inside Building
Methanol	Photocopiers
Nitropyrenes	Photocopiers
Oxalic Acid	Blue Prints
Ozone	Photocopiers
Particulates	Dust, Soot, Ash, Carpet Fibers, Something from Ceiling
Perfumes, Hairspray, Lotion	Humans in Building
Pesticides	Surfaces Sprayed
Petroleum Distillates	Gasoline, Aerosols, Furniture Polish
Photographic Chemicals	Graphics Section
Photomapping Chemicals [potentially harmful substances]	Photomapping Section
Toluene	Cleaners, Rubber Cement
Toner	Photocopiers, Printers
Trichloroethane	"White-Out"
Vinyl Chloride	Plastics, Carpet

List of substances in employee's workplace.

Specific Worksite of _name of claimant_ from Month, Year to Month, Year

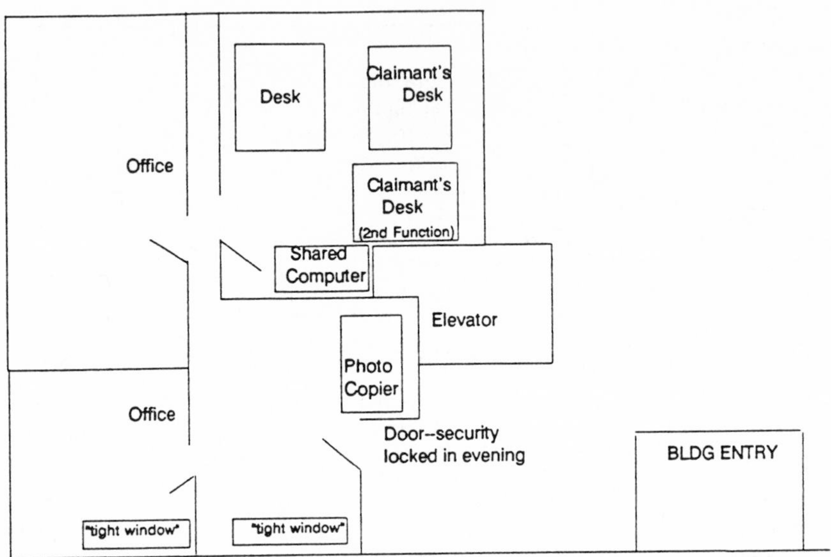

Note: Due to sensitive nature of information, all doors were locked at night and special security locked system was installed on door opening to the three office areas.

Materials in use in these areas include:

Paper Mate office products **correction fluid** (Note: avoid contact with clothing. Advise professional dry cleaner to handle as if paint stain. Inhaling contents can be harmful or fatal.)

Correction fluid solvent #163 ("inhalation of contents can be harmful or fatal").

Slyde lubricating spray compound (silicone spray aerosol: isobutane-propane propellant).

Glass cleaner (isoproponal glass cleaner).

Cleaner (general purpose detergent "Do not take internally; rinse hands; keep away from flame").

Toner (Savin Duplicator—isoparaffinic petroleum solvent—combustible).

Pens (white board pens [acetone?] and felt-tipped pens for charts).

Perfume, cologne, hair spray, lotions (worn in heavy amounts by both men and women).

Workplace map.

has been conducted with TMA and other toxics. The numbers of toxics screened are not even the tip of the potential iceberg. It is possible that some immunoglobulin readings are identifying toxic exposure to something other than the specific chemical being tested. What is known is that demonstration of these immunoglobulins is a marker of toxic exposure with a certain degree of predictability. For example, people with Ig readings relating to toxics with blood tests demonstrating full blown immune response patterns plus poor neuropsychological assessment scores will show some degree of toxic encephalopathy on PET scans and brain topography analyses of the brain's electrical function. It is perhaps also significant that these immunoglobins are not found in unpoisoned populations. Failure to understand the significance of the antibody (Ig) tests is a function of ignorance, not test invalidity. The National Research Council proposes antibody tests as a marker for CS.[453a]

The CS patient suspected of having organic brain syndrome should be referred for neuropsychological assessment. That testing can identify very subtle intellectual dysfunction even before evidence would show on MRI or standard EEG tests. Records of this assessment are important documents in the CS patient's file.

Pinpointing the Source

Trimellitic anhydride, or TMA, isn't something most people recognize. At this point the chemical sensitive undertakes a fact-finding mission. What is TMA? What are its uses? What is the effect on human health of this chemical? The CS patient will want to know the source (or probable source) of his exposure to this chemical.

Tracking down this chemical is important and may be critical "proof" of workplace injury, but it should be kept in mind that in tight buildings, it is highly likely that other chemicals are involved. At this point, however, it is important to follow any lead, and this chemical sensitive's test shows that TMA exposure four times greater than the most expected for the "normal" population has occurred. One very helpful article dealing with asthma symptoms and a variety of chemicals, including TMA, is "State of Art—Occupational Asthma" by Moira Chan-Yeung and Stephen Lam.[136] From this and other literature* the chemical sensitive in our case was able to learn about possible sources of TMA exposure. He kept summaries of important information in his document file.

**The following items in the Bibliography deal with TMA: 46, 60, 61, 62, 63, 65, 89, 92, 135, 136, 205, 212, 234, 271, 351, 352, 353, 354, 356, 360, 376, 395, 462, 465, 476, 477, 481, 484, 485, 493, 562, 585, 591, 592, 658, 694, 718, 720, 750, 801, 802, 803, 804, 805, 806, 807, 808.*

Calling local chemical consultants or industrial hygienists and discussing TMA (or another chemical) with those who perform air quality testing can also help the person who has CS identify the source. In this particular case, numbers of contacts resulted in the following information:

1. The first place to look for the source of TMA is not the air ("air study") but the carpet—any new carpet, especially glued-down carpet. Off-gassing is fairly fast. The problem comes from TMA in the fibers of the carpet. Drop a box on the carpet, or vacuum it, and the particulates become airborne. The particulates are inhaled and fall into the lower lungs. Vinyl and upholstery are additional sources of TMA and TMA is used in paint and glue to make them flow smoothly.

2. The place to seek the source is where the symptoms are worse. If it's at work, look there. If the person feels better at home, it would be a waste of money to perform a study there.

3. Respiratory problems are the known adverse health effects of TMA. There have been no neurotoxicity studies of the chemical, according to EPA.

In our case study, the source was easy to identify. A new, glued-down carpet installed in the entire secured area (illustrated in the workplace maps) during the spring of the year in which the employee was hired poisoned the worker over a period of about a year and a half. The cause and effect had been established. The three physicians who followed the case agreed. The employee had to leave the workplace. Based on the condition of the employee at that time, it was unlikely that another location would prove any better. The employee was experiencing severe reactions to "road fumes" and other substances by that time. With physicians' letters, the employee used the information gathered during documentation and filed for workers' compensation, disability retirement, and Social Security.

Sample

Our employee secured a letter from each of three physicians, stating his problem and each physician's recommendations. The letters ranged from simple, as in the first example below, to quite detailed, as in the second.

Dear (name of patient):

It is my opinion that you have Multiple Chemical Sensitivity Syndrome. This is a medical impairment. You need to be in a clean air environment in order to be symptom free, including travel to work location.

Realistically, therefore I recommend you do not return to work.

Thank you,
(name of doctor)

TO WHOM IT MAY CONCERN:

(Name of patient) has multiple chemical sensitivity syndrome due to poor air quality at work. . . .

Immune evaluation reveals that he does have positive IgE antibodies to TMA. . . .

He also has the presence of autoimmunities with anti-parietal cell of the stomach antibody and anti-brush border of the kidney antibodies present. This is not expected in a normal person but is present in patients with chemical sensitivity. He also has an elevated interleuken 1 generation which is typical of people with chemical sensitivity. He also has elevated T-1 positive cells which are also present in chemical sensitivity.

At this time, his condition is not medically stable. He is not medically free to work anywhere. He will have to work in a very limited environment that does not involve commuting. Any building that he would have to work in would have to be free of offending chemicals. Possibly he could find something to do at home where at least he could attempt to control the environment. . . .

Sincerely yours,
(name of doctor)

With the documentation provided and the concurrence of the employer as to cause and effect, it took two weeks for approval of disability retirement. It took nine months for approval of the workers' compensation medical expense and wage loss payments due to work-related "multiple chemical sensitivity syndrome" (MCSS). Because the worker had worked only four of the last five years on a covered plan, Social Security was denied.

To chemical sensitives, this resolution might appear uncharacteristically—indeed, unbelievably—quick and easy. Nine months was quick? Yes indeed, given the current situation with CS claims. Frustration is much more common than quick resolution. In some cases, benefits are paid when the claim is filed, but that money must be repaid if the claim is not accepted. In other cases, such as this one, no compensation is paid until the claim is formally accepted. Then there is a back pay check, and monthly payments follow. There aren't that many people who are capable of surviving financially for that length of time. Unemployment compensation does not apply.

Workers' Compensation

Workers' compensation is intended as no-fault insurance for on-the-job injury. Providing workers' compensation avoids employee-employer lawsuits. It works well for cut-and-dried cases such as broken bones, but claims administrators tend to be cautious when dealing with an injury that cannot be seen and does not have a time frame for recovery. There is reason to believe that CS claims are intentionally refused in some cases despite medical records indicating severe disabling conditions. A CS claimant who inquires why his case is taking so long to resolve may be given a story about an employee who claimed a back injury and was later seen painting the second story of his home; this "Injured Worker Seen Painting" story seems to be standard in the repertoire of claims administrators. What it means is that they have to be sure the injury is real and work-related. This is one reason documentation is so important, but unfortunately even thorough documentation does not guarantee a favorable outcome for the CS patient. Sadly, since there is no oversight on entitlement programs, administrators may choose to ignore even judicial orders, or apply guidelines arbitrarily. This type of conduct is so standard that there is a term for it: non-acquiescence.[350]

Oddly, initial claims approval may increase the CS patient's stress level. With the expectation that medical expenses will be reimbursed, the claimant will submit his self-paid medical bills for reimbursement, if he had not already done so. None may be reimbursed; some may be reimbursed, while others are not; or they may all be reimbursed. This confusing situation only makes things more difficult for the CS patient. He may attempt to communicate and discover that the sought-after answers never really come. The advice "Take what you can get, and don't make waves" may be given by others who have had experience with the program.

Some chemical sensitives will accept the "don't make waves" advice; others will reject it and pursue any route to reach their objectives (e.g. secure entitlements). Whether workers' compensation programs are administered by the federal government or state government or another self-insured program, there is recourse open to the CS claimant. That recourse is the legislature and the executive office at either federal or state level. When problems arise, state programs provide easier access to the courts than federal programs.

Workers' compensation programs are an administrative function of government. Even those self-insured programs of a non-governmental nature (e.g. those provided by employers) are authorized through government. The executive office (the office of the president of the United States, if the program is federal, or the office of the governor, if the program is not federal) is where the buck stops for administrative functions.

The legislature first authorizes the programs through law, and then approves funding for the program's administration. When he feels wronged by his program administrators, the chemical sensitive can appeal for help to the appropriate executive officer or senators and representatives in the responsible legislative body. Normally, the contact is made in writing. The addressee contacts the responsible official, and the claimant eventually receives some reply. Anytime a reply is not forthcoming, the CS patient should be prepared to appeal to the next higher level.

When a response does arrive, it may represent a sincere effort to help the claimant. It may be a request for further information; it may be a standard reply that sounds great but utterly fails to answer the question. These are some of the possible responses from legislators or executives. The claims administrator will have his own range of responses toward the claimant who pursues his appeal in such a manner. He may resolve the issue; he may resolve the issue but incorporate some form of retribution; he may ignore the issue but respond to further action with retribution. In such cases, the CS patient may be sidetracked from the real issue to the point where his appeals are seen as the actions of a disgruntled claimant—which they may be. Chemical sensitives have a tendency to have accompanying organic brain syndrome with impaired thought processes. Sometimes chemical exposure generates rage. Add that to poor communication or what appears to be denial of entitlements, and the CS claimant may react without thinking clearly. Government officials may have no idea what "set off" the claimant, and their behavior may further "set off" the claimant. When CS is better understood, some of these problems may diminish, and understanding and patience may increase.

Even when the claim is approved on a temporary or even permanent basis, there is another reason why the work-related CS claimant cannot relax: He may be too busy attending medical appointments. Not only does he continue to see his own physicians, but also the workers' compensation program administrators may send him to a variety of appointments. Documenting this process is valuable as a preface to the CS patient's medical file.

Special Problems

Because CS is not well known, there are special problems for which physicians may be unprepared. Challenge testing, for example, is potentially dangerous for some chemical sensitives. In our case study, a pulmonary physician participating in an IME chose to administer a methacholine challenge test to determine whether the patient had asthma. This particular case demonstrates one of the problems with IMEs: The normal doctor-patient relationship does not exist, and it may be impossible for the patient to report adverse reactions. This physician had ordered the same test for a CS patient about eight months prior, but the barrier between the patient and IME physician perhaps prevented the physician from learning that the previous patient had an adverse reaction to the challenge, sharply increasing his dependence on asthma medications. Indeed, this physician administered the same test to yet another CS patient later on. All three patients experienced irreversible bronchoconstriction following the test.

Any time a CS patient has a significant adverse reaction to drugs assumed safe, it is important to call the local Food and Drug Administration (FDA) office and report an adverse reaction to a drug. Patients as well as physicians may do this. The FDA is part of the U.S. Department of Health and Human Services, and the phone number is listed by the department under the FDA subheading. The next page shows a copy of the initial report on the adverse reaction of our case-study patient. It is important to report these reactions, because there will never be a warning until people know there is a problem. This is the manner in which adverse drug reactions are identified. There is no time limit. Several of the people with adverse reactions to methacholine experienced increased bronchoconstriction. In one case the response had not resolved after six years.

When a workers' compensation program administrator sends a CS claimant to a physician, and there has been a problem such as the methacholine challenge, it is advisable to obtain a protection letter from treating physicians. This may sound absurd, but the effect is a good one.

Sample

These two examples from our case-study patient's file show how physicians might phrase protection letters.

TO WHOM IT MAY CONCERN:

(Name of patient), a patient of mine with Chemical Sensitivity Syndrome, should not be subjected to any invasive procedures, especially those using any chemical or drug.

He is still recovering from the ill effects of a Methacholine Challenge test administered several weeks ago.

Sincerely,
(name of doctor)

TO WHOM IT MAY CONCERN:

(Name of patient) is under my care. He has allergy to inhalants including dust. He also has a severe problem with multiple chemical sensitivity syndrome and sick building syndrome because of exposure to poor air quality at work. . . .

DEPARTMENT OF HEALTH AND HUMAN SERVICES
PUBLIC HEALTH SERVICE
FOOD AND DRUG ADMINISTRATION (HFN-730)
ROCKVILLE, MD 20857

ADVERSE REACTION REPORT
(Drugs and Biologics)

Form Approved: OMB No. 0910-0230.

FDA CONTROL NO.

ACCESSION NO. 5/30/90.

I. REACTION INFORMATION

1. PATIENT INITIALS (In Confidence)	2. AGE YRS.	3. SEX	4.-6. REACTION ONSET MO.	DA.	YR.
			04	26	90

7. DESCRIBE REACTION(S)

Irreversible bronchoconstriction

13. RELEVANT TESTS/LABORATORY DATA

8.-12. CHECK ALL APPROPRIATE:

- [ ] PATIENT DIED
- [ ] REACTION TREATED WITH Rx DRUG
- [ ] RESULTED IN, OR PROLONGED, INPATIENT HOSPITALIZATION
- [x] RESULTED IN PERMANENT DISABILITY
- [ ] NONE OF THE ABOVE

II. SUSPECT DRUG(S) INFORMATION

14. SUSPECT DRUG(S) (Give manufacturer and lot no. for vaccines/biologics)

Methacholine

15. DAILY DOSE

16 ROUTE OF ADMINISTRATION

17. INDICATION(S) FOR USE
Test for asthma

18. DATES OF ADMINISTRATION (From/To)
4/26/90

19 DURATION OF ADMINISTRATION

20. DID REACTION ABATE AFTER STOPPING DRUG?
[ ] YES [X] NO [ ] NA

21. DID REACTION REAPPEAR AFTER REINTRODUCTION?
[ ] YES [ ] NO [X] NA

III. CONCOMITANT DRUGS AND HISTORY

22. CONCOMITANT DRUGS AND DATES OF ADMINISTRATION (Exclude those used to treat reaction)

23. OTHER RELEVANT HISTORY (e.g. diagnoses, allergies, pregnancy with LMP, etc.)

Patient had been diagnosed as having asthma 4 times prior to the administration of the test on 4/26/90.

IV. ONLY FOR REPORTS SUBMITTED BY MANUFACTURER

24. NAME AND ADDRESS OF MANUFACTURER (Include Zip Code)

24a. IND/NDA NO. FOR SUSPECT DRUG

24b MFR. CONTROL NO.

24c. DATE RECEIVED BY MANUFACTURER

24d. REPORT SOURCE (Check all that apply)
[ ] FOREIGN [ ] STUDY [ ] LITERATURE [ ] HEALTH PROFESSIONAL [ ] CONSUMER

25 15 DAY REPORT?
[ ] YES [ ] NO

25a. REPORT TYPE
[ ] INITIAL [ ] FOLLOWUP

V. INITIAL REPORTER (In confidence)

26.-26a. NAME AND ADDRESS OF REPORTER (Include Zip Code)

Food & Drug Administration
P.O. Box 3012

26b. TELEPHONE NO. (Include area code)
(206) 486-8788

26c. HAVE YOU ALSO REPORTED THIS REACTION TO THE MANUFACTURER?
[ ] YES [X] NO

26d. ARE YOU A HEALTH PROFESSIONAL?
[ ] YES [X] NO

Submission of a report does not necessarily constitute an admission that the drug caused the adverse reaction.

NOTE: Required of manufacturers by 21 CFR 314.80

FORM FDA 1639 (7/86) PREVIOUS EDITION MAY BE USED

Adverse reaction report form.

> His reactions to drugs are unpredictable and potentially serious for him because of his sensitivity to chemicals. He should not have any further invasive or challenge procedure without approval of his treating physician. . . .
>
> Sincerely yours,
> (name of doctor)

Another reason for post–claims approval stress is that the CS claimant may be investigated by workers' compensation administrators. The general reaction is to feel invaded. This is particularly true when the CS patient either discovers the investigation by accident, or discusses it with a physician who asks whether the patient perceives himself as paranoid. It is not possible to prove, but workers' compensation officials will tell others off the cuff that negative reports (those making it appear that the case is fraudulent) are filed, and positive reports (those indicating the claimant has a valid disability) are usually destroyed. Investigation may occur in the absence of notice to the claimant. Patients should be prepared to be videotaped, monitored over the phone, visited by investigators, and so on.

The sad fact is that the post–claims approval period is full of stressful influences, and there will probably be times in the CS patient's life when it seems that the whole world is at war with him. Even professionals whose services may at first glance seem appropriate for the chemical sensitive may actually contribute to the patient's stress level through their actions. One such category of professionals comprises certain medical specialists. While it may seem logical to seek out specialists for the bizarre symptoms CS patients experience, one must remember that CS is a systemic disease, affecting many parts of the body. It is vitally important for a CS patient to pursue a generalist medical approach to his initial diagnosis. Otherwise, entitlements, if secured, may cover only a portion of his condition.

Finding the right diagnostician is often difficult. For one thing, doctors most likely to recognize CS are in the field of environmental medicine—but many orthodox doctors have attempted to discredit that field, and their prejudice can backfire on the CS patient. Another problem is that some doctors who claim to recognize CS actually view it, and treat it, as a psychogenic disorder. A CS patient may spend precious financial resources to see a CS "specialist" only to receive a report stating that his condition is resolved and he is free to work—whereas a non-specialist recognizes severe medical impairment and counsels against return to the workplace.

To avoid these pitfalls it is wise when CS is suspected to identify the experts and get referral from doctors known to diagnose and treat CS *as* CS, not as a psychiatric problem. The experts cited in Appendix B and the Bibliography may be helpful in this regard.

In other situations, professionals who should be helpful to the chemical sensitive can be adversaries when they perform their jobs incompletely or even unethically. For example, the CS patient in our case study asked for an air study in his workplace, in order to identify the source of TMA exposure as well as to identify the contents of a white powder that continually rained from the ceiling under which the employee worked. The company's personnel officer ordered the air study and indicated repeatedly that the industrial hygienist performing the study was not to make any comments about the employee.

Nevertheless, the report contained a number of remarks about the employee's medical data and even disputed the physician's claim that his medical tests demonstrated allergies or autoimmune disease. The study also referred to a supposed "history of 'asthma'," though the physician's report states that no such history existed prior to TMA exposure. The report also concentrated on the fact that the employee was a smoker and opined that smoking (as well as "emotional stress") was probably the reason for his health problems. The hygienist disregarded the fact that the employee's symptoms perfectly paralleled the known toxic effects of TMA poisoning, as well as the evidence in current literature[136, 255, 270, 783] that smoking is unrelated to SBS or CS symptoms. A recent National Research Council publication[453a] found that studies are not bias free when dealing with the assumption that tobacco use figures as a cause of carcinogenic disease.

Meanwhile, as for seeking out the TMA exposure source, the hygienist reported as follows:

> Analyzing collected samples for the presence or absence of tri-mellitic anyhydrides (TMA) is not provided by our contract laboratory and many other laboratories and was, therefore, not performed in these initial evaluations.... The level of TMA anti IgE globulin reported by the "Antibody Assay Laboratories" is regarded as inconclusive evidence of an allergic response by one of our occupational medicine consultants.... It seems doubtful that TMA exposure would either, 1) occur at the worksite or, 2) be related to his office-based symptomatology.

As for the white powder from the ceiling, the ceiling panels were "tested for the presence of asbestos" (for which they proved negative); the report contained no further remarks on this subject.

Finally, the report contained misleading conclusions about the volume of "fresh outside air" in the office, as follows:

> The Society of Heating, Refrigeration and Air Conditioning Engineers recommended ... that for nonsmoking office areas there should be a minimum of 5 cfm of fresh outside air per person. The two areas of concern had 15 and 19 cfm per person of fresh outside air.... The carbon dioxide concentration of 300–400 ppm showed that there is an adequate supply of fresh air to the area.

The hygienist did not explain how this "fresh outside air" entered the office; a second hygienist later stated that the only path for entry or exit of air in the office was through the unvented fluorescent light fixtures in the ceiling, and that no other ventilation existed. Further, the hygienist did not mention that the quality of the "fresh outside air," as measured by a local pollution control agency which has a monitoring station in the parking lot of the building, was far from satisfactory. The particulate matter and sulfur dioxide levels measured in that location could bring into the building substances which are capable in combination of doing respiratory damage. Failure to consider sources of ventilation and the quality of the outside air demonstrate the sort of incomplete staff work that can cause problems for the CS claimant.

One of the major failures with workplace air studies is the inability of equipment to measure zero. Equipment was designed for industrial environments. The levels they can measure are too high to detect the presence or absence of indoor office pollution.[595].

One more professional who must perform his job well or risk further injuring of the CS patient is the claimant's attorney. The attorney who accepts CS cases knows that the client may have extremely limited resources and that the work required to resolve that client's problems through legal or administrative channels is demanding, seemingly endless, frustrating, and not financially rewarding. It also requires him to deal with clients who may have considerable mental difficulty. As a result, CS cases may be viewed as very undesirable. Numbers of attorneys, though qualified to take them, flatly refuse.

Most CS patients need an attorney who specializes in their need: personal injury, workers' compensation, and so on. It is legitimate to ask, at the initial interview, about the attorney's track record. How long has he dealt with CS cases? How many have concluded successfully? How many have not? When a client calls his office to speak with the attorney, does his call get referred to a paralegal? Will he return calls?

The significant issue to most CS patients is finding an attorney who is willing to take the case, but that does not assure getting a good one. One hazard in attorney selection is that the CS case may be shoved to the back burner. As a result, a case, particularly an entitlement case, may be lost due to overlooked action dates. If this occurs, legal malpractice becomes yet another issue for the CS patient. In such cases documentation of legal unprofessional activity is critical. In Chapter 5 there are resources that may direct the CS patient to a professional attorney and help prevent legal problems. Referral to experts is important. Advocacy and support groups may provide helpful referrals. In some cases physician referrals are valuable, particularly when the physician has been used as a witness for CS patients in court or administrative hearings.

Additional Documentation

Journal Keeping

Keeping a daily journal is a task that chemical sensitives and some physicians may find distasteful. The CS patient may find journal keeping an unpleasant reminder of symptoms, and something that is tiring at the end of the day. Some physicians may perceive it as requiring too much symptom focus. Nevertheless, for physicians who work with CS patients to identify specific exposures which need to be avoided, journal keeping is critical. Even if a physician does not require journal keeping, it still has merit. The person with CS can use it to identify exposures to avoid, and, in the case of those CS patients who are followed by benefits claims examiners, journal keeping shows whether and when a condition has stabilized. Some benefit programs pay a certain amount monthly and then, when the condition becomes stable, there is a larger one-time amount paid for settlement. The journal-keeping exercise can be a valuable tool to identify stabilization.

The next page shows an example of how journal keeping can be done with minimal effort. The symptoms characteristic to the specific patient are catalogued in the column on the left. To the right is a week's worth of space for data gathering. A numbering system grades severity of symptoms (1 = no interference with activity; 2 = moderate interference with activity; 3 = prevented activity; 4 = required medical intervention). The patient lists exposures on a daily basis at the top of each column on the right. On a −3 to +3 continuum, the CS patient lists an emotional score for the day. A zero indicates apathy. Medicine used is listed just beneath the symptom column. At the very bottom of the chart, the patient evaluates the day. On a day when the patient is too sick to record the day's experiences in the journal, he can write "too sick to record" on the daily entry space.

Any method of journal keeping that is preferred by the CS patient is useable. There may be some value in a more narrative approach by some CS people. Some physicians may provide charts of their own as useful tools for computerized input, which ultimately facilitates analysis.

Record Keeping

It is critically important that the CS patient establish a filing system to contain all reports, correspondence, medical expenses, information gathered, and so on. How to organize depends on the individual, but the

DATE 1989	S (5/6)	M (5/7)	T (5/8)	W (5/9)	T (5/10)	F (5/11)	S (5/12)
CONDITIONS ENVIRONMENTAL	AT HOME	DENTIST	FAMILY DOCTOR	AT HOME	DOWN-TOWN HOSP.	IN TOWN (BUS)	IN TOWN (BUS)
EMOTIONAL Low -3 -2 -1 0 +1 +2 +3 High	+2	+1	0	0	+1	+1	+1
	FEEL LIKE SOMETHING LEFT ON BEACH AFTER TIDE GOES OUT						
SYMPTOMS							
HEADACHE	3	3	3	3	3	3	3
BACK OF HEAD/NECK ACHE	2	2	2	2	3	3	3
BRAIN FOG	3	3	3	3	3	3	3
MEMORY LAPSES	3	3	3	3	3	3	3
DIZZINESS OR FAINTING	2	3	3	2	2	2	3
ELECTRICAL PROBLEMS (PARESTHESIAS)	2	2	2	2	2	2	3
IRRITATION		1	2	2			
HYPERACTIVE							
FATIGUED	3	3+	(4)	3+	3	3+	3
SLEEPLESSNESS							
SLEEPINESS		3	3	3	3	3	3
LOSS OF SENSE OF SMELL	1	1	1	1	1	1	1
ACUTE SENSE OF SMELL	1				1		
SWOLLEN INSIDE MOUTH							
LOSS OF HEARING	1	1	1	1	1	1	1
RINGING EARS	V Loud	VL	VL	VL	VL	VL	VL
NUMB FINGERS	1	2 (all 5)	1	2	2	2	2
MOTOR SKILL DIFFICULTY	2	2	2	2	2	2	2
MUSCLE ACHES		1	1	1	1	1	1
JOINT PAIN							
HEAVY ARMS AND LEGS		2	2	2	2	2	1
VISION (DIFFICULTY FOCUS)			1		1	1	1
VISION (BLURRED)							
ITCHING EYES							
HIVES						1	
SHORTNESS OF BREATH	3	3	3	3	2	2	3
CHEST PAIN	2	3	(4)	3+	3	3	3+
ASTHMA (W = LOUD WHEEZING)	3 W	3 W	3 W	3 W	2	2	2
BRONCHITIS			2	2	2	2	2
SORE THROAT							
LARYNGITIS	1	1	1	1	1	1	1
NAUSEA	1						
DIARRHEA	1 (RB)	1 (RB)				1 (RB)	1
LIVER PAIN	1	2	2	2	2	2	2-3
SPLEEN(?) PAIN							
HAIR LOSS	1	1	1	1	1	1	1
VORACIOUS APPETITE	1	1	1	1	1	1	1
DEFORMED NAILS	1	1	1	1	1	1	1
INFECTION							
OTHER: COUGH (TIGHT)	2	2	2	2	2	2	2
TACHYCARDIA	1	1	1	1	1	1	1
RED SKIN & BLEEDING BLISTERS	1	1	1	1	1	1	1
medicine etc	VENTOLIN	VENTOLIN →	→	→	→	→	→
			COUGH SYRUP	→	→	→	→
OVERALL EVALUATION OF DAY	Okay	Okay	Tolerable	Okay	Okay	Okay	Okay

Comments:

5/8 - Saw family doctor. In addition to reduced ability to breathe, I have bronchitis. Home bound. Rest. Steam. Cough syrup. Call if I cough up anything yellow.

Symptom Experience Code
1 = no interference with activity
2 = moderately (interfered somewhat with activity)
3 = significantly (prevented activity)
4 = very significantly (required medical intervention)

MCSS Journal

Sample journal page for recording CS symptoms.

manner of organization should take into account the need for information retrieval. Examples of things to file including the following:

Workers' compensation data
  wage loss claims
  medical expense claims
  original claim filed—master copy
Disability retirement data
Social Security data
Attorney correspondence
Appeal (complaint/inquiry) correspondence—by addressee
Complete medical report/test file
Protection letters
FDA—adverse reaction correspondence
Chemical information
CS organizations publications (e.g. newsletters)
EPA—indoor air pollution information
Article files—by subject (e.g. asthma, environmental illness, immune system)
Medical studies
Local air pollution control agency data summaries

Hanging file folders with manila file inserts are helpful. For CS patients who have a tendency to drop things, metal clips designed for two-hole punch devices can be very helpful in keeping papers together and in order. Another alternative is a three-ring binder with tab page inserts. Vinyl binders can cause problems for some people, but there are cloth-covered or paper-covered binders available.

Despite the forces apparently arrayed against him, the CS patient is not without defenses. The keys to success are *documentation, communication,* and *persistence.* Treating physicians need to see and document the damage. That documentation serves as evidence which the CS patient and his attorney can communicate through hearings, in court, and to legislators at state or federal levels, whichever applies. It should be kept in mind that workers' compensations programs operate as a result of legislation. Legislative investigations may be difficult to obtain but not impossible. That's one place where persistence comes in.

Persistence may contribute serendipitous value. In one case the problem of proving the link between workplace carpet installation and CS development was solved. For a brief description of this toxic carpet issue, see Appendix D.

6. Society and the Chemical Sensitive

Issues in Chemical Sensitivity

Anyone with CS will face a variety of problems beyond the effects of the disease. Without major changes in society, these problems will be very difficult to handle. In addition to an overall belief by much of society that the chemical sensitive is a malingerer out to abuse the system, there are three other sources of problems: economic impacts on society, medical disagreements about the condition, and legal or ethical issues. All the problems can't be neatly attributed to a single source; some have multiple sources. Having said that, let's look at some of the issues.

Belief That Chemical Sensitives Are Abusing the System

In times of tight budgets, taxpayers look for a way to cut government expenses. One favorite place to suspect abuse is within the welfare, disability retirement, and workers' compensation systems. Many people suspect that these recipients are too lazy to work and are milking the system of hard-earned tax dollars. A chemical sensitive who applies for government benefits may be lumped into this category of unproven welfare cheats.

To apply for benefits, chemical sensitives often must overcome a personal reluctance to ask for the help to which they are legally entitled. To receive benefits, they must prove they can't work—an additional blow to their self-esteem. When family, friends, coworkers, supervisors, doctors, and welfare administrators then accuse or suspect them of "faking" their symptoms, they often struggle to work even after they suspect it is dangerous for them.

The suspicion that the chemical sensitive is faking illness is pervasive in society. Without a major change in attitudes throughout all segments of society, diagnosis and treatment will not advance. Financial and moral support for victims will be denied. The problem will escalate.

Economic Impacts of Recognizing Chemical Sensitivity

Over 37 million Americans may have environmentally related illness, and that number is expected to double in the next few years. Many contracted CS at work. If workers' compensation paid their claims and medical costs, the United States would face higher budget deficits. Typically, patients visit about 15 doctors before their condition is diagnosed. Testing and treatment are not cheap. The PET scan, one of the best diagnostic tests for toxic encephalopathy, costs about $2500. Brain topography (qEEG) with evoked potentials can more than double that amount. Since the equipment isn't available in all communities, patients may have interstate travel and living costs to pay in addition to the test costs. Multiply the cost of one test—one of many—by 37 million people and the economic impact of CS is devastating. Doubling that figure can lead one to understand why it so often seems easier to ignore or deny CS.

Because it is so expensive to test for and treat CS, many institutions have an economic interest in delaying or denying recognition of the disease. For example, a manufacturer might fight in court to avoid product liability claims. An insurer might refuse to pay medical claims by saying the problem had no work-related causes. When the chemical sensitive contacts benefits program administrators, the problems compound.

Although many workers' compensation programs recognize Multiple Chemical Sensitivity Syndrome (MCSS), administrators legitimately expect the worker to prove causation, i.e., that there is a medical condition and that the cause at least in part came from the workplace. Workers' compensation is no-fault insurance. In some instances, workers' compensation administrators will shift from the perspective of causation into one of proving fault. Such a position additionally burdens the CS worker and is definitely inappropriate.

The employee is not allowed to test the air without employer permission. How can the chemical sensitive prove poisoning occurred if testing is not allowed? Even if permitted to test, the individual faces the same problems as industrial hygienists: In the 1980s, the Environmental Protection Agency listed 65,000 known toxic chemicals and each year adds 1,500 more chemicals to the list. The number of individual chemicals—not to mention synergistic combinations—is too exhaustive to contemplate. Further, the equipment for low level testing of the potential toxics does not exist.

If by some stroke of good fortune and cooperation, the employee can document workplace poisoning, administrators of benefits programs—federal, state, and private workers' compensation programs; Social Security; and disability retirement programs—still have other routes to avoid or delay payment. They can require the CS patient to go to doctors they select for independent evaluation. More will be said about this in the next section.

Federal programs can agree that the chemical sensitive has a case but still refuse to pay. This is called federal non-acquiescence.[350] The person with CS must then go to federal court. The court can order payment, but the agency may find it cheaper to pay repeated court costs than to pay medical costs. Therefore, it can refuse payment again and force the patient back to court. Meanwhile, the patient's funds are being drained by having to pay both medical and legal expenses. The federal government can outlast the individual.

A diagnosis of CS does not have to mean economic disaster for everyone involved. Many workers with CS are, or were, "workaholics." What if their condition were diagnosed correctly at early stages? They might be able to make arrangements with enlightened employers to work at home or in some other chemically safe environment. Being removed from the immediate cause of poisoning might slow the development of CS. The worker might not develop reactions to other chemicals, might not increase the number of systems involved in CS, and might experience less neurological damage. This could reduce medical and welfare costs while retaining the chemical sensitive worker in a productive role.

In most cases it is more cost-effective to protect people from injury than to pay for the cost of that injury. This is known in the legal community as the Learned Hand formula, after the influential American jurist who developed it. That is, if the cost of eliminating a hazard is less than the cost of paying for the damage, safety measures should be taken. The usual approach is to wait until there is a very clear problem with many, many people affected before taking remedial action. Unfortunately, remedial action may be taken by employers and bureaucrats while they deny that the problem for which they took corrective action ever existed.

Medical Disagreements and Their Effects on Chemical Sensitives

As mentioned earlier in the book, there is a split within the medical community. Since orthodox physicians have been slow to recognize chemical sensitivity, others have filled the void—specialists in environmental medicine (formerly clinical ecology). Some orthodox doctors insist on rigorous testing that can do irreversible damage to CS patients.

Some medical specialists move so rapidly they may use inadequately tested treatments that don't help or may even harm the patient by using procedures or treatment considered standard. Meantime, the chemical sensitive incurs medical expenses with no easing of the condition and often legal expenses without resolving conflicts.

Chemical sensitivity is just beginning to be recognized by the medical community and society at large. It isn't even known by a single name. Few doctors practicing today have studied about it in medical school. Most are specialists who focus on one body part or system. CS involves many systems. What does this mean to the patient? Several things:

1. The family physician who can't figure out what the patient's symptoms mean will commonly refer the patient to a specialist. Specialists will focus on their specialty and see only one tree instead of the whole forest of symptoms. They might even prescribe medicine containing something else the patient reacts to, thus complicating the problem.

2. If the doctors involved are seeking the respect of their peers, they may hesitate to diagnose chemical sensitivity. After all, they may not want to be known as recognizing or legitimizing something whose existence is questioned by others in their profession.

3. Most referrals for consultation or evalution are made to specialists who treat patients with the suspected problem. However, because of the split within the medical community, chemical sensitives are often referred to or evaluated by doctors who deny the existence of their condition. This is totally against good medical practice in other specialties but quite normal for IMEs. Should there be a prohibition against a doctor's evaluating a patient for a disease when that doctor neither diagnoses nor treats patients with the given disease?

4. Some doctors have published articles that imply or state that chemical sensitivity is all in the patient's mind. Yet they are still on the list of doctors who might be asked to evaluate people for benefits. Perhaps, if they deny claims by denying the disease, they can get additional referrals from the agencies? This is a safe source of income because they can't be sued for malpractice if their diagnosis is wrong. They cannot be sued if the tests they order before diagnosing the patient cause harm. They could only be sued if they treated the patient and used the wrong treatment.

All this means the patient must work at finding a physician who takes a generalist view of the body and its systems. That physician should have an open mind and be willing to consider all the facts. The physician also needs the courage of independent thought and the willingness to say, "I might be wrong," or, "This might be poisoning and not a play for sympathy." In other words, the patient may have to select a physician with extreme caution—or help educate one. The physician who recognizes CS may also have to spend significant time testifying in depositions, hearings, and court. This factor provides countless disincentives toward overt recognition of CS.

Legal, Constitutional, and Ethical Challenges Facing the Chemical Sensitive

Many people with occupational diseases fight tremendous economic and political pressure to have their condition recognized. Coal miners with black lung, Vietnam-era veterans with concerns about Agent Orange, and World War II asbestos workers are some examples. The chemical sensitive finds similar resistance. Here are some of the problems:

1. Federal workers' compensation includes a number of entitlement programs: Federal Employees' Compensation Act (FECA), the Longshore and Harbor Workers' Act, the Jones Act, Nonappropriated Funds Instrumentalities Act, and so on. Few attorneys are willing to handle FECA cases. Why? Because in most personal injury cases, the attorney can work for a percentage of the award. In FECA cases, however, the government sets limits on the kinds of services an attorney can charge for and the amounts that can be charged. There is no direct access to the court. The Secretary of Labor is the final appeal. Absolute power from claims administration to final remedy kept within a single federal agency is invitation to corruption, regardless of how well intentioned the officials may be. Accountability can become irrelevant when no external oversight exists. Attorneys spend countless hours for minimal results. Consequently, people may find there are no attorneys in their town willing to take a FECA case. Other federal programs, though perhaps better planned, have their problems. Even if the case is won in court, the agency can refuse to pay, and the process begins again.

2. Access to medical care, an assumed right, is restricted. Medical costs are high and must be paid. If there is doubt about whether or when bills will be paid, medical care may be denied. Insurance companies may deny claims saying the disease was caused by workplace exposure and should be covered by workers' compensation. Workers' compensation may deny claims because "it's not work-related," leaving the claimant

caught in the no-man's-land between group insurance and workers' compensation. Or the workers' compensation administrators can deny a claim because one of their "independent" medical examiners denied the existence of the disease. The patient may have spent all his savings and be unable to afford uninsured treatment. If reduced to financial assistance (welfare), many CS patients discover that many of these programs view allergy treatment as experimental, and treatment of immune system disorder or dysfunction as less than experimental. The term "experimental" is a basis for refusal to pay. Due to economic forces, the patient loses the right to equal access to medical care.

3. Freedom of speech is often compromised. The chemical sensitive who speaks out to legislators or the press in an effort to cut through red tape and payment delays may irritate program administrators, the people who can decide not to acquiesce to court-ordered payments. Yet not speaking may convince those same administrators that this patient won't make waves if payment is denied. Whether the patient speaks out or remains silent, the results may be the same: non-payment of legitimate claims.

4. America was founded on the belief that everyone is entitled to "life, liberty, and the pursuit of happiness." Due to administrative rules, chemical sensitives can be denied the right to life. Any time they are involved in litigation or in entitlement or benefit programs, they can be required to go to an Independent Medical Examination (IME). An IME can be performed by one doctor or by a panel. The patient has no say in who is selected to conduct the IME (even when they know the IME doctor is biased and will produce a negative report before even seeing the doctor); the opponent does have a say. The doctor selected may work in an environment that has harmful effects on the patient, may require challenge tests (even ones that other doctors say will harm the patient), and will render an opinion, often from a known biased position that CS is illusory. The patient is to have no further contact with the doctor, thus protecting the doctor from knowledge of delayed reactions to the tests and causing some doctors to repeat the harmful tests with other patients. In some cases, patients have suffered irreversible damage from IME-ordered tests or the environments in which they are administered. Legally, no crime has been committed.

A serious ethical problem is requiring a challenge test during an IME. A challenge test is similar to an allergy test. During allergy testing, patients are subjected to small doses of natural substances—dust, pollens, and so on. A challenge test subjects the patient to man-made or natural substances the patient has reported as harmful and toxic in the past. Test results—whatever they may be—can be discounted. For instance, if the patient has a bad reaction, it can be accepted as a legitimate physical reaction or dismissed as a hysterical reaction to fear. If the patient has no immediate reaction, it can be concluded that the test dose wasn't high enough, that the reaction may be delayed and not occur until after the test time, or that it was "all in their head." Since test results can be interpreted according to the doctor's predisposed views and since patients have been irreversibly damaged by challenge tests, many people question the ethics of conducting such human experimentation.

Where Do We Go from Here?

Considering the presumed extent of chemical sensitivity and the overwhelming issues faced by patients and their families, one would expect more attention to be paid to the condition. What kind of attention is needed? Here are some practical suggestions:

1. Form support groups and link them in a national network. Possible goals for such groups could include providing information about the condition to patients, families, and doctors; campaigning for changes in federal and state workers' compensation to provide (1) external oversight and a dedicated ombudsman to assist patients with problems, (2) to prevent the practices of federal non-acquiescence and of IME referrals to doctors who don't diagnose or treat chemical sensitives, and (3) to develop means to assure accountability among medical professionals who injure patients through practices other than treatment (i.e., testing and other procedures as well as making unfounded judgments); and working with employers to encourage flexible work rules that might allow chemical sensitives to work at home or in other safe locations.

2. Contact elected representatives. Can they encourage employers to be more flexible in work rules, finding ways the chemical sensitive can work in a safe location? This could slow the progress of the disease, keep the patient working in some capacity, and reduce the burden on government benefit programs. To the extent that elected representatives can influence rules of federal compensation programs, ask that they seek an end to federal non-acquiescence.

3. Encourage more health research into the disease. Possible researchers include universities, medical schools, government organizations, and professional organizations. Sources of funding could include government, pharmaceutical firms, or private endowments. Directions

for research could include these ideas: Is there a biological marker for susceptibility to the disease? Is there a link between chemical sensitivity and other conditions? Are there diagnostic tests that cause less stress and harm to patients? Is there a treatment other than avoidance? What will longitudinal studies show about the progress of the disease?

4. Emphasize education about chemical sensitivity. Patients with CS and those around them need to change attitudes and behavior. It is acceptable and appropriate to apply for legitimate benefits. Through formal and informal education efforts, lessons learned can be passed on to others.

It is possible to solve problems created by these issues. Doing so would not require significant time. In the long run, it would not be of substantial comparative cost. What is required is a federally funded study devoid of university or other special interests. The study should be conducted by or at the direction of physicians (a mix of orthodox and environmental, to initiate a ceasefire and begin to build through communication) who meet the following qualifications:

1. They diagnose and treat CS patients. This qualification excludes physicians who take CS patients while rejecting the concept of CS [e.g. references 40, 101, 609, 613, 629, 682] and or any with recognized bias or lack of scientific credibility.[174a]
2. They have on-going, current experience with a minimum patient pool of 100 to 200.
3. They have been diagnosing and treating these patients for a minimum of five years or they have made significant progress in understanding CS.

These physicians should ask for study volunteers from their patient pool so that the study data would consist ultimately of 5,000 to 10,000 patients.

Patient qualification should consist of the following:

1. Evidence of toxic exposure (e.g. IgE, IgM, IgG to a toxic, or other toxicological data demonstrating toxic exposure).
2. Evidence of an activated immune system if available during or within two weeks of the period of exposure.
3. Neuropsychological assessment characteristic of toxic exposure, or other evidence of toxic encephalopathy or other forms of organic brain syndrome.
4. A well-documented medical file.

Funding should cover the following:

1. Initial physician meetings to design the study, determine how and by whom it will be conducted, and decide how the data will be published.

2. Copying of initial patient data and gathering of the following data every year or two for a period of from six to ten years:
   a. immunological profiles
   b. neuropsychological assessment
   c. PET scan
   d. brain topography with evoked potentials with wave averaging and frequency analysis (also called quantitative EEG [qEEG] with evoked potentials)
   e. other.

It would be enlightening to provide standard environmental medicine treatment (e.g. detoxification, nutritional planning and supplementation, and so on) to half of the group so that the efficacy of such treatment could be compared to the group not provided such treatment.

To bring such a study about, individuals can lobby their federal senators and representatives to do something positive to settle the issues. A multiple-agency approach would be helpful. These agencies could be involved: the Environmental Protection Agency, the Consumer Products Safety Commission, and the National Institute of Environmental Health Sciences, plus the National Academy of Sciences, OSHA, and NIOSH, with a liaison from the Senate Committee on Environment and Public Works and the House Committee on Science, Space, and Technology. The combined agencies and committees could provide funding, coordination, and study review. Such a study would be appropriate federal action in the 1990s, the Decade of the Brain.

Appendix A: Chapter 1 Charts

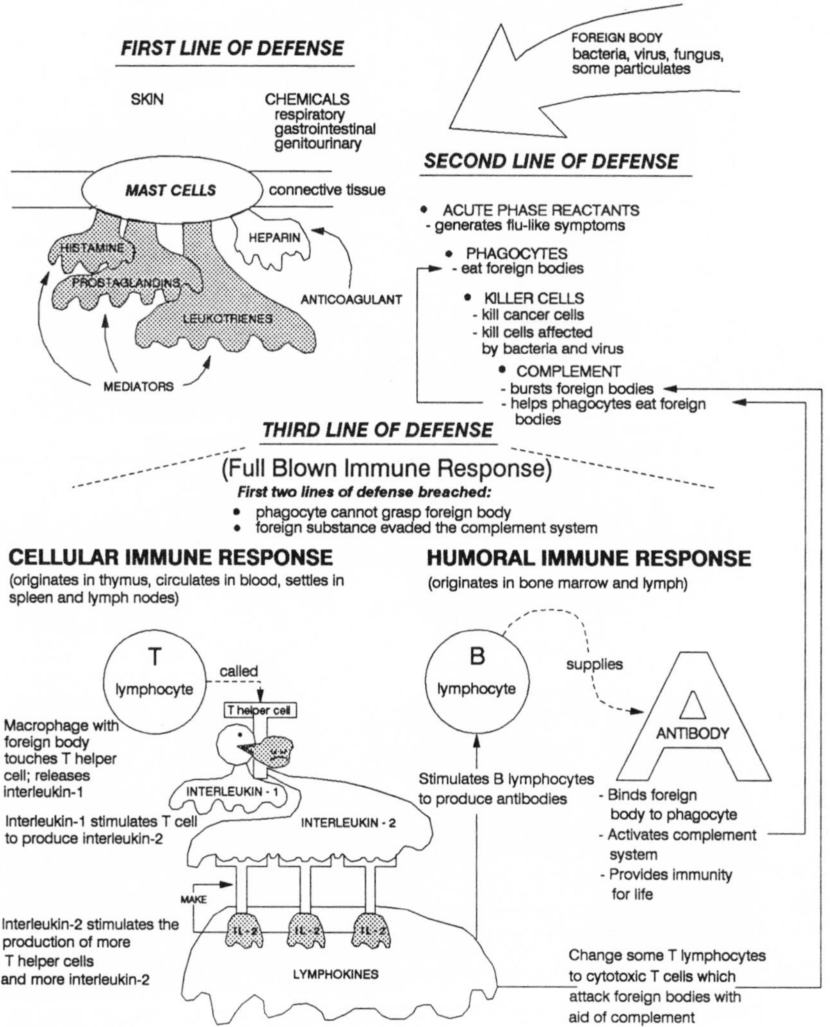

IMMUNE SYSTEM BASICS
The immune system is not designed to handle man-made toxic chemicals.
The immune system is designed for invasion by:
FOREIGN BODY
bacteria, virus, fungus, some particulates
FIRST LINE OF DEFENSE
SKIN
CHEMICALS
respiratory
gastrointestinal
genitourinary
MAST CELLS
connective tissue
HISTAMINE
PROSTAGLANDINS
LEUKOTRIENES
HEPARIN
ANTICOAGULANT
MEDIATORS
SECOND LINE OF DEFENSE
• ACUTE PHASE REACTANTS
- generates flu-like symptoms
• PHAGOCYTES
- eat foreign bodies
• KILLER CELLS
- kill cancer cells
- kill cells affected by bacteria and virus
• COMPLEMENT
- bursts foreign bodies
- helps phagocytes eat foreign bodies
THIRD LINE OF DEFENSE
(Full Blown Immune Response)
First two lines of defense breached:
• phagocyte cannot grasp foreign body
• foreign substance evaded the complement system
CELLULAR IMMUNE RESPONSE
(originates in thymus, circulates in blood, settles in spleen and lymph nodes)
T
lymphocyte
called
T helper cell
Macrophage with foreign body touches T helper cell; releases interleukin-1
INTERLEUKIN - 1
Interleukin-1 stimulates T cell to produce interleukin-2
INTERLEUKIN - 2
MAKE
IL-2
Interleukin-2 stimulates the production of more T helper cells and more interleukin-2
LYMPHOKINES
HUMORAL IMMUNE RESPONSE
(originates in bone marrow and lymph)
B
lymphocyte
supplies
ANTIBODY
Stimulates B lymphocytes to produce antibodies
- Binds foreign body to phagocyte
- Activates complement system
- Provides immunity for life
Change some T lymphocytes to cytotoxic T cells which attack foreign bodies with aid of complement

COMPONENTS IN NEUROENDOCRINEIMMUNE INTERACTION

exert control over

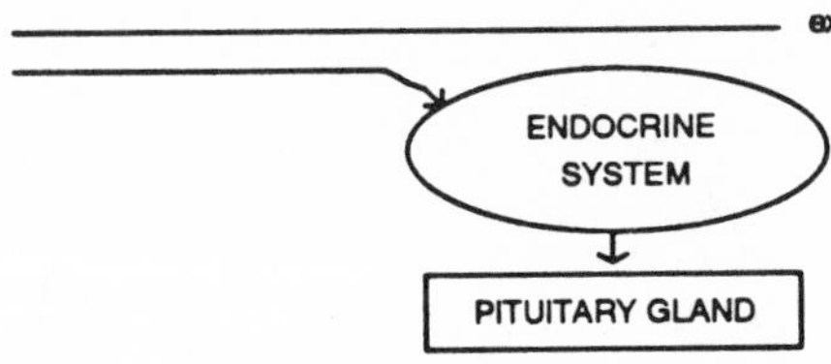

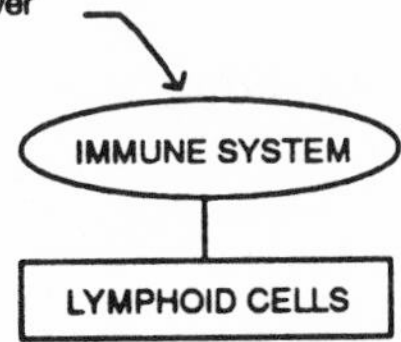

PITUITARY GLAND

Function: secretes hormones with regulatory activity on growth, reproduction, and various metabolic processes

Releases:
* proteins
* enzymes
* vasopressin
* oxytocin
* adrenocorticotropic hormone (ACTH)
* growth hormone
* thyroid stimulating hormone (TSH)

ADRENAL GLAND

Function: synthesizes and stores catacholamines (dopamine, epinephrine, norepinephrine)

☐ Cortex

Function: secretes hormones manufactured from cholesterol

Releases:
* Glucocorticoids (cortisol, corticosterones)
  Function: required for immunogenesis and suppression; acts on carbohydrate metabolism; anti-inflammatory agents; long-term - catabolism
* Mineralocorticoids
  Function: affect electrolytes (sodium and potassium)
* Androgens, estrogens, progestins

☐ Medulla

Function: controlled by and functions in concert with sympathetic nervous system

Releases: - norepinephrine,
- epinephrine

LYMPHOID CELLS

Structure: Lymphocytes have receptors for neurotransmitters

Neurotransmitter effect:

* epinephrine and norepinephrine - don't penetrate cell but change functional state of cell by acting on adrenoreceptors through adenylcyclase and cAMP on cell metabolism
* acetylcholine acts through cholinoreceptors and on cell metabolism through cGMP
* steroid hormones penetrate cell membrane

Function: antibody forming cells decrease level of norepinephrine in vicinity of cell

STIMULI
* bacteria, virus, fungus
* natural particulates
* toxic chemicals
* synthetic particulates
* exogenous toxins
* endogenous toxins
* fear, anxiety
* chronic immune system activation

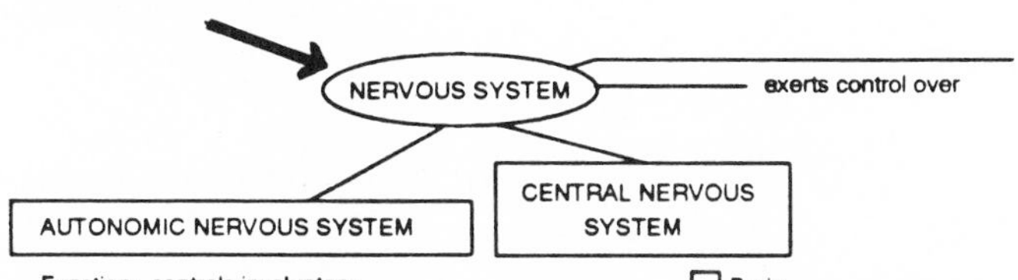

Function: controls involuntary bodily functions (glands, smooth muscle, heart), secretions may provide immunomodulation

☐ Sympathetic Nervous System
Function: prepares body for emergency (increased cardiac output, increased blood pressure, dilates pupils, bronchodilation, suppressed tone and motility of GI tract)
Releases: * somatostatin,
* vasoactive intestinal peptide,
* enkephalins, * acetylcholine,
* epinephrine, * norepinephrine

☐ Parasympathetic Nervous System
Function: prepares body for sedentary activity (reverse effect of sympathetic nervous system: constricts pupils, contracts GI tract muscle, constricts bronchioles, slows heart rate, increases gland secretions)
Releases: * substance P,
* vasoactive intestinal peptide,
* enkephalins, * somatostatin,
* cholecystokinin, * TRH

☐ Peripheral Nervous System
Structure: cranial and spinal nerves plus their branches to all parts of the body, it includes sensory nerves (olfactory and optic) but not central nervous system.
Releases:
* Neurotransmitter
  - acetylcholine
  - epinephrine
  - norepinephrine
* neuroregulatory peptides
  - somatostatin
  - vasoactive intestinal peptide
  - substance P

☐ Brain

Releases:
* vasopressin
* oxytocin
* neurophysin
* somatostatin
* neurotensin
* endothelial growth factor
* brain growth factor
* neural tissue (pineal gland)
  - melatonin

Openings in blood-brain barrier:

* median eminence of hypothalamus
* subfornical organ
* organum vasculosum of the lamina terminalis
* pineal gland
* subcommissural organ
* area postrema of the fourth ventricle and
* cerebrospinal fluid via arachnoid villi in superior sagittal sinus
* third ventricle to blood vessels of the median eminence

Hypothalamus

Function: Neurons continually process incoming information of various types from various sources; controls homeostasis; reacts to antigens by specific firing patterns from immunogenesis to immunosuppression

Releases:
* neurosecretory function: metabolism-water balance; sugar and fat metabolism; body temperature;
* endocrine gland secretions
  - vasopressin
  - oxytocin
* neuroendocrine transducers
  Function: change neuron signals to chemical signals
* corticotropin releasing factor
* growth hormone releasing factor
* thyroid releasing factor
* somatostatin

Hippocampus

Function: participates in process of new learning; inter-brain information transfer site

Examples of Neuroendocrine Immunomodulation

STIMULUS	RESPONSE
Learned helplessness	Immunosuppression: Decreased immune response; reduced T & B lymphocytes
Anxiety	Immunosuppression: Release of corticosterone from adrenal cortex corticosterone---> decreased T & B cells; enhanced tumor growth
Parasympathetic nervous system secretions	Immunoenhancement: increased immune response; increased antibody formation
Hypothalamus-corticotropin releasing factor; Neurotransmitters: epinephrine, norepinephrine, acetylcholine; histamine; seratonin	Stimulates pituitary release of ACTH
ACTH	Release of Glucocorticoids (corticosterone, cortisol)
Glucocorticoids	Inhibit release of TSH Influence lymphokine production
Corticosterone	Immunosuppression Affects switch from IgM to IgG
Cortisol	Inhibits release of ACTH
Hypothalamus - Growth hormone releasing factor	Release of growth hormone from pituitary
Growth Hormone	Immunoenhancement: increases immune response
TSH	Contributes to inflammatory response in eye muscles and connective tissue
Chronic immune system activation	Immunopotentiation Decreased neurotransmitter levels
Decreased neurotransmitter levels	Increased receptor sites
Low molecular weight, fat soluble chemicals	Can enter neurological system through circulating blood and act as neurotransmitter
Production of antibody	Decrease norepinephrine level in cell vicinity
Presence of antigen	Increase firing in hypothalamus

NEUROTRANSMITTER	IMMUNE RESPONSE
Elevated serotonin	Decreased B cells
Elevated dopamine	Decreased B cells, increased T cells & macrophages
B-Adrenergic stimulation	Decreased B cells, T cells, macrophages
A-Adrenergic stimulation	Increased B cells, T cells
Cholinergic stimulation	Increased B cells, T cells
Elevated morphine	Decreased T cells
Elevated enkephalin	Increased T cells

Appendix B: Detoxification

Background—There are two types of toxics: *exogenous* (those originating outside the human organism) and *endogenous* (those originating inside the human organism). Exogenous toxics can become endogenous when they enter the human system. Those which are water soluble can be eliminated with comparative ease and are not likely to become endogenous; those which are fat soluble tend to accumulate for years in human fat tissue (e.g. the brain, nervous system, breast, and other tissues). More than 300 fat-stored toxics have been identified, including some carcinogens.[11] Once stored in human fat, toxics do not necessarily remain in the location in which they are initially stored. Fat in human organisms is released intermittently to circulating blood. Releasing triggers are (1) exposure to stresses of heat, illness, and emotion, and (2) sleep, during which time the toxic(s) stored and the effects of the toxic(s) can migrate from location to location.[1, 6, 12] Whether symptoms are a response to endogenous toxics stored in fat is clinically determined by trained physicians.

Rationale—For the patient experiencing symptoms from fat-stored toxics, detoxification may provide appropriate therapy by reducing the levels of exogenous toxics which have become endogenous, thereby reducing symptoms. Successful detoxification therapy has three objectives: (1) to mobilize toxics from stored fat, (2) to channel the toxic(s) to excretory exit points, and (3) to enhance excretion (breathing or sweating out toxics, or elimination through urinary or GI tracts).

Caution—The human organism in which systemic integrity has already been compromised depends even more critically on carefully maintained balances (of water, electrolytes, etc.). For that reason only a trained, experienced physician should conduct detoxification therapy. Patients with CS or untrained doctors should not attempt to initiate detoxification.

Detoxification Therapy (Hubbard Technique)—This therapy is based on a technique developed in the 1970s for treating toxic drug cases.

To meet the first objective—to mobilize toxics from stored fat—therapeutic aerobic (cardiovascular) exercise and controlled doses of vitamin B-3 (nicotinic acid) are used. The means used to meet the second objective—to channel toxics to excretory exits—is the increased blood circulation from exercise and vitamin B-3. The method to meet the third objective—to enhance excretion—is therapeutic sauna (160°) to activate water- and oil-based skin excretion. Exposure to heat stress (10 to 30 minutes) alternates with cool-down rest periods during which vital signs are monitored. Daily exercise and therapeutic sauna can require up to five hours' time commitment a day. The third objective also includes administration of cold-pressed polyunsaturated oils to retard re-assimilation of toxics through intestines and to assist excretion through the colon.

To maintain systemic balance, water, potassium, and salts are administered to replace what is lost in concentrated sweating. Because the dose of vitamin B-3 is increased during therapy, adjustments are made in vitamins and minerals to avoid deficiency states.

The patient follows a daily schedule, not missing sessions, and gets adequate sleep during the period. Dietary change is not necessary except for more emphasis on fiber and leafy green vegetables. Treatment length averages 25 days, though length depends on individual patients.

References

1. Findlay, G.M., deFreitas, A.S.W.: "DDT movement from adipose to muscle cells during lipid utilization." *Nature*. 1971; 229: 63–65.

2. Kilburn, K.H., Warsaw, R.H., Shields, M.G.: "Neurobehavioral dysfunction in firemen exposed to polychlorinated biphenyls (PCBs): possible improvement after detoxification." *Archives of Environmental Health*. Nov/Dec 1989; 44(6): 345–350.

3. Randolph, T.G., Wisner, R.M.: "Detoxification: personal survival in a chemical world." *HealthMed*. 1988.

Provides an overview of detoxification.

4. Root, D.E., Lionelli, G.T.: "Excretion of a lipophilic toxicant through the sebaceous glands: a case report." *Journal of Toxicology—Cutaneous and Occular Toxicology*. 1987; 6(1): 13–17.

Hubbard technique of detoxification enabled a woman to return to work after exposure to soot and ash from exhaust stack and filter pads of an oil fired electrical generator. It was her job to clean equipment with washwater corrosive enough to dissolve paint.

5. Shields, M., Beckman, S., Cassidy-Brinn, G.: "Improvement in perception of transcutaneous nerve stimulation following detoxification in firefighters exposed to PCBs, PCDDs, and PCDFs." *Clinical Ecology* 6(2).

Continuing neurologic symptoms following toxic exposure may be due to storage of the toxic in fat in some patients. Neuropathologic symptoms may be partially reversible through detoxification therapy.

6. Schlierf, G., Dorow, E.: "Diurnal patterns of triglycerides, free fatty acids, blood sugar, and insulin during carbohydrate induction in man and their modification by nocturnal suppression of lipolysis." *Journal of Clinical Investigation* 1973; 52: 732–740.

7. Schnare, D.W., Ben, M., Shields, M.G.: "Body burden reductions of PCBs, PBBs, and chlorinated pesticides in human subjects." *Ambio*. 1984; 13(5–6): 378–380.

Reduction in fat-stored xenobiotics occurred using Hubbard technique. Follow-up study demonstrated that reduction was not a matter of moving stored toxics from one body location to another.

8. Schnare, D.W., Denk, G., Shields, M., Brunton S.: "Evaluation of a detoxification regimen for fat stored xenobiotics." *Medical Hypotheses*. September 1982. 9(3): 265–282.

9. Schnare, D.W., Robinson, P.C.: "Reduction of hexachlorobenzene and polychlorinated biphenyl human body burdens." International Symposium on Hexachlorobenzene, International Agency for Research on Cancer, Lyon, France, June 24–28, 1985.

Detoxification reduced measurable levels of endogenous toxics.

10. Tretjak, Z., Shields, M., Beckman, S.L.: "PCB reduction and clinical improvement by detoxification: an unexploited approach." *Human and Experimental Toxicology*. 1990; 9: 235–244.

11. U.S. Environmental Protection Agency: "Broad scan analysis of the FY82 national human adipose tissue survey specimens." EPA-560/5-86-035, December 1986. Characterization of HRGC/MS unidentified peaks from the analysis of human adipose tissue. EPA-560/5-87-002A, May 1987.

12. Wirth, A., Schlierf, G., Schettler, G.: "Physical activity and lipid metabolism." *Klinische Wochenschrift*. 1979; 57(22): 1195–1201.

Appendix C: Opinions of Experts

The author mailed a request for opinions from more than 80 national experts who have or have had something to say regarding chemical sensitivity, though different terms for the illness may be used. Some of the following individuals responded to the author's request for their "opinions regarding the issues of (1) chemical sensitivity and (2) functional mental illness or organic brain syndrome or other involvement of the central nervous system." Each was asked to use his own terminology. The following opinions are printed with the understanding that the study of chemical sensitivity is new and that the opinions are subject to change. In those cases where persons contacted did not respond, some of their opinions from published comments and references are cited here. Some quoted comments are broader than the personal communications, but the opinion tends to come through. It is, perhaps, worth mentioning that there was only one response from any of the individuals contacted who have or had a known expressed negative opinion of the existence of chemical sensitivity and in that case the opinion given expressed none of the expected negativism.

American Federation of Government Employees
80 F Street NW
Washington DC 20001

[From the statement of David Schlein on behalf of the American Federation of Government Employees before the Committee on Environment and Public Works, United States Senate, 101st Congress, 1st Session, May 3, 1989.]

Just two months ago our union released the preliminary results of a survey of Federal and Washington, D.C. government employees. More than 90% reported experiencing physical symptoms often associated with indoor air quality. There is a serious cost to the Government in not addressing these problems. These costs result from increased use of sick leave, decreased productivity, health care and workers' compensation costs.

While the search for new knowledge about the causes of health effects of indoor air quality are laudable, we would like to see a balanced approach to the problem with equal emphasis on three issues of research, remediation, and compensation for victims. [page 34]

American Lung Association
National Headquarters
1740 Broadway
New York NY 10019-4374

[From the statement of Dr. Philip Bromberg on behalf of the American Lung Association before the Committee on Environment and Public Works, United States Senate, 101st Congress, 1st Session, May 3, 1989.]

Outside the workplace, air pollution in the past has been perceived as primarily an outdoor problem with the indoor environment providing a so-called refuge.... The indoor environment is often even more polluted than the outdoor environment.

A rapidly enlarging body of literature has described sources of pollutants and exposures ... in the indoor environment. While many putative health effects of indoor pollutants remain controversial, some effects have been described with certainty and should be considered clinically relevant. [pages 22–23]

[From the statement of Dr. Philip Bromberg on behalf of the American Lung Association before the Committee on Science, Space, and Technology, U.S. House of Representatives, 101st Congress, 1st Session, July 20, 1989.]

ALA believes that the primary obstacle to federal action to control indoor air pollution is ... lack of clear regulatory authority. [page 165]

American Psychological Association
1200 Seventeenth Street, NW
Washington, DC 20036

[From the statement of Robert Balster on behalf of the American Psychological Association before the Committee on Environment and Public Works, United States Senate, 101st Congress, 1st Session, March 6, 1989.]

There are many, many chemicals that can affect the nervous system. Obviously, the nervous system is a very sensitive organ to chemical exposure. [page 40]

Exposure to chemical substances can result in adverse effects on the nervous system, including impaired sensory and motor function, cognitive and intellectual performance, and emotional well-being. In severe cases some substances can cause paralysis and death. [page 152]

In written testimony accompanying the statement, there is some additional information. Table 1 provides the following information: **Neurobehavioral Effects Following Exposure to Toxic Substances** Motor Effects: convulsions, weakness, tremor/twitching, lack of coordination/unsteadiness, paralysis, reflex abnormalities, activity changes. Sensory Effects: equilibrium changes, vision disorders, pain disorders, tactile disorders, auditory disorders. Cognitive Effects: memory problems, confusion, speech impairment. Mood/Personality Effects: sleep disturbances, excitability, depression, irritability, restlessness, nervousness/

tension, delirium, hallucinations. General Effects: loss of appetite, depression of neuronal activity, narcosis/stupor, fatigue, nerve damage. [page 168] *Table 3 provides information, the following of which are examples:* **Industries in Which Neurotoxic Chemicals Are Found** Agricultural services and hunting, special trade contractors, food and kindred products, tobacco manufacture, apparel and other textile products, furniture and fixtures, paper and allied products, printing and publishing, petroleum and coal products, rubber and plastic products, leather and leather products, fabricated metal products, electrical equipment and supplies, transportation by air, food stores, automotive dealers and service stations, eating and drinking places, personal service, auto repair/services/garages, medical and other health services. [page 173]

There is a very small amount of data on the neurotoxic potential of chemicals in the work place. [page 41]

Zoltan Annau, Ph.D.
Department of Environmental Health Sciences
The Johns Hopkins University
School of Hygiene and Public Health
615 N Wolfe Street
Baltimore MD 21205

In my opinion chemical sensitivity is the reaction of a sensitive sub-population to chronic exposure to either one or a mixture of chemicals. It is a real disease of unknown etiology and is associated with industrial chemicals. Because it seems to involve a sensitive population, and in many cases has no clear exposure history, it is very difficult to study and reproduce in the laboratory. The lack of recognition of the symptoms by medical personnel and the discomforts of the victim may give rise to secondary "mental" symptoms that eventually send these patients to the psychiatrist, who in turn does not recognise the disease and mistreats it. I have not seen evidence that chemical sensitivity results in nervous system disease directly, although in theory this could also occur.

[Personal communication]

Nicholas Ashford, Ph.D.
Director and Associate Professor of Technology and Policy
MIT Center for Policy Alternatives
77 Massachusetts AV
Cambridge MA 02139

[From the Preface, *Chemical Sensitivity: A Report to the New Jersey State Department of Health,* December 1989, © Nicholas A. Ashford and Claudia S. Miller.]

Sufficient "proof" is not available to satisfy the most skeptical critic that chemical sensitivity exists as a physical entity; nor is there convincing proof that it does not. We, however, are persuaded that the collective evidence, in part anecdotal and in part based on good scientific studies, does present a sufficiently compelling case to warrant further study. We can assert that millions of people are affected, although exposure to many chemicals is ubiquitous and is expected to continue. The size of the public health problem is unknown, but the scale of potential exposure suggests that the problem could be significant.

Gordon P. Baker, M.D.
14203 Ambaum Blvd., SW
Seattle, WA 98166

The rapid proliferation and intrusion of new chemical compounds into almost every aspect of our lives has brought not only the benefits of these new materials, but also new diseases due directly to adverse effects of these substances on the human body. The first man-made chemical was created in Germany in 1856, when Perkins produced an aniline dye, mauvinc. By 1895, the first three cases of bladder cancer were found in exposed workers. DuPont built a factory to produce this dye in southern New Jersey in 1916 and by 1931 the first cases of bladder cancer were seen in workers in this factory.

The first case of shortness of breath due to asbestos was reported in 1899, yet even 50 years later a Harvard medical faculty scientist said there was no problem with asbestos in U.S. Navy shipyards. This doctor had examined people who had worked in the shipyards for less than three years and did not realize there was a long latent period before symptoms develop from asbestos exposure.

Chemical sensitivity has been termed the "asbestoses of the '90's." Given the lack of appropriate action on the part of industry, government, organized science, and labor groups, it may take years before the magnitude and impact of the problems of exposure to chemicals are widely appreciated and appropriate action taken.

My first encounter with organic brain syndrome caused by toxic chemical exposure was when, as a U.S. Naval flight surgeon, I was asked to evaluate an air traffic controller who had abandoned his duty post because of unbearable frustration and anxiety. Six aircraft were calling for landing and takeoff instructions. He later had episodes of fainting, and falling from his motor scooter on at least two occasions. It turned out that he had an after-hours job loading pesticides into crop duster airplanes, and developed what I would now recognize as an organic brain syndrome due directly to pesticide exposure. His abandoning his duty station was the result of cognitive difficulties, inappropriate frustration, and inability to perform tasks previously easily fulfilled, resulting in his inability to function in a demanding job.

In 1956, the first case of poisoning from toluene di isocyanate was reported in this country. By 1961 about 250 cases of isocyanate poisoning were reported in the *New England Journal of Medicine*. Among other symptoms, isocyanates cause a chemically induced asthma. In 1965 I saw my first patient with isocyanate induced asthma. He eventually died, and his widow has never received compensation. Isocyanates were the cause of thousands of deaths and chronic disease in the chemical spill in Bouphal, India, more recently. I have seen patients with the multiple chemical sensitivity syndrome induced by isocyanates.

Today it is possible to recognize patients with both acute and chronic chemical poisoning. Immune tests are available that aid in this diagnosis. Many of unfortunate patients have memory loss and deficiencies of cognition, that are discovered on neuropsychologic testing. Some patients will have objective findings on MRI, or PET scans, or other procedures described in this book. With a good history, appropriate laboratory studies, and neuropsychological tests performed by a competent neuropsychologist, a proper diagnosis can be made. The patient can be observed in and away from the offending environment, and can be seen to be better or worse depending upon different environmental exposures. Then the diagnosis on chemical sensitivity can be established and differentiated from other diseases. What happens to the patients? Some can find the resources to get their lives together and remain productive. Some give up completely and end up on welfare, after having been productive people. Some are fortunate enough to have families to support them. Others fall through the cracks held wide open by the system and end up with broken families, destroyed lives, and even in some cases, suicide.

Unfortunately, this is not a problem that will go away. We can only hope that with the efforts of dedicated people, it will not take a half century, as it has taken in the disgraceful asbestos saga, to properly deal directly with the problem of chemical poisoning and the multiple chemical sensitivity syndrome.

[Personal communication]

Rebecca Bascom, M.D., MPH
Assistant Professor, The Johns Hopkins School of Medicine
615 N Wolfe Street
Baltimore MD 21205

[From the testimony of Rebecca Bascom, M.D., MPH, before the Committee on Science, Space, and Technology, United States House of Representatives, 101st Congress, 1st Session, July 20, 1989.]

First of all, as I have seen and as the literature has documented, many Americans do have a variety of health concerns linked to their indoor home and their work places, and I think the respiratory effects are very common. But I would agree that there are other long-range concerns such as fatigue—people describing their thinking as being off a cog; by Monday, they're okay; by Wednesday, they just can't think straight; they take Thursday off; they feel better; they go back to work Friday, and then they kind of can put in a day, and then they recover over the weekend. I think that's a real problem with productivity, particularly for the individuals I see who very much rely on clear thinking for their work.

The second reason I think there is concern is the TEAM study of the EPA that shows the multitude of volatile organics in the indoor environment that are clearly present in higher concentrations than the outdoor environment, and I believe they have grouped them into several different groups of exposure categories. One is building materials, like carpets, and paneling, and upholstery; one would be automobile emissions that are entrained in the ventilation; and then the other would be consumer products, things that are used as part of the office work.

And then I would also underscore the problem of the bio-aerosols. There are clearly people that have very specific and serious hypersensitivity responses to substances coming from the ventilation system. . . . So the specific hypersensitivity responses can be tremendous and are both in the work place and in the home.

The medical community do not—and other individuals, don't have good ways of precise diagnoses identifying the specific component. We make educated guesses now. If there's a big water leak and the ventilation system has been dripping, we think it's probably a bio-aerosol. If it's a newly remodeled building and people are having a lot of irritant symptoms, we think it's probably a VOC type of a problem. But that is kind of the level of our approach at this time.

And, finally, there's no good source for information for individuals, and so many people who get referred to me have already made 10 or 20 phone calls to a variety of Government agencies, and the person on the other end of the phone says, "Well, I don't know about that, but I could tell you about radon," or, "I don't know about that, but I could tell you about asbestos." So there's a gap between what people, I think, are needing and what agencies are currently able to provide. [pages 171 and 172]

In response to questions: In the work place setting, you get a material safety data sheet to see what it is that the worker is using. In the indoor environment, we can't really get a material safety data sheet for our carpet or for our glue, and there is a lot—the components that are a minority of the product may be either not included in the MSDS or may be a trade secret material, and it is often difficult to get that information. [page 180]

Iris R. Bell, M.D., Ph.D.
University of Arizona Health Sciences Center, Department of Psychiatry
1501 N. Campbell Ave.
Tuscon AZ 85724

Chemical sensitivity is a chronic multisystem, multi-symptom disorder, including CNS symptoms, that is triggered in susceptible individuals by low dose chemical exposures once established. Susceptibility patterns are not established, but previous vulnerability to depression and somatization disorders may play a role. The etiology is not likely to be biological only or psychological only. Kindling phenomena in the brain's limbic system may contribute to the development of these problems. As with other chronic medical illnesses, depression from psychological causes can also occur but cannot be used as the sole explanation of the phenomena, as research in biological psychiatry clearly indicates biological mechanisms for many types of depression. Responsivity to biological or psychological treatments also does not establish etiology, as an illness with an initial etiological factor can respond to interventions in a different modality (e.g. cancer, heart disease—both biological *and* psychological interventions are helpful).

Until research that is adequately designed looks at biological and psychological factors rigorously, the above issues cannot be settled.

[Personal communication]

Dr. David W. Brandes
Northridge Neurological Group
18433 Roscoe Blvd., Suite 207
Northridge CA 91325

1) Due to genetic factors (many as yet undescribed), some people are more sensitive to various chemicals, medicines, skin preparations, etc. These sensitivities then result in clinical symptomatology.

2) Organic brain syndrome may develop in persons subjected to chronic low-level toxic exposure due to:

(a) Build up of chemicals over time due to the body's inability to excrete or detoxify a chemical.

(b) Hypersensitivity of certain people to certain chemicals, such that smaller amounts than "normally" tolerated cause such a reaction. This would probably be genetically determined."

[Personal communication]

Dr. Peter Breysse
University of Washington SC-34
Department of Environmental Health
Seattle WA 98195

[Testimony of Dr. Peter A. Breysse, Industrial Hygienist, before the Committee on Environment and Public Works, United States Senate, 101st Congress, 1st Session, March 6, 1989.]

The occupational health standard is not designed to protect all the workers. A review of the preamble states that the standards are developed to protect most of the workers.

Secondly, the standard is really not designed to evalute complex mixtures that might involve possibly 60 or 70 different compounds.

Thirdly, the standard is not directed toward a seven-day work week with one day off a month. That certainly extends the exposure period.

Furthermore, almost all of the occupational health data for exposure to workers is based on white males. There is little or no information based on exposure of chemicals to females, as far as the adverse effects are concerned.

Other problems we face in the composites is that the fibers and the dust of the composites are important. The fibers, if they are respirable, durable, and have the same length to diameter ratio as asbestos, are carcinogenic in animal experiments.

Many of the fibers and the dust particles may also contain various chemicals that have attached themselves to the dust and the fibers which may very well add additional hazards to the toxicity of inhaling those dust and fibers, complicating factors.

One of the chemicals, formaldehyde, has a number of studies indicating that workers and non-workers exposed to formaldehyde develop neurobehavioral aspects as a result of exposure. [pages 36–37]

The Building Owners and Managers Association International
1201 New York AV NW
Suite 300
Washington DC 20006

[From the statement of Allan S. Bisk, representing The Building Owners and Managers Association International, before the Committee on Environment and Public Works, United States Senate, 101st Congress, 1st Session, May 3, 1989.]

Where building related indoor air problems exist, they are often sensationalized. . . .

Buildings which experience air quality problems are the exception, not the rule. Where complaints exist, they may be attributable to discomforting temperature or humidity levels, objectionable odors or poor air circulation. Some of these are within the capability and resources of the building owners and managers to address.

Many general working conditions which affect an employee's level of workplace satisfaction are beyond the purview of the owner or manager, but the responsibility of tenants, design professionals, contractors, suppliers, and others. [pages 32–33]

HVAC systems, tobacco smoke, carbon monoxide, ceiling tiles, wall paper, carpeting, furniture, flush toilets, humidifiers, pressed wood products, insulation, and textiles are all sources of airborne contaminants. We know that." [page 39 in response to questions by Senator Lautenberg]

Business Council on Indoor Air
1225 19th St NW, Suite 300
Washington DC 20036

[From the statement of Paul Cammer, President, Business Council on Indoor Air, before the Committee on Environment and Public Works, United States Senate, 101st Congress, 1st Session, May 3, 1989.]

I think yes and no. I think, yes, there are some bad situations. There are bad substances. There are bad contaminants.

I think those are relatively few in number. [page 40]

Chemically Injured United Coalition
P.O. Box 26054
Encino CA 91426

[From the testimony of Beth Gausman, President, Chemically Injured Coalition, before the Committee on Environment and Public Works, United States Senate, 101st Congress, 1st Session, March 6, 1989.]

The medical evidence is building and we do know that this is a factor in the immune breakdown. These chemicals cause immune function breakdown and the individual as in my case becomes more and more sensitive to everyday household chemicals and substances and chemicals that are part of our lives. Many people who have this hypersensitivity are ostracized, told that it is all in their heads, that it is psychological in nature. The evidence is clear that these chemicals cause neurological problems, organic brain syndrome, memory loss, and these are not psychological problems, rather, they are neurological problems. [page 72]

This may be the most important learnings of the century. We have turned the corner to the chemical age. We are now seeing the ensuing results. [page 73]

Consumer Federation of America
1424 16th Street NW
Suite 604
Washington DC 20036

[From the statement of Stephen Brobeck, Executive Director, Consumer Federation of America, before the Committee on Environment and Public Works, United States Senate, 100th Congress, 1st Session, April 24, 1987.]

...the Consumer Federation sees indoor air pollution as the nation's number one hidden health threat. Individual pollutants ranging from radon to asbestos to secondary tobacco smoke, to formaldehyde and methylene chloride may well kill tens of thousands of Americans every year and injure millions more.

...when Oak Ridge Laboratories examined 40 homes, they found between 20 and 150 hazardous chemicals in concentrations between 10 and 45 times greater than is found in the outdoors.

That is why the EPA, in its recent reassessment of 31 environmental hazards ranked radon first and indoor air pollution from other sources fourth as a threat to public health.

Despite these findings, most of the public is still not fully aware of the hazards to their health. Recently a national pollster asked a random sample to rate the health risk of indoor air pollution, and they rated it low....

My second point is that in part because of this lack of public awareness, the Federal Government is not giving indoor air quality adequate attention. [page 37]

Morton Corn, Ph.D.
Professor and Director
Division of Environmental Health Engineering
The Johns Hopkins University
School of Hygiene and Public Health
615 N Wolfe Street
Baltimore MD 21205

I believe it exists, that it reflects a response of the immune system in selected individuals, that we are very inefficient at identifying susceptible individuals and that a great deal of investigation will be needed to sort out the categories of response and associated mechanisms of action now designated & addressed by "chemical sensitivity."

[Personal communication]

Mark R. Cullen, M.D.
School of Medicine
Yale University
Yale New Haven Occupational Medicine Program
333 Cedar Street
New Haven CT 16510

(1) My view on the nature of MCS remains unchanged from the 1987 monograph—a *syndrome* of *unknown cause* characterized [by] *acquired* symptoms related to *multiple organ-systems* precipitated by *diverse environmental factors* in the *absence of a recognizable pathologic process* which could explain the symptoms.

(2) Almost all MCS patients have symptoms referable to the CNS. No organic pathology of the CNS has yet been demonstrated in these patients by any test—X ray, MRI, neuropsychological tests, etc. It is *unclear* at present whether the symptoms are psychological in origin and, if so, whether this is the *cause* of MCS or its *consequence*.

[Personal communication]

Devra Davis, Ph.D., MPH
Director, Board on Environmental Studies and Toxicology
National Research Council
National Academy of Sciences
2101 Constitution Avenue
Washington DC 20418

The absence of evidence that there is an effect should not be construed as a lack of effect. Is it possible that there is a group of people who are reacting to the environment? Certainly. Can we measure it? Unlikely, given the tools we have at this time. Serious research needs to be done.

[Personal communication]

Mr. Earon S. Davis, JD, MPH
643 Hibbard Road
Wilmette IL 60091

[Testimony of Earon S. Davis before the Committee on Environment and Public Works, United States Senate, 101st Congress, 1st Session, May 3, 1989.]

. . . People with Chemical Sensitivity Disorders. These little understood disorders represent an illness within an illness. First, something affects the central nervous and/or immune systems to create an increased sensitivity to chemically induced damage, even at amazingly low concentrations and from a widening range of substances. Second, each further miniscule exposure appears to cause transitory but disabling symptoms which may cascade into total disabling and even life threatening illness.

Many afflicted people, such as some EPA personnel exposed to new carpeting and poor ventilation, require major accommodations and lifestyle change in order to keep these "reactions" under control. Some are totally disabled. This illness was identified more than 30 years ago and is the subject of hundreds of scientific articles. However, government agencies, academic institutions, and industry have, for various unfortunate and unacceptable reasons, avoided the entire topic. [page 189]

MCS is most likely a product of man's misuse of his environment; his reckless polluting of our planet—not just by emission into the air and water—but through the very products and materials we are producing to make our lives more convenient, safe, and healthful. A growing proportion of our population is succumbing to chemical sensitivity disorders and we had better do something about it. [page 194]

Environmental Defense Fund
National Headquarters
257 Park AV S
New York NY 10010

[From testimony by Ellen K. Silbergeld, Ph.D., Senior Scientist, Environmental Defense Fund, before the Committee on Science, Space, and Technology, United States House of Representatives, July 1989.]

It is now undeniable that the condition often called "sick building syndrome" exists. Several well controlled studies, primarily in England, have established that definable, objective signs and symptoms occur in persons working in certain indoor environments. These signs and symptoms involve the respiratory and nervous systems primarily; they are a cause of lost work days, decreased productivity, worker dissatisfaction, and increased employer costs.

The factors associated with indoor air pollution and "sick building syndrome" are—*inadequate ventilation and air exchange, *improper maintenance of ventilation and air handling systems, *poor building design and ergonomics, *unsafe products—furniture, carpets, etc., *contaminated water (in AC systems). [page 148]

. . . if ventilation and air handling systems are not properly maintained, then increasing the rate of ventilation may actually *increase*, rather than *decrease* the problem by increasing input of contaminants (microbiological and other) from the contamination source. Poor workplace design and ergonomics may add to the stresses upon workers, accentuating neurotoxic symptoms. Unsafe products were identified in the Danish studies as sources of contamination—these products included furniture, draperies, wall coverings, and carpeting, and taken as a whole they can produce hundreds of different toxic substances primarily from offgassing. Cleaning products can leave residues on surfaces and equipment. Assessments of hazard based upon compound-by-compound or product-by-product analysis may fail to detect the overall presence of unacceptable levels of exposure. . . . [page 149]

Richard H. Kropschot, Associate
Lab. Director for Energy Sciences
Lawrence Berkeley Laboratory
1 Cyclotron Rd
Berkeley CA 94720

[From the testimony of Richard H. Kropschot before the Committee on Environment and Public Works, United States Senate, 101st Congress, 1st Session, May 3, 1989.]

Our substantial experience has made us well aware of the exposures and health effects occurring inside different types of buildings. We strongly support a concerted effort to understand the behavior of indoor air pollutants and the resulting degree of risk, along with the development of a plan for responding, where appropriate, to these risks by developing guidelines and methods for control. The risks from indoor pollutants are often larger than those deemed acceptable in outdoor air, and thus deserve substantial attention. In fact, the risks attributed to indoor pollutants approach those from accidents in our homes, cars, and industrial workplaces, or from industrial exposures to toxic chemicals. [page 213]

Mary Lamielle, President
National Center for Environmental
Health Strategies
1100 Rural Avenue
Voorhees NJ 08043

[From the statement of Mary Lamielle, President, National Center for Environmental Health Strategies, before the Committee on Science, Space, and Technology, United States House of Representatives, 101st Congress, 1st Session, September 27, 1989.]

Scientific studies by government, industry, and university researchers have established that indoor air is contaminated by many substances. Bacteria, fungi, and dust particles may be present in ventilation ducts and air conditioning systems. These pollutants may include legionella and aspergillus bacteria, both implicated in the development of serious respiratory illnesses.

Even more insidious is the witch's brew of gaseous pollutants which harbor in our homes and buildings. With over 60,000 chemicals in daily use in the U.S. today and hundreds of new ones introduced each year, the intensity of these contaminants is an ever-growing problem. These chemicals, for the most part, have not been tested for their individual, cumulative, or synergistic effects. Meanwhile, scientists at the Congressional Office of Technology Assessment have indicated that there is "increasing evidence that many chemicals have neurotoxic effects." Accordingly to NIOSH most solvents in everyday use have never been tested for neurotoxic or neurobehavioral effects. [page 410]

Tens of thousands of individuals are so debilitated by chemical sensitivity disorders that they have had to make major lifestyle changes to cope with the illness. These are just the tip of the iceberg. There are hundreds of thousands more—the walking wounded—people trudging along, trying to get by from day to day, having great difficulty at work, at home, or during other activities. Many are unaware that their chronic complaints are either caused or exacerbated by their own surroundings.

From classrooms in North Dakota to metropolitan hospitals, from Fortune 500 companies to EPA Headquarters, and in private residences across America, people are becoming ill from the complex array of chemicals in building materials, furnishings, and consumer products. Some people with chemical sensitivity disorders become ill from a specific contaminant in the indoor environment—from particle board, or new carpeting and adhesives, or home insulation, or termite treatments. Many others have chronic exposures, a slow and subtle poisoning. Regardless of the triggering contaminant(s), known or unknown, most indoor environments are a nightmare for those who have sensitivity disorders.

Individuals with this illness suffer from a wide variety of mild to life-threatening symptoms from every day chemical exposures. Plastics, particle board, adhesives, carpeting, dry cleaning chemicals, paint, varnish, natural gas, detergents, cleaning products, moth balls, room deodorizers, pesticides, tobacco smoke, fragrances and fragranced items are some of the many indoor items which can cause debilitating reactions.

Symptoms from chemical sensitivity disorders include multiple complaints such as fatigue, confusion, memory loss, headache, migraine, seizures, and other neurological difficulties, respiratory involvement with bronchitis, asthma, and shortness of breath; and muscle and joint pain and weakness. Gastrointestinal problems such as food intolerances, nausea, and indigestion; hives, rashes, eczema and flushing; and cardiovascular complaints such as vasculitis, hypertension, and irregular or rapid pulse are also common. Many individuals have allergic rhinitis, sinusitis, dizziness, vertigo, and visual disturbances.

Chemically sensitive people come from all walks of life: from laborers to professionals. The ranks of the chemically sensitive include professionals in areas such as medicine, law, architecture, journalism, academia, and government. . . . Even indoor air pollution specialists have succumbed to his devastating illness. [pages 401 through 413]

Eileen R. McCarty, Clinical Psychologist
901 Boren, Suite 701
Seattle WA 98104

(1) Chemical sensitivity is a toxic reaction to low levels of chemicals (airborne, ingested, absorbed) following an overexposure to a chemical. The overexposure may be to a massive single exposure or to daily exposure to toxic chemicals over time. Intensity of reaction (symptoms) appears to vary with individuals. The reason for this is more hypothetical than known fact. Sensitization to one chemical frequently expands to sensitivity to a broad spectrum of chemicals. Sensitivity does not appear to be reversible.

(2) In my opinion chemical overexposure (single massive exposure or prolonged low dose exposure) may cause organic brain syndrome. It is speculated that neurotransmitter function is impaired so that CS individuals may experience any and all of the following: impaired concentration, memory lapses, word aphasia, difficulty in acquiring new information, visual-spatial impairment,

loss of executive function, loss of interest in usual pursuits, loss of energy and fatigue, emotional lability. Some of these difficulties remit partially when the CS individual remains in a toxic free environment. Restoration of pre-illness level of function is rare even if a non toxic environment is maintained.

Chemical sensitivity is an illness that does not limit itself to emotionally stable people or to those who are free of unhealthy personality traits or disorders. When one is less able to function, personality disorders become more manifest and emotional control is less operable. In addition CS patients must adapt to a new way of life, frequently with significant limitatons. Many cannot work; others must seek less taxing and complex careers. Anger, frustration and adapting to a new life style are all feelings with which CS patients must learn to cope. Frequently counseling or psychotherapy is advised to help sort pre-illness issues from present issues and to aid in adaptation/resolution of both sets of issues.

CS patients complain of numbness, tingling, weakness, pain in arms, legs and back. These reactions tend to come and go. They are frequently more noticeable following re-exposure to chemicals. Living with these neurological symptoms also requires adaptation/adjustment.

[Personal communication]

Minnesota Dept. of Health
717 SE Delaware Street
P.O. Box 9441
Minneapolis MN 55440

[From testimony by Laura Oatman, Minnesota Department of Health, before the Committee on Environment and Public Works, United States Senate, 100th Congress, 1st Session, April 24, 1987.]

. . .the health risks associated with the exposure to an indoor air contaminant must be considered when determining the nature of a government's response to a problem. [page 103]

. . .the air quality standards of the Occupational Safety and Health Administration (OSHA) for industrial settings have been adopted to protect healthy workers over an eight hours per day interval. They should not be applied to employees located in a non-industrial workplace. Many people are using the terms "sick building syndrome" or "tight building syndrome" to describe the air quality problems that can occur in office settings. Even though the workplace includes both industrial and office settings, the health status of some individuals in non-industrial settings may make them more susceptible to adverse health effects from exposure to air contaminants. A different set of standards or guidelines needs to be used for air quality in non-industrial workplaces. [page 108]

Susan Molloy, Editor
Reactor Newsletter for the Environmentally Sensitive
2 Park Circle, #202
Marin City CA 94965

In Spring of 1990 the California State Attorney General's Commission on Disability issued a 140-page report delineating measures essential to access for people with disabilities including Environmental Illness/Multiple Chemical Sensitivity. The Final Report calls for, among other accommodations to this disability, providing access to medical facilities, which should be built and maintained with chemically safe materials, and requiring safe access to all facilities housing tax-supported programs including psychiatric wards. The Final Report concludes that people with E.I./M.C.S. are not receiving from state agencies even those services necessary for survival. Conformance to such decorating conventions as wall-to-wall carpet, for example, and exposing us to the tobacco smoke of other patients at the expense of our access to medical and psychiatric care is exceedingly cruel and discriminatory.

Many of us, myself included, have severe movement disorders resulting from exposures to synthetic chemicals and other environmental elements. Others among us have behavioral problems of self-destructive behaviors which occur following exposures and not otherwise. All of us undergo a process of adjustment to this disability, which necessitates radical lifestyle changes as do certain other disabilities. For these and many reasons, we should get (and are legally entitled to) expert psychological and psychiatric care. However, at this stage, it's too risky to permit most mental health professionals to take positions of authority in our lives. Most professionals are too distracted and perturbed by our disability and its resultant symptoms to get on with the business of helping us with our personal adjustment issues.

[Personal communication]

National Foundation for the Chemically Hypersensitive
Attn: Fred Nelson
101 Harbor Village Drive
Hampstead NC 28443

I call this malady "Chemical Hypersensitivity" with a subtitle of "Toxic Response Syndrome." It is a toxic insult that is more than the body can process. It usually starts with a significant exposure to a toxic chemical that impairs future exposure to groups of chemicals: petroleum products, phenols, pesticides, detergent enzymes, synthetic fragrances and flavors (products in small amounts). It can and does affect most any tissue or organ system. It manifests itself as an inappropriate inflammatory process. It affects the immune system and can lead to extensive autoimmunity.

[Personal communication]

Richard A. Nelson, M.D.
1001 South 24th Street West
Creekside Two, Suite 202
P.O. Box 1152
Billings MT 59103-1152

If we are to use the concept of multiple chemical sensitivites as defined by Dr. Mark Cullen of Yale in his *Occupational Medicine State of the Art*

Review, vol. 2 #24 Oct.–Dec. 1987, it would be defined as an acquired disorder characterized by recurrent symptoms referable to multiple organ systems occurring in response to demonstrable exposures to many chemically unrelated compounds at doses far below those established in the general population to cause harmful effects. The systems that are involved here are primarily the nervous system, the immune system, liver and kidneys. From the neurological point of view there are over 5,500 chemicals which have been found to be toxic to the nervous system.

The most commonly found toxins that we deal with on a clinical basis are those associated with pesticides and herbicides as well as solvents of industrial origin and chemicals that produce anoxic or hypoxic episodes such as iocyanates, cyanides, hydrogen sulfides, carbon monoxide, etc.

It has been quite difficult for us to apply until recently any of the biological markers which may help support the neuropsychometric testing in our discussions of the chronic mental syndromes that may be associated with chemical sensitivity and intoxication cases. We have seen papers coming through the literature associated with diagnostic studies including PET scanning and quantified EEG, otherwise known sometimes as brain mapping studies, which indicate that almost invariably when we have an abnormality in neuropsychometric testing associated with concentration, attention, memory, visual spatial memory, psychomotor functions, and hand dexterity abnormalities that there will also be abnormalities reflected in the PET scanning as well as in the quantified EEG studies.

If one couples the findings of PET scanning, psychometric testing, and quantified EEG with the immune studies which show abnormalities in activation or suppression of the immune system in the subsets of lymphocytes and generation of Interluken I and II, one has a fairly significant cross section of abnormalities generated in both the nervous system and the immune system. They will need to be further quantified and characterized as larger numbers of cases are brought to this type of study, but certainly this is the opening of a window that may be utilized to begin the analysis of these cases, using organic parameters rather than psychometric parameters only.

We have, therefore, established a beachhead of methodological techniques which will be of significant value in further evaluating the relationships of chemical sensitivities or organic mental syndromes and the structures of the brain which are very likely to be involved.

[Personal communication]

Dr. James Repace
U.S. Environmental Protection Agency
ANR 443, M2814A
401 M Street SW
Washington DC 20460

I have been working in the field of indoor air pollution since 1979, and have had contact with many persons who have been subject to significant indoor air pollution episodes from all over the country. Some of these individuals report multiple chemical sensitivity syndrome which they attribute to these exposures. Within the last two years, a cluster of individuals at EPA headquarters has also developed this syndrome; EPA's Waterside Mall building has been extensively studied as a result of numerous indoor air quality problems. Based upon these extensive anecdotal reports from widespread parts of the country, I have concluded that MCS syndrome may occur in some individuals as a result of indoor air pollution. I have helped initiate ongoing studies in EPA's research laboratories in North Carolina to study this phenomenon, which is currently, and incorrectly, classified by the American College of Physicians, as a "somatiform disorder" having its roots in mental illness.

[Personal communication]

Noel Rose, M.D., Ph.D.
The Johns Hopkins University
School of Hygiene and Public Health
4013 Hygiene
600 N Wolfe Street
Baltimore MD 21205

My personal views of this topic:

1. The importance of CSS should not be underestimated, qualitatively or quantitatively. The number of individuals who have, or believe they have, this syndrome is large and growing. Moreover, they are often *really sick*. Whether the symptoms have a physical or an emotional basis, they have a significant impact on the health of the individuals and their ability to function in society.

2. This syndrome is not a single disease. There are no constant sets of signs and symptoms, no reliable laboratory tests and no historical findings that distinguish these patients as a group.

3. A number of different diseases, organic or psychological, account for overlapping symptoms in some patients.

4. It is unlikely that a single causative agent, or even related group of agents, will be found to produce these symptoms. Diverse agents producing particular components of the symptom complex are probably involved.

5. Some symptoms in some patients may be due to allergy to particular inhalants or ingestants. If so, the agent should be identified with certainty by accepted methods of testing including elimination and reexposure.

6. In most cases, there is no evidence of clincially significant immune disorder, dysregulation or insufficiency. Were such disorders to account for any of the cases, it should be possible to identify the particular agent and the particular immune impairment by the tools available to the clinical immunologist.

In brief, then, it is my opinion that we are dealing with a number of different diseases with different etiologies. Confusion will continue to reign until they are sorted out clinically, their epidemiological characteristics distinguished and the respective causative agents identified. Only then will it be possible to diagnose, treat and prevent these illnesses. Clearly, more fundamental and clinical research are needed.

[Note: Dr. Rose is Professor and Chairman, Department of Immunology and Infectious Diseases at the Johns Hopkins University.]

[Personal communication]

Stephen A. Schacher, M.D.
Washington Institute of Neurosciences, Inc.
2825 Eastlake Avenue East, Suite 333
Seattle, WA 98102

Happy, indeed, is the patient whose illness fits into the current realm of medical knowledge. Today's epileptic fares far better than did those earlier unfortunates who were told that demons caused their illness. Today's patient with temporal lobe epilepsy is no longer considered crazy, but medically impaired. The "mad hatter" is no longer insane but the victim of mercury poisoning.

But sad and outcast is the soul whose disease lies outside of what is currently known or accepted. This is the way that I see the patients whom I have examined with Multiple Chemical Sensitivities. They complain of an inability to complete thoughts following exposure to common chemicals. Memory is challenged; they become fatigued. They cannot complete sustained mental or physical work.

They may feel emotionally labile. They may have headaches, muscles aches, joint aches, rashes, or diffuse body pain. Exposure to common items like newsprint, carpet glues, perfumes, deodorants, and toner from copy machines may trigger symptoms completely out of proportion to the seemingly benign nature of the substances themselves.

They have reason to see an allergist, because of their reactions. Yet most allergists are unable to accept their complaints as valid. Their sensitivities may precipitate asthma, and so they are sent to a pulmonologist. They complain that their brain does not work; they are sent to a neurologist. When nothing is found, they are sent to a psychiatrist. They are considered to be depressed or histrionic, perhaps malingering, or perhaps hysterical.

Finally an occupational medicine specialist is asked to decide their fate, because they claim that the damage to their health happened in the workplace and that they can no longer work.

We are an advanced medical society. We have sophisticated methods for examining the body. These patients have multi-system complaints. We apply very sophisticated tests that have worked for all of yesterday's diseases, and there is no trace of illness. The only possible conclusion is that the patient must be making it up, because if they were sick certainly our technology would reveal it.

The MCS patient does not rest. He/she pursues newer technologies (such as PET scans, evoked potentials, unusual antibody testing). These tests *do* show abnormalities, but the technology is not yet mainstream. The results are suspect.

I am a doctor of internal medicine in a group practice that specializes in separating the psychological from the physical and treating either or both. Because we have performed brain evoked potentials that we feel reveal damage in chemically sensitive patients, we have recently seen a significant number of such individuals. Several results have emerged from this experience:

i. When people who deal primarily with the body (general internists, allergists, neurologists) are unable to make a physical diagnosis, they tend to diagnose "multiple somatic complaints." They recommend a psychiatric consultation.

ii. Psychiatrists usually diagnose "depression" in these same patients.

iii. *Rarely* are any of these diagnoses based on an actual diagnostic instruments (such as neuropsychological testing or depression scales), but usually on "clinical impressions."

iv. When diagnostic instruments *are* used, such as the MMPI (Minnesota Multiphasic Personality Inventory) or depression scales, an odd phenomenon occurs. Since the results are interpreted by a psychologist (or by a computer), *no attempt is made to correlate these findings with the clinical course of the patient.* Here is what I mean by that.

Sometimes the MMPI will show a high Somatization score. Yet if one reads any psychiatry text, somatization disorder will be found to be an extremely different disorder from the clinical course presented by these patients. Unlike true somatization disorder, these patients do *not* have a lifelong history of somatic complaints; they *rarely* complain of the most typical symptoms of this disorder; and they rarely have complaints outside a few specified body systems. Similar comments can be made for conversion disorder, hypochondriasis, and malingering.

There is another possibility. These patients have an illness that we do not understand, *but which is giving us an opportunity to understand.* Even though I realize that industry is already overwhelmed with OSHA requirements, the lives of these patients are telling us that we need to continue to balance our chemical inventiveness with a need for biological protection.

By having neuropsychological symptoms, they are highlighting the fact that emotional symptoms can sometimes have a physical basis.

By having immunological abnormalities, they challenge us to realize that we may not understand what it means to be hypersensitive to formaldehyde or to the styrenes of photocopier ink.

By having the inability to tolerate the modern workplace, they challenge our notion of the office, like the mines and foundries of the last century, may not be safe for everyone.

And by being incapacitated, they frighten us that we will have to support them financially.

They are a source of stress to us, whether we are in medicine, in government, or in industry, and like any stressed organisms, we respond thoughtlessly in anger and in fear. It's their fault, and we want them to go away.

The way out of this stress, as any stress, is to take a breath, relax, turn the thinking mind back on, and become interested in the problem.

These patients present with an identifiable clinical syndrome with symptoms involving the immune system, the lungs, and the limbic systems. Antibodies we don't completely understand are found in abnormal amounts. PET scans of the hippocampus do not look normal and correspond to lesions found in animals experimentally exposed to similar chemicals. Evoked potential testing of the brain is not normal. The areas of damage correspond to areas where inhaled chemicals would be thought to settle, the old "smell brain" of the animal kingdom. Pulmonary function tests are frequently abnormal.

Nothing is served by saying, as I have so often seen on expert opinion reports, that the "neurological exam is normal." Does this mean that the expert examined the hippocampus in detail, did a careful sensory exam worthy of a neurologist, reviewed the PET scans, looked at the evoked potentials, and checked the special senses? Usually not.

In my opinion, we are letting the index cases (the first cases of an epidemic) go undiagnosed and untreated, because we think to diagnose them is impossible and to treat them too expensive. Yet Nature is leading us, through them, to new knowledge. Plague didn't go away because the victims scourged themselves; and yellow fever did not fall until the Aëdes mosquito was identified and eradicated.

Chemical sensitivity won't go away because we do not examine it or indemnify its victims, but only when we understand what chemicals cause it, what mechanisms perpetuate it, and what we must do to prevent it. It is a call to intelligence and creativity, not to burying our heads in the sand. And when we respond to it, we will be excited by the new knowledge it has given us.

[Personal communication]

Dr. John C. Selner
From article "Chemical Sensitivity" in *Current Therapy in Allergy, Immunology and Rheumatology* (1988, B.C. Decker, Inc.)

[In reference to universal reactors]:

Psychologic interaction has tended to reveal a disturbing incidence of life threatening physical abuse and sexual abuse in early childhood among these patients. [page 51]

Gregory Simon, M.D.
Center for Health Studies ZF-10
University of Washington
Seattle WA 98195

Multiple chemical sensitivity (MCS) is an acquired syndrome of severe sensitivity to a variety of chemically unrelated substances. Offending substances typically include solvents or volatile organic compounds and reported symptoms typically involve multiple organ systems, especially the central nervous system. Proposed mechanisms of sensitivity include immunologic abnormality, nervous system toxicity, and psychological conditioning. At present, all of these are interesting hypotheses without firm scientific support. Existing data on the mechanism of sensitivity is mostly anecdotal and convincing data on effectiveness of various treatments is nonexistent. Many MCS sufferers report cognitive symptoms (memory loss, impaired concentration) and emotional symptoms (depression, moodiness, irritability). Even with sophisticated neuropsychologic testing, it is not possible to crisply separate "organic" cognitive impairment from the effects of emotional state on mental performance. At this point, it is unclear whether reported emotional symptoms represent neurotoxic effects, psychological effects of disabling physical illness, or pre-existing psychological distress which has contributed to sensitization.

[Personal communication]

John D. Spengler, Ph.D.
Professor of Environmental Health
Harvard University
School of Public Health
Boston MA 02115

[From testimony of John D. Spengler, Ph.D., before the Committee on Environment and Public Works, United States Senate, 100th Congress, 1st Session, April 24, 1987.]

There is growing evidence that there are chemically sensitive individuals in our society. Many, it is believed, may have acquired the sensitivity due to chronic exposures. But even without the frank illness, the syndrome of irritation, fatigue, shortness of breath and nausea associated with building-related problems results in lost productivity and wasteful investigations and litigation. [page 84]

WASHPIRG
(The Washington Public Interest Research Group)
Richard Bunch, Executive Director
340 15th E
Seattle WA 98112

My knowledge of chemical sensitivity is anecdotal but frightening. Over the past couple of years, I have met or talked to many people who believe they have chemical sensitivity problems. Several of these people have had to change their lifestyles drastically because of their inability to tolerate exposure to chemicals. Chemical sensitivity seems to build up with continued exposure, that is, it is not cured by minimizing exposure, only alleviated; unlike allergies, it seems to be accumulative.

[Personal communication]

George C. Zerr, M.D.
111 5th NE
Auburn WA 98002

After having seen some 250 plus patients that had been exposed to toxic chemicals, I have come to the conclusion that chemicals have the capacity to create multiple physical problems for people. At this time, I think it is reasonably well documented, both in the literature and in my own experience, that individuals immune systems are affected by chemicals yielding asthma and other kinds of respiratory and bowel symptomatology. However, in my own experience, which has been mostly in dealing with individuals that are displaying intellectual and neurological symptomatology secondary to that exposure, there is no question in my mind that significant neurological damage can be inflicted by chemicals. They have all of the earmarks of a dementia with memory loss, irritability, loss of interest in things previously interesting, etc. I could go into a good deal of elaboration on the subject but simplistically put, there is no question in my mind that exposure to chemicals yields chemical sensitivity and organic brain syndromes.

[Personal communication]

Grace Ziem, M.D., DrPH
1722 Linden AV
Baltimore MD 21217

Multiple chemical sensitivity is a condition in which illness reactions are triggered by relatively low exposures to combustion products and petrochemicals, including pesticides. Prominent symptoms often include confusion, impaired thought, concentration, and memory, as well as fatigue. Other organ involvement may also occur. Reactions commonly occur within a few hours of exposure and symptoms last for several hours to several days or more. If exposures are frequent, the person can present as a chronically ill individual. Adequate reduction of exposures which trigger symptoms often results in symptom improvement, and the underlying condition may then gradually improve over several years or more. It is not known whether "cure" ever occurs. At this time, there is no epidemiologic evidence that persons with multiple chemical sensitivity have more psychologic dysfunction than other chronically ill individuals or that psychologic dysfunction precedes or predisposes to MCS.

[Personal communication]

Appendix D: Solving the Toxic Carpet Question

In "toxic carpet" cases across the country there is significant correlation between poisoning and findings of TMA antibody in the patient's blood. Scientists were beginning to suspect, though they lacked the confirming data, that although TMA exists in small amounts of carpets and could serve as an initial sensitizer, the other substances in the benzene family of chemicals—which are involved in carpet manufacture and are part of the adhesive used to secure carpets to the floor—were cross reacting in the blood test. The reason for the suspected cross reaction is that the metabolites of TMA and a chemical called 4-PC are so similar chemically that the test could mistake 4-PC for TMA. 4-PC is the unpleasant odor of new carpets and it occurs as a byproduct of the styrene-butadiene adhesive. There are two basic glue forms for carpets: the latex (styrene-butadiene) form with no known health hazards and the toluene form for which health hazards are listed. To identify whether a specific patient's symptoms were related to carpet glue and whether the glue would generate the TMA antibodies, a test was designed which consisted of the following:

1. brain mapping which consisted of a quantitative electroencephalogram (qEEG) with challenge to the chemicals suspected of causing the problem and evoked potentials (auditory, visual, upper and lower somatosensory) which would demonstrate residual damage, if any, in those areas. (The first challenge used the toluene glue. The second challenge used the styrene-butadiene glue.)
2. blood testing for TMA antibodies would precede and follow the second challenge test. Blood testing was scheduled one day prior to the challenge (day zero) and after the challenge on the following schedule: day 3, day 7, day 13, day 17.

Two qEEG's with challenge were administered to the patient. The first challenge was performed January 1992. Chemicals involved in this challenge consisted of: toluene, carbonic acid calcium salt (471-334-1), kaolin (1332-58-7), solvent naphtha light aliphatic (64742-89-8), petroleum distillates hydrotreated light (64742-47-8), hexane (110-54-3), ethylene glycol, and diallyl phthalate. The second challenge, performed February 1992, consisted of exposure to a small piece of carpet with a noxious odor and styrene-butadiene glue, a combination thought to be quite safe. Challenge was administered in a room approximately 8′ × 10′. The lid was removed from a quart jar of carpet glue which was not stirred. The patient was exposed to fumes at about 2 feet for 15 to 20 minutes.

Both qEEG's with challenge demonstrated that after a significant delay of an hour or two, bursts of alpha and delta wave activity occurred. This activity saturated the major portion of the brain, leaving little room for normal activity. The effect of these bursts is narcotic in nature. The first challenge caused profound brain fog such that the patient appeared to be in the end stages of a dementing illness. Untreated the condition continues for weeks. In this case nasal administration of thyrotropic releasing hormone (TRH)[30a, 34a, 292] on the day after the first challenge and shortly after the second challenge caused the effects of brain fog to mitigate within two to three hours. TRH is a natural bain hormone. It is effective in reducing damage but is not adequate to prevent further damage or improve the present condition.

The evoked potentials demonstrated significant results also. In terms of visual function, the electrical impulse from vision was directed to the visual and also to the auditory center of the brain. This finding links the damage to the workplace in that one of the initial symptoms is a "constant ringing in ears." The visual signal sent to the auditory part of the brain is the scientific explanation of the ringing in the ears. The patient literally hears visual signals. The cause is not illusory.

The visual mapping shows additional information which occurs subsequent to the initial poisoning and is no longer dependent on toxic stimuli. Bright visual images flood the patient's brain with voltage. When viewing the map on a computer screen, the signal followed appears white while other signals are other colors which vary from green to red to blue. In the case of flooding, the entire area of the brain viewed is white, wiping out all other color.

Auditory evoked potential results are equally significant. The auditory signal is very weak and the speed with which it reaches the part of the brain involved with short term memory is too late for storage in memory. This explains memory problems identified on neuropsychological assessment. When coupled with PET scan data showing a hippocampal lesion, the hippocampus being involved in short term memory storage, memory problems are not only to be expected, they should become the rule.

The visual and auditory evoked potentials demonstrate a condition in the patient called Wernicke's aphasia. This is a serious brain related communication problem which impairs ability to communicate verbally and in writing. It explains the patient's difficulty in oral and written communication.

The somatosensory evoked potentials examine electrical impulses from the hands and feet to and inside the brain. In this case these impulses arrive at the brain without difficulty. Once they reach the brain the impulses bounce all over the brain without touching the part of the brain to which they should be directed, the motor cortex. There is one exception. One foot transmits to the hand part of the motor cortex on the wrong side of the brain. These evoked potentials are significantly unusual. They explain the patient's lack of knowledge of position of hands and feet, balance problems, ataxia, dropping things held in hands, and so on. It should be noted that prior to working in the office in which the employee was poisoned, the individual had exceptionally good balance, having performed in intricate dance in the past and having climbed 400 foot rock walls and walked across piled boulders which moved as they were crossed. Those abilities have been destroyed.

Overall what the qEEG and evoked potentials demonstrate is that the systemic integrity of the individual has been seriously compromised. Further toxic exposure (and what is toxic to the patient, due to chemical sensitivity of the brain, might be undetected by non-poisoned individuals) could render the patient incapable of communicating or moving.

Having the complete medical record, the doctors were able to compare other tests. The finding that the neuropsychological assessment, MRI, PET scan, and the qEEG with evoked potentials all show the same picture is significant. The MRI, PET, and qEEG all show the same three brain lesions as if they were taken with the same camera. The cognitive symptoms identified in neuropsychological assessment match hand-in-glove with the MRI, PET, and qEEG objective evidence. Essentially the patient has structural, metabolic, electrical, and cognitive damage.[19a]

Results of blood testing with the second challenge on day zero were negative. It would appear, then, that toluene glue from the first challenge did not set off TMA antibody production. Day three and day seven following the challenge also produced negative results. On day 13, however, a scientific breakthrough occurred. The results were positive with a TMS IgM titer of 32, as high as the test goes. Day 17 results were positive with 16 IgM to TMA. The TMA antibody was a result of patient exposure to styrene-butadiene glue which contained no TMA. The test demonstrated a cross reaction, probably due to the close chemical relationship between metabolites of TMA and styrene-butadiene.

The qEEG and the blood tests together certainly explode the discriminatory belief of some doctors that CS symptoms are a result of illusory psychiatric problems and or that symptoms following low level, chronic exposure to low level toxics do not result in any permanent residual damage. Bursts of alpha and delta brain wave activity are not illusory. Development of antibody after chemical exposure is not illusory.

This test does not, however, discount TMA as a factor in CS development. It is possible and likely that during the days just following the carpet installation, while the carpet was still wet, the initial sensitization occurred. Some office workers remove their shoes while at their desks. This employee did so routinely. Otherwise there would have been no knowledge that the carpet was wet. During the period of carpet drying, the employee easily inhaled and absorbed through the skin a number of chemicals with known health hazards. TMA is a known sensitizer. Since the 4-PC produced by carpet and carpet glue is so close chemically, once the body metabolizes it, there is no reason to assume that the body will distinguish between the two any better than the blood test did. Any synergistic effect between TMA and styrene-butadiene glue is anybody's guess. What is certain is that once sensitized, lower and lower amounts of the chemical to which one is sensitized can produce the same reaction. While TMA completes off-gassing fairly readily, styrene-butadiene glue can take much longer, the difference being one of days as opposed to months. The exposure in this case may have been substantially prolonged by the lack of ventilation in the office and the daily carpet vacuuming during work hours.

That the individual became sensitized to glued carpet in the workplace is clear. Neither before, during, nor after the individual's employment was new carpet installed in the home. In fact symptoms subsided when the person remained at home. That pattern was consistent during employment and continued after medical removal from the workplace.

The hope is that these data will finally establish the severity and permanency of the disability that may occur as a result of glued carpet exposure and cause the "no known health hazards" label to be removed from styrene-butadiene glue cans to protect the public. Since styrene is known to cause CNS disturbance, how styrene-butadiene ever qualified as a substance of "no known health hazard" is a mystery.

Glossary

acute exposure a single contact with toxic substance(s)

acute phase reactants chemicals released into the blood following an acute exposure (the effect is flu-like symptoms)

adaptation developed ability to tolerate toxic substancs to a certain extent

addiction substance dependency, either physical, psychological, or both

adversarial physician a physician not chosen or paid by the patient; usually selected by entitlement or benefits administrators or opposition in a lawsuit

aerosols solid or liquid particles suspended in gas (for example, industrial aerosols are visible in the plumes rising from smokestacks, the smoke of burning wood, insecticide and hairsprays)

anaphylaxis a systematic hypersensitive reaction to a substance to which the subject has been previously exposed (can produce serious shock)

antibodies immunoglobulins produced in reponse to antigens to counter antigen effects

antigen a foreign substance which induces the formation of antibodies

asthma difficulty breathing resulting from constriction of airways and or swelling of mucous membranes

atopic not poisonous

autoantibodies an antibody which attacks parts of the body rather than invasive substances

autoimmunity disorderly immunologic response to self

blood-brain barrier a layer of closely positioned cells in the walls of blood vessels which permit some substances to pass through while preventing the passage of others

blood cells red blood corpuscles (erythrocytes), white blood corpuscles (leukocytes). There is variety in leukocytes: granulocytes (having granules in cytoplasm) and agranulocytes (lacking granules in cytoplasm). Granulocytes include neutrophils, basophils, and eosinophils. Agranulocytes include lymphocytes and monocytes. Blood counts measure proportion of each type of cell relative to another to identify bacterial or viral infection. White cell counts may be quite high during the appearance of symptoms of the actual poisoning level being reached

brain fog a non-medical term used to describe the mental confusion and other intellectual dysfunction as well as impaired consciousnes after neurotoxic exposure

bronchoconstriction contraction of muscles which results in narrowed bronchi (air passages from trachea to lungs)

bronchodilator medicine, usually in aerosol form, which opens constricted airways

catecholamines chemicals such as norepinephrine and dopamine which function as hormones or neurotransmitters. They affect the nervous and cardiovascular systems, metabolic rate, temperature, and smooth muscle

cellular immune response the T cell (delayed sensitivity) response mediated by T lymphocytes

central nervous system (CNS) one of two major divisions of the nervous system; composed of brain and spinal cord

chemical sensitivity following an initial toxic exposure, a disease which has systemic symptoms due to lack of tolerance to one or a variety of chemicals in such a way that one or more symptoms develop from increasingly lower levels of further exposure

chronic exposure repeated contact with toxic substance(s)

complement protein in blood which bursts invading foreign bodies and helps phagocytes eat the foreign bodies

conditioning (Pavlovian conditioning) association of response to stimulus. For example, when trained to associate food with the ringing of a bell, the dog will salivate at the sound of the bell even in the absence of food

connective tissue tissue which supports and connects other tissues (mucous, fibrous, reticular, adipose, cartilage, bone)

cytotoxic chemical which destroys cells

cytotoxic T cells cells changed by lymphokines to work with complement to destroy foreign bodies

delayed hypersensitivity reactions which occur hours or days after exposure to a substance to which the individual is sensitive (cellular immune response)

detoxification a process of removing toxic substances from the body

disease a condition of mind or body in which there is structural or functional change with identifiable clinical signs and symptoms (generally but not always associated with microbial cause)

disorder a condition of mind or body in which there is structural or functional change (generally but not always associated with mental conditions)

double blind study a method of investigating in which neither the subject nor the investigator knows the method of treatment. It is useful in drug testing, for example, where individuals in a group receive either a drug or placebo (something which appears to be a drug but is not). Neither subject nor investigator knows which the individual receives, though records are maintained. The purpose of the double blind studies is to remove bias from the subjects being tested and from the investigator. In applying this investigative technique to the study of CS, there are ethical issues, because of the toxic nature of substances that generate reactions

edema excess fluid accumulation

encephalopathy wasting away of brain matter, leading to fluid-filled spaces in the brain associated with motor disorders and impaired mental function

etiology cause of disease or injury

euphoria exaggerated sense of well-being

excitotoxicity a process by which a neurotransmitter floods cells, weakens their membranes, and leads to cell death

fibrosis tissue which can be separated into fibers (e.g. scar tissue)

functional mental problem inappropriate or non-adaptive behavioral pattern not related to any physical injury or illness

histamine a substance released from mast cells in response to the signal that an antigen is present

histiocyte *see* phagocyte

histrionic dramatic

humoral immune response the antigen-antibody response mediated by B lymphocytes (this response also activates complement and provides life-long immunity)

hyperosmia increased sensitivity to odor

illness sickness, usually associated with long-term condition

immune complexes antigen + antibody + complement

immune system a system designed to provide protection and resistance for the body against disease or disorder originating inside or outside the body

immunological disease dysfunction of the recognition or memory of, response to, or clearance of foreign substances in the body or those diseases which arise within the body (malignancies)

interleukin 1 a chemical released by a macrophage with foreign body when it contacts (literally touches) a T helper cell (this substance causes the T helper cell to release interleukin 2, activating a full blown immune system response). Interleukin 1 generates flu-like symptoms

interleukin 2 a chemical released by T helper cells which stimulates production of T helper cells

intoxicant poison

intoxication poisoning by drug or toxic substance (also, too much of something non-toxic, such as water intoxication from too much intake or retention)

killer cells cells which search for and destroy cancer and cells affected by bacteria and viruses

leukotrienes internally produced, extremely active substances which have inflammatory and bronchoconstrictor properties

lymphatic system the body's filtering and drainage system for excess fluids from the circulatory system

lymphokine a chemical produced by T helper cells which (1) communicates to B lymphocytes to supply more antibodies, and (2) causes some T cells to change to cytotoxic T cells to join with complement to destroy foreign substances

macrophage *see* phagocyte

mast cells early warning system for the detection of entry into the body of foreign bodies (they are located in connective tissue)

mediators chemicals released from mast cells in response to the recognition of a foreign body (these are called mediators, because their function is indirect, rather than direct)

metabolism chemical changes in living cells by which energy is provided and material is assimilated

microphage *see* phagocyte

myelin a fatty substance serving the purpose of electrical insulation in a living body

neurotoxicity adverse change in structure or function of the nervous system as a result of a chemical reaction. (Note: There is some disagreement over the term *adverse* here. Clearly adverse are memory loss, permanent neurological damage [lesions, seizures, toxic generated abnormal electrical patterns], death, reduced intellectual function. More questionable are brief headaches and temporary drowsiness. At present the standard method of assessment is neuropsychologic.)

neurotransmitter a chemical substance released from presynaptic neurons that acts on postsynaptic neurons

neurotransmitter system disease malfunction in neurotransmission process resulting from structure failure in blood-brain barrier

non-acquiescence a policy employed by federal agencies to ignore or partially or temporarily implement a court decision

organic brain syndrome brain damage including altered sensory and behavioral function, interference with integration of normal thought, impaired consciousness, and altered motor function. It results from an organic cause as opposed to emotional causes.

paresthesia sensation without apparent cause such as tingling, prickling, mild shocking, heightened sensitivity

particulates small fragments (examples are dust, flour, and wood particles from sanding)

peripheral nervous system (PNS) one of two major divisions of the nervous system; composed of nerves linking spinal cord and sensory organs, glands, blood vessels, and muscles

phagocyte cell which eats foreign bodies and dead tissue (macrophages eat dead tissue, cells, and particulates; microphages eat bacteria; histiocytes eat particulates)

plasticizer a chemical substance that makes plastics bend

prostaglandins extremely active chemicals which affect every cell in every organ system

reaginic having to do with antibodies associated with atopic reactions

sick building syndrome a set of symptoms which result from intolerance to low level indoor air pollution. The symptoms are reversible by eliminating, reducing, or avoiding the source.

somatization the development by an individiual of symptoms of an illness in the absence of the illness

spreading phenomenon after chemical sensitivity has developed, the addition of other chemicals to which the individual also reacts adversely

symptom observable alteration in structure or function that indicates presence of disease and aids in the diagnosis

symptomizer label attached to individuals who develop symptoms in the absence of disease (an identical label is *somatizer*)

synchronicity non-random electrical firing in the brain; except while the brain in engaged in new learning, this is normal

syndrome a group of symptoms related by anatomic, physiologic, or biochemical characteristics

synergy combined effort or operation of two or more agents in which the combined effect is greater than that of the sum of the single agents not acting together

systemic affecting the whole body rather than a part, or a whole system rather than a part

T suppressor cells cells that turn off the immune response by inhibiting the macrophage–T helper cell reaction

temperature inversion a weather condition in which warm air moves over colder, ground level air. The effect is to reduce wind flow and trap pollutants near the ground

threshold limit value (TLV) the term for the part-per-million levels which the Environmental Protection Agency has used as guidelines to non-hazardous air quality (EPA presently recognizes that these levels are set too high)

TLV *see* threshold limit value

tolerance capacity for enduring a large amount of a substance without adverse reaction

toxic substances materials which have the potential to poison

toxin a protein (this term is often used incorrectly as the equivalent of *toxic*)

VOCs *see* volatile organic compounds

volatile a substance which vaporizes at relatively low temperature

volatile organic compounds (VOCs) chemicals which give off airborne vapors (TLVs are for measuring the amount of these chemicals in air)

xenobiotics strange substances in the environment

Bibliography

This section should help to dispel the myth that chemical sensitivity is little known and poorly understood. There are reasons why few know about or understand the disease, but lack of literature is not one of them. This list contains about half the literature available to the author. Major sources or controversial ones are included here. The purpose of this section is to provide those who look for answers or arguments with selections which may apply to their specific area of interest.

Items starred in the following list are used with the kind permission of the state of Maryland, Department of the Environment, from the comprehensive overview *Chemical Hypersensitivity Syndrome Study*, by Rebecca Bascom, M.D., M.P.H. That study was prepared for the State of Maryland, Department of the Environment, March 1989. Annotations for the starred items are reproduced just as they appeared in that publication; italic type indicates that the source is directly quoted. Annotations in non-starred items are the work of the author, except where italic type or quotation marks indicate that an abstract or computer database is being quoted.

Abbreviations

Acta Derm Venerol (Stockh)	*Acta Dermato-Venereologica (Stockholm)*
Acta Med Scand	*Acta Medica Scandinavica*
Acta Neurol Scand	*Acta Neurologica Scandinavica*
Acta Ophthal	*Acta Ophthalmologica*
Acta Otolaryngol (Stockh)	*Acta Otolaryngologica (Stockholm)*
Adv Exp Med Biol	*Advances in Experimental Medicine and Biology*
Adv Immunol	*Advances in Immunology*
Adv Neurol	*Advances in Neurology*
Agents Actions	*Agents and Actions*
Allergy Proc	*Allergy Proceedings*
Am Ind Hyg Assoc J	*American Industrial Hygiene Association Journal*
Am J of Clin Nutr	*American Journal of Clinical Nutrition*
Am J of Ind Hygiene	*American Journal of Industrial Hygiene*
Am J of Ind Med	*American Journal of Industrial Medicine*
Am J of Med	*American Journal of Medicine*
Am J of Psych	*American Journal of Psychiatry*
Am J of Pub Hlth	*American Journal of Public Health*
Am Rev Resp Dis	*American Review of Respiratory Diseases*
Am Soc Rev	*American Sociological Review*
Anal Chem	*Analytical Chemistry*
Anat Anz	*Anatomischer Anzeiger/Perspectives in Anatomical Research*

Ann Allergy	*Annals of Allergy*
Ann Clin Lab Sci	*Annals of Clinical and Laboratory Science*
Ann Int Med	*Annals of Internal Medicine*
Ann Ist Super Sanità	*Annal: dell Istituto Superiore di Sanità*
Ann Neurol	*Annals of Neurology*
Ann NY Acad Sci	*Annals of the New York Academy of Science*
Ann Occ Hyg	*Annals of Occupational Hygiene*
Ann Otol Rhinol Laryngol	*Annals of Otology, Rhinology and Laryngology*
Ann Psychol	*Année Psychologique*
Ann Rev Med	*Annual Review of Medicine: Selected Topics in the Clinical Sciences*
Annu Rev Pharmacol Toxicol	*Annual Review of Pharmacology and Toxicology*
Appl Indus Hyg	*Applied Industrial Hygiene*
Appl Occ Env Hyg	*Applied Occupational and Environmental Hygiene*
Arch Env Contam	*Archives of Environmental Contamination*
Arch Env Hlth	*Archives of Environmental Health*
Arch Gen Psych	*Archives of General Psychiatry*
Arch Int Med	*Archives of Internal Medicine*
Arch Int Pharmacodyn	*Archives Internationales de Pharmacodynamie*
Arch Invest Med (Mex)	*Archives of Investigative Medicine*
Arch Neurol	*Archives of Neurology*
Arch Otolaryngol	*Archives of Otolaryngology*
Arh Hig Rada Toksokol	*Arhiv za Higizenu Rada i Toksokologiju*
Bacteriol Rev	*Bacteriological Review*
Biochem Biophys Acta	*Biochimica et Biophysica Acta*
Br J of Haematol	*British Journal of Haematology*
Br J of Ind Med	*British Journal of Industrial Medicine*
Br J of Psych	*British Journal of Psychiatry*
Br Med Bull	*British Medical Bulletin*
Br Nutr	*British Journal of Nutrition*
Brain Behav Immun	*Brain, Behavior and Immunity*
Brit Med J	*British Medical Journal*
Bull Entomol Soc Am	*Bulletin of the Entomological Society of America*
Bull Env Contam Toxicol	*Bulletin of Environmental Contamination and Toxicology*
Bull Eur Physiopathol Resp	*Bulletin Européen de Physiopathologie Respiratoire*
Bull Hist Med	*Bulletin of the History of Medicine*
Can J of Physiol Pharmacol	*Canadian Journal of Physiology and Pharmacology*
Can Med Assoc J	*Canadian Medical Association Journal*
Clin Allergy	*Clinical Allergy*
Clin Encephalogy	*Clinical Encephalography*
Clin Exp Immunol	*Clinical and Experimental Immunology*
Clin Immunol Allergy	*Clinical Immunology and Allergy*
Clin Immunol Immunopathol	*Clinical Immunology and Immunopathology*
Clin Nephrol	*Clinical Nephrology*
Clin Toxicol	*Clinical Toxicology Review*
Compr Psychiatry	*Comprehensive Psychiatry*
Curr Psych Ther	*Current Psychiatric Therapies*
Derm Beruf Umwelt	*Dermatosen in Beruf und Umwelt*
Dev Pharmacol Ther	*Developmental Pharmacology and Therapeutics*
Dis Nerv Syst	*Diseases of the Nervous System*
Drug-Saf	*Drug Safety*

Env Hlth News	*Environmental Health News*
Env Hlth Persp	*Environmental Health Perspectives*
Env Intl	*Environment International*
Env Law Reporter	*Environmental Law Reporter*
Env Mutagenesis	*Environmental Mutagenesis*
Env Research	*Environmental Research*
Env Trends	*Environmental Trends*
Exp Pathol	*Experimentelle Pathologie*
Fund Appl Toxicol	*Fundamental & Applied Toxicology*
Horm Res	*Hormone Research*
Hum Toxicol	*Human Toxicology*
Immunol Rev	*Immunological Reviews*
Immunol Today	*Immunology Today*
In Vitro Toxicol	*In Vitro Toxicology*
Int Arch Allergy Appl Immunol	*International Archives of Allergy and Applied Immunology*
Int Arch Occ Env Hlth	*International Archives of Occupational and Environmental Health*
Int J of Neurosci	*International Journal of Neuroscience*
J of Abnorm Soc Psychol	*Journal of Abnormal and Social Psychology*
J of Allergy	*Journal of Allergy*
J of Allergy Clin Immunol	*Journal of Allergy and Clinical Immunology*
J of Am Water Works Assoc	*Journal of the American Water Works Association*
J of Anal Toxicol	*Journal of Analytical Toxicology*
J of Appl Physiol	*Journal of Applied Physiology*
J of Biol Chem	*Journal of Biological Chemistry*
J of Biosocial Res	*Journal of Biosocial Research*
J of Chromatog	*Journal of Chromatography*
J of Clin Exp Neuropsychol	*Journal of Clinical and Experimental Neuropsychology*
J of Clin Immunol	*Journal of Clinical Immunology*
J of Clin Invest	*Journal of Clinical Investigation*
J of Clin Lab Immunol	*Journal of Clinical and Laboratory Immunology*
J of Env Hlth	*Journal of Environmental Health*
J of Exp Med	*Journal of Experimental Medicine*
J of Hepatol	*Journal of Hepatology*
J of Immuno	*Journal of Immunology*
J of Int Acad Prev Med	*Journal of the International Academy of Preventive Medicine*
J of Lab Clin Med	*Journal of Laboratory and Clinical Medicine*
J of Natl Cancer Inst	*Journal of the National Cancer Institute*
J of Neurol Neurosurg Psych	*Journal of Neurology, Neurosurgery and Psychiatry*
J of Neurol Sci	*Journal of Neurological Science*
J of Neuropsych	*Journal of Neuropsychiatry*
J of Nutr	*Journal of Nutrition*
J of Occ Med	*Journal of Occupational Medicine*
J of Orthomol Psych	*Journal of Orthomolecular Psychiatry*
J of Ped	*Journal of Pediatrics*
J of Person Soc Psychol	*Journal of Personality and Social Psychology*
J of Pest Reform	*Journal of Pesticide Reform*
J of Resp Dis	*Journal of Respiratory Diseases*
J of Tenn Med Assoc	*Journal of the Tennessee Medical Association*
J of Toxicol Clin Toxicol	*Journal of Toxicology-Clinical Toxicology*

J of Toxicol Cut and Ocular Toxicol	*Journal of Toxicology: Cutaneous and Ocular Toxicology*
J of Toxicol Env Hlth	*Journal of Toxicology and Environmental Health*
JAMA	*Journal of the American Medical Association*
Jap J of Ophthalmol	*Japanese Journal of Ophthalmology*
Lab Invest	*Laboratory Investigation*
Med Clin North Am	*Medical Clinics of North America*
Med Econ	*Medical Economics*
Med J Aus	*Medical Journal of Australia*
Med Hist	*Medical History*
Med Hypoth	*Medical Hypotheses*
Med Lav	*Medicina del Lavoro*
Microcirc Endothelium Lymphatics	*Microcirculation, Endothelium and Lymphatics*
Milbank Q	*Milbank Quarterly*
Milit Med	*Military Medicine*
N Engl Reg Allergy Proc	*New England and Regional Allergy Proceedings*
Nat Law J	*National Law Journal*
Ned Tijdschr Geneeskd	*Ned Tijdschrift voor Geneeskunde*
Neurotoxicol Teratol	*Neurotoxicology and Teratology*
Nord Med	*Nordisk Medicin*
Occ Hlth Safet	*Occupational Health & Safety*
Occ Med	*Occupational Medicine*
Otolaryngol Clin North Am	*Otolaryngology Clinics of North America*
Otolaryngol Head Neck Surg	*Otolaryngology—Head & Neck Surgery*
Pediatr Clin N Am	*Pediatric Clinics of North America*
Person Soc Psychol Bull	*Personality & Social Psychology Bulletin*
Persp Biol Med	*Perspectives in Biology and Medicine*
Proc Natl Acad Sci	*Proceedings of the National Academy of Science*
Prog Brain Res	*Progress in Brain Research*
Prog Clin Biol Res	*Progress in Clinical and Biological Research*
Psych Ann	*Psychiatric Annals*
Psychosom Med	*Psychosomatic Medicine*
Recenti Prog Med	*Recenti Progressi in Medicina*
Residue Rev	*Residue Review*
Rev Fr Allerg	*Revue Française d'Allergologie*
Scand J of Soc Med	*Scandinavian Journal of Social Medicine*
Scand J of Work Env Hlth	*Scandinavian Journal of Work and Environmental Health*
Southern Med J	*Southern Medical Journal*
Toxicol Appl Pharmacol	*Toxicology and Applied Pharmacology*
Toxicol Ind Hlth	*Toxicology and Industrial Health*
Toxicol Let	*Toxicology Letters*
West J of Med	*Western Journal of Medicine*
Yale J of Bio Med	*The Yale Journal of Biological Medicine*

1. *ABC News Nightline*: "The Stealth Fighter's Toxic Secret," show #1914, air date Sept. 22, 1988. Transcript from Journal Graphics, Inc.
2. *Ad Hoc Committee on Environmental Hypersensitivity Disorders: Office of the Minister of Health, Toronto, Canada, 1985, pp. 17–18.
3. *Adams, R. M.: *Occupational Skin Disease.* 1983; Grune and Stratton, New York; 477 pp.
4. Ader, R. (editor): *Psychoneuroimmunology.* 1981; Academic Press, New York. Collection of insightful and valuable writings from various authors regarding the interactions between the nervous, endocrine, and immune systems plus factors in the dynamic process such as psychosocial, stress, disease, conditioning, and mind-body interaction. Contains a number of comments regarding the illusory perspective of the disease among which are the following:

   The mechanism(s) by which psychological factors contribute to the etiology of any given disease is largely speculative [page 6].

   The term "psychosomatic disease" . . . loses its meaning, and justifiably so [page 7].

   Many physicians who fail to understand a set of symptoms and signs prescribe tranquilizers, dismiss the problem (and the patient) by labeling the patient a "crock," or by labeling the disease "psychosomatic." This leaves the drug company richer and the patient sicker. To these practitioners, "psychosomatic" does not mean what the term originally was designed to describe (i.e., the unity of "psyche" and "soma"). To them, the term means: having "psychological" and therefore illusory character [page 468].

5. *Adkinson, N. F.: "Environmental influences on the immune system and allergic reactions." *Env Hlth Persp* 1977; 10: 97.
6. Ahmad, D., W. K. C. Morgan, R. Patterson, T. Williams, C. R. Zeiss: "Pulmonary haemorrhage and haemolytic anaemia due to trimellitic anhydride." *The Lancet* 1979; Aug. 18: 328–330.
7. *Air Quality Data Summary for the Counties: King, Kitsap, Pierce, Snohomish.* Puget Sound Air Pollution Control Agency, 1987, 1988, 1989.
8. *Akiyama K., J. J. Pruzansky, R. Patterson: "Hapten-modified basophils: a model of human immediate hypersensitivity that can be elicited by IgG antibody." *J of Immunol* 1984; 133: 3286–3290. Fascinating paper from a highly respected research group providing evidence for a new model of hypersensitivity resulting from human exposure to chemicals capable of combining with autologous proteins. The mechanism may explain immediate-type hypersensitivity reactions in which IgG antibody has not been demonstrated. Much more work is needed to determine whether this is a common or uncommon mechanism.
9. Albers, J. W., L. R. Kallenbach, L. J. Fine, G. D. Langolf, R. A. Wolfe, P. D. Donofrio, A. G. Alessi, K. A. Stolp-Smith, M. B. Bromberg: "Neurological abnormalities associated with remote occupational elemental mercury exposure. *Ann Neurol* 1988; Nov. 24(5): 651–659. "Although exposure was not age dependent, several neurological measures showed significant age-mercury interaction, suggesting that natural neuronal attrition may unmask prior exposure-related subclinical abnormalities."
10. *Aldrich, F. D., A. W. Stange, R. E. Geesaman: "Smoking and ethylene diamine

sensitization in an industrial population." *J of Occ Med* 1987; 29: 311–314. A clinical report from scientists at IBM describing respiratory sensitization to ethylene diamine in an industrial population. Cigarette smokers appeared to have an increased risk of sensitization. Ethylene diamine has been implicated as a sensitizer in paints, lacquers, lubricants, cosmetics, and household products. The mechanism is unknown.

11. Allen, N.: "Chemical neurotoxins in industry and environment." In *The Nervous System*, Vol. 2, D. B. Tower (Ed), 1975, Raven Press, New York.
12. American Academy of Allergy and Immunology: "Position statements: allergen standardization." *J of Allergy Clin Immunol* 1980; 66(6): 431.
13. *American Academy of Allergy and Immunology, Executive Committee: "Position statements: controversial techniques." *J of Allergy Clin Immunol* 1981; 67: 333–338.
14. *______: "Position statements: clinical ecology." *J of Allergy Clin Immunol* 1986; 78(2): 269–271.

> *The idea that the environment is responsible for a multitude of human health problems is most appealing. Yet, to present such ideas as facts, conclusions, or even likely mechanisms without adequate support is poor medical practice.*
>
> *The theoretical basis for ecological illness in the present context has not been established as factual, nor is there satisfactory evidence to support the actual existence of "immune system dysregulation" or "maladaption."*
>
> *There does remain the problem of the patient with multiple symptoms who does not clearly fit any disease category and whose illness fails to respond to conventional therapy. These patients are often labelled as psychosomatic, a concept that many patients and physicians have trouble accepting and managing. That dilemma may lead the patient to seek out the clinical ecologist.*
>
> *An objective evaluation of the diagnostic and therapeutic principles used to support the concept of clinical ecology indicates that it is an unproven and experimental methodology. It is time-consuming, and places severe restrictions on the individual's lifestyle. Individuals who are being treated in this manner should be fully informed of its experimental nature. Advocates of this dogma should provide clinical and immunologic studies supporting their concepts, which meet the usually accepted standards for scientific investigation.*

15. *______: "Position statements: candidiasis hypersensitivity syndrome." *J of Allergy Clin Immunol* 1986; 78(2): 271–273. Review of what is termed "candidiasis hypersensitivity syndrome" as proposed by Truss and Crook. The proponents argue that many common symptoms are due to candida overgrowth and require treatment with antifungal agents. The committee concluded that the entire concept was speculative, that no published evidence existed to support the diagnosis or treatment plan, and that important potential risks included overgrowth with resistant forms of candida, and untoward effects of antifungal agent. General good health principles of exercise, mental health programs and good nutrition were supported, but the use of antifungal agents or allergenic extracts should be used in an experimental setting with informed consent only.
16. *American Broadcasting Companies: "Much ado about nothing." Transcript of *ABC News 20/20*, show #810, interview with Dr. Bruce Ames, broadcast March 18, 1988. Biochemist Ames takes issue with popular misconception that

man-made is inherently harmful and natural is inherently safe. He points to the introduction of thousands of new chemicals, but the unchanged cancer rate (except for lung cancer secondary to cigarettes and skin cancer secondary to sun exposure). He advocates cancer risk assessments which rank risks in order to make rational decisions. Dr. Ames states, "We're so healthy and life is so clean compared to what it used to be. And a lot of that healthiness is due to modern technology."

17. American College of Physicians: "Clinical Ecology." *Ann Int Med* 1989; 111(2): 168–178. (See entry 453a.)
18. *American Conference of Governmental Industrial Hygienists: *Threshold Limit Values and Biological Exposure Indices for 1988–1989.* Cincinnati OH, American Conference of Governmental Industrial Hygienists. Appendix C, Threshold Limit Values for Mixtures:

> *When two or more hazardous substances, which act upon the same organ system, are present, their combined effect, rather than that of either individually, should be given primary consideration. In the absence of information to the contrary, the effects of the different hazards should be considered as additive. That is, if the sum of the following fractions,*
>
> $C_1/T_1 + C_2/T_2 + Cn/Tn$
>
> *exceeds unity, then the threshold limit of the mixture should be considered as being exceeded.* C_1 *indicates the observed atmospheric concentration and* T_1 *the corresponding threshold limit.*
>
> *Exceptions to the above rule may be made when there is a good reason to believe that the chief effects of the different harmful substances are not in fact additive, but independent....*
>
> *Synergistic action or potentiation may occur with some combinations of atmospheric contaminants. Such cases at present must be determined individually. Potentiating or synergistic agents are not necessarily harmful by themselves. Potentiating effects of exposure to such agents by routes other than that of inhalation is also possible, e.g. imbibed alcohol and inhaled narcotic (trichloroethylene). Potentiation is characteristically exhibited at high concentrations, less probably at low.*
>
> *When given operation or process characteristically emits a number of harmful dusts, fumes, vapors or gases, it will frequently be only feasible to attempt to evaluate the hazard by measurement of a single substance. In such cases, the threshold limit used for this substance should be reduced by a suitable factor, the magnitude of which will depend on the number, toxicity and relative quantity of the other contaminants ordinarily present.*
>
> *Examples of processes which are typically associated with two or more harmful atmospheric contaminants are welding, automobile repair, blasting, painting, lacquering, certain foundry operations, diesel exhausts, etc.*

19. *American Medical Association: *Guides to the Evaluation of Permanent Impairment,* 2nd edition. 1984; Amerian Medical Association, Chicago IL.

19a. American Psychiatric Association Official Actions: "Quantitative electroencephalography: a report on the present state of computerized EEG techniques." *Am J of Psych* 1991; 148(7): 961–964. Indications are that qEEG has value with mapped evoked potentials and producing high quality EEG records. Of particular value is detection of slow wave abnormalities (stroke, dementia, delirium, intoxication). Findings have greater value when used in conjunction with other brain imaging tests.

20. *Ames, B. N., et al: "Ranking possible carcinogenic hazards." *Science* 1987; 236: 271–280.

20a. Anderson, R. C.: "Measuring the effects of indoor pollutants testing toxins." In "Science and the Law" *Indoor Pollution Law Report* 1991: May 4(12).

21. *Andreoni D.: "The cost of occupational accidents and diseases." Number 54, Occupational Safety and Health Series. 1986. Geneva, Switzerland. International Labour Office. Provides a framework for assessing the cost of "Chemical Sensitivity Disorder."

22. Angier, N.: "Environmental illness may be mental." *New York Times*, Dec. 26, 1990.

> *In a report being published today in the Journal of the American Medical Association, Dr. Donald W. Black and his colleagues . . . said they found that when they evaluated a group of patients in whom environmental illness has been diagnosed the patients were much more likely to meet the criteria of a current or past psychiatric problem than were a group of normal people selected from the community.*
>
> *Dr. Leo Galland [an internist in New York] said the study might have been worthwhile had it compared patients in whom environmental illness has been diagnosed with people who suffer from asthma or some other disease considered to be organic by the medical community. As it is, he said, "the study is a waste of time."*

23. **Annals of the American Conference of Governmental Industrial Hygienists: Protection of the Sensitive Individual*, Vol. 3. 1982; American Conference of Governmental Industrial Hygienists, Cincinnati OH. Proceedings of a symposium addressing the scope of the problem, design and assessment of office building ventilation, and assessment of ventilation problems.

24. "Architect, heal thyself" (author unidentified). From *Science and Technology* 1989; May 13: 89–90.

25. *Arlien-Soborg P., P. Bruhn, C. Gyldensted, et al. "Chronic painters' syndrome: chronic toxic encephalopathy in house painters." *Acta Neurol Scand* 1979; 60: 149–156.

26. Ashford, N.: "New scientific evidence and public health imperatives." *Environmental Impact Assessment Review* 1987; 7: 203–206.

27. ______, C. Miller: *Chemical Exposures: Low Levels and High Stakes* 1990; Van Nostrand Reinhold, New York. Up to date review of populations, terminology and concepts, sources of chemical sensitivity and effects, mechanisms, diagnosis and treatment, and recommendations.

28. ______, C. Miller: "Chemical sensitivity: a report to the New Jersey State Department of Health." December 1989. Review of the literature—focus on orthodox and environmental medicine.

29. ______, C. Spadafor, C. Caldart: "Human monitoring: scientific, legal and ethical considerations." *Harvard Environmental Law Review* 1984; 8(2): 263–364.

30. ASHRAE Standard 62-1989: "Ventilation for Acceptable Indoor Air Quality." 1989; American Society of Heating, Refrigerating and Air-conditioning Engineers, Inc., Atlanta, Georgia.

30a. Aslanov A. S., G. I. Lavretskaya: "Effect of TRH on the Central Nervous System." Translated from *Problemy Endokvinologii* 1987; 33(4): 51–55.

31. *Atwood, S. (GNS): "Real or imagined." *Gannett Westchester Newspapers*, Health Section, Aug. 4, 1987: C1-27. Newspaper article describing the symptoms and practical problems of people with environmental illness. Highlights the controversy between traditional allergy and Dr. William Rea.
32. *Bach, B., L. Molhave, O. F. Pedersen: "Human reactions during controlled exposures to low concentrations of organic gasses and vapors known as normal indoor air pollutants." Performance tests. In: B. Berglund, T. Lindvall, J. Sundell (editors): *Indoor Air: Proceedings of the 3rd International Conference on Indoor Air Quality and Climate. Sensory and Hyperreactivity Reactions to Sick Buildings*. 1984: 397–402; Swedish Council for Building Research, Stockholm, Sweden. Describes a study of 62 subjects suffering from "indoor climate symptoms." Subjects were exposed to clean air or 5 mg/m^3 and 25 mg/m^3 of a mixture of 22 common indoor air pollutants (VOC). These concentrations were the average and maximum indoor air concentrations of VOCs found in new Danish homes. Memory, as assessed by the digit span test, was altered by VOC exposure, and the authors concluded that "indoor air pollution seems to impair mental performance." The authors noted that the digit span test can be altered by situational anxiety and stress. Attention and concentration, as measured by the graphic continuous performance test was not altered, and two new tests of trigeminal sensitivity, the Stinger's test and nasal spray test, showed wide individual variability and no effect of exposure. (See note 432.)
33. Bahn, A., J. Mills, P. Synder, P. Gann, L. Houten, O. Bialik, L. Hollman, R. Utiger: "Hypothyroidism in workers exposed to polybrominated biphenyls." *New England Journal of Medicine* 1980; 302(1): 31–33.
34. Bahura, J.: "Medical theories on multiple chemical sensitivities (MCS)." *Env Hlth News* 1990; 1(3): 4–8.
34a. Bajorek, J. G., R. J. Lee, P. Lomax: "Neuropeptides: anticonvulsant and convulsant mechanisms in epileptic model systems and in humans." *Adv Neurol* 1986; 44: 489–500.
35. *Balla, J. I., S. Moriatis: "Knights in armour: a follow-up study of injuries and legal settlement." *Med J Aus* 1970; Aug. 22.
36. Baranowski, Z.: *Free Radicals, Stress, and Antioxidant Enzymes*. Pamphlet (source unidentified).
37. *Bardana, E. J.: "Formaldehyde: Hypersensitivity and irritant reactions at work and in the home." *Immunology & Allergy Practice* 1980; 2: 60.
38. *______: "Office epidemics. Why are Americans suddenly allergic to the workplace?" *The Sciences* 1986; 26: 39–44.
39. *______, A. Montanaro: "Tight building syndrome." *Immunology & Allergy Practice* 1986; 8: 17–31. A good review of current information on tight building syndrome. Dr. Bardana states he hopes "the data will stimulate well designed studies in this emerging and important field." He urges allergists to become involved in the evaluation of these problems.
40. ______, A. Montanaro: "Chemically sensitive patients: avoiding the pitfalls." *J of Res Dis* 1989; 10(1): 32–45. Authors reject low level chemical exposures as triggering agents in medical conditions "commonly presenting as toxicity or hypersensitivity to environmental exposure." Bardana encourages physicians not to reject patients who "believe" they are chemically sensitive because it "encourages these patients to seek non-traditional approaches."
41. *Barnes, J. M.: "Assessing hazards from prolonged and repeated low doses of toxic substances." *Br Med Bull* 1975; 31: 196.

42. Barnes P. J.: "Asthma as an axon reflex." *Lancet* 1986; 242.
43. *Barsky A. J., G. L. Klerman: "Overview: Hypochondriasis, bodily complaints, and somatic styles." *Am J of Psych* 1983; 140: 273–383.
44. *Bascom R., D. Green, L. Sauder, A. Kagey-Sobotka: "Rhinitis symptoms and increased posterior nasal resistance in subjects with a history of environmental tobacco smoke sensitivity." *Am Rev Resp Dis* 1988; 137: A230 (abstract).
45. Bastomsky, C.: "Polyhalogenated aromatic hydrocarbons and thyroid function." *Clinical Ecology* 1985; 3(3): 162–163.
46. Batyrova, T. F., E. R. Uzhdavini: "The toxicology of trimellitic acid and trimellitic anhydride." *Institut Neftekhim Proizvod* 1970; 2: 149–154. "They can lead to chronic intoxication in the event of frequent absorption through the lungs."
47. Becker, C. E., A. Lash: "Detecting subtle human CNS dysfunction: challenge for toxicologists in 1990's" (editorial; comment). *J of Toxicol Clin Toxicol* 1990; 28(1): vii–xi.
48. Beebee, G.: *Toxic Carpet II.* 1988; Glenn Beebee, P.O. Box 399086, Cincinnati OH 45239 (independent publisher).
49. Bekesi, J., J. Holland, H. Anderson, A. Fischbein, W. Rom, M. Wolff, I. Selikoff: "Lymphocyte function of Michigan dairy farmers exposed to polybrominated biphenyls." *Science* 1978; 199: 1207–1209.
50. Belkin, L.: "Seekers of Clean Living Head for the Texas Hills." *The New York Times National,* Sunday, Dec. 2, 1990: 1 and 21. People seeking extreme chemical avoidance discover there's no safe place.
51. Bell, I.: "Environmental illness and health: the controversy and challenge of clinical ecology for mind-body health." *Advances* 1987; 4(3): 45–55.
52. *______: *Clinical Ecology 1982.* Common Knowledge Press, Bolinas CA. Introduced by Theron Randolph, M.D., as an "excellent presentation of clinical ecology." Dr. Bell summarizes the key concepts of clinical ecology and acknowledges the lack of evidence supporting them. "A major challenge to clinical ecologists and researchers in environmental medicine is to test the fundamental clinical observation of CE with controlled studies and to explore mediating mechanisms within the body."
53. *______, D. S. King: "Psychological and physiological research relevant to clinical ecology: overview of current literature." *Clinical Ecology* 1982; 1: 15–25.
54. Bellinger, D., A. Leviton, C. Waternaux, H. Needleman, M. Rabinowitz: "Longitudinal analyses of prenatal and postnatal lead exposure and early cognitive development." *New England Journal of Medicine* 1987; 316: 1037– 1043.
55. Belson, M.: "EPA to remove troublesome carpet at Waterside." *The Washington Times,* Sept. 15, 1989; B6.
56. *Bennett, W. R. (editor): "Chronic fatigue syndrome." *Harvard Medical School Health Letter* 1988; 13: 1–3. Description of the approach being used to study another elusive syndrome, using strict criteria and a working group of experts. The author comments:

    The current popularity of chronic fatigue syndrome as a diagnosis has created the hazard that both doctors and their patients will too hastily assume that fatigue is the result of this syndrome and neglect to look for other, treatable causes. On the other hand, there appear to be people with a real illness that can be called chronic fatigue syndrome; they may suffer not only from their symptoms but from lack of appropriate sympathy for their situation.

57. *Berglund, B., I. Johansson, T. Lindvall: "A longitudinal study of air contaminants in a newly built school." *Env Intl* 1982; 8: 111–115.

58. *Bernade, M. A., E. W. Mayerson: "Patient-physician negotiation." *JAMA* 1978; 239: 1413.
59. Bernard, A., R. Lauwerys: "Epidemiological application of early markers of nephrotoxicity." *Toxicol Let* 1989; Mar 46 (1–3): 293–306. "With the exception of microproteinuria observed in chronic cadmium poisoning, no epidemiological data are available on the prognostic value of subclinical renal effects caused by nephrotoxic chemicals."
60. Bernstein, D. I., J. S. Gallagher, L. D'Souza, I. L. Bernstein: "Heterogeneity of specific-IgE responses in workers sensitized to acid anhydride compounds." *J of Allergy Clin Immunol* 1984; 74(6): 794–801.
61. ______, R. Patterson, C. R. Zeiss: "Clinical and immunologic evaluation of trimellitic anhydride- and phthalic anhydride–exposed workers using a questionnaire with comparative analysis of enzyme-linked immunosorbent and radioimmunoassay studies." *J of Allergy Clin Immunol* 1982; 69(3): 311–318.
62. ______, D. E. Roach, K. G. McGrath, R. S. Larsen, et al: "The relationship of airborne trimellitic anhydride concentrations to trimellitic anhydride-induced symptoms and immune responses." *J of Allergy Clin Immunol* 1983; 72 (6): 709–713.
63. ______, C. R. Zeiss, P. Wolkonsky, D. Levitz, et al.: "The relationship of total serum IgE and blocking antibody in trimellitic anhydride–induced occupational asthma." *J of Allergy Clin Immunol* 1983; 72(6): 714–719.
64. *Bernstein, I. L. : "Occupational asthma: coming of age." *Ann In Med* 1982; 97: 125–127 (editorial). Notes the increase in the occurrence of occupational asthma in the chemical, plastics, and pharmaceutical industries since World War II, and the importance of collaborative efforts between occupational health professionals, clinical immunologists, physiologists and asthma specialists in developing ground rules for diagnosis and management. In 1982, occupational asthma was not recognized as a reportable disease in any state, making prevalence information difficult to obtain. Dr. Bernstein also alludes to the "uncertainty many industrial safety and medical officers have in distinguishing between the chief varieties of obstructive airways disease," and the need for "reliable and practical in vitro methods . . . for early diagnosis and prevention of occupational asthma."
65. ______, D. I. Bernstein: "Respiratory allergy to synthetic resins." *Clin Immunol Allergy* 1984; 4(1): 83–101. "A study of trimellitic-anhydride suggests that workers develop immunological mediated respiratory symptoms."
66. Bernstein, J.: "New perspectives on immunologic reactivity in otitis media with effusion." *Ann Otol Rhinol Laryngol* 1988; 97 (3 Part 2), Supplement 132: 19–23.
67. Bertschler, J., et al: "Psychological components of environmental illness: Factor anlaysis of changes during treatment." *Clinical Ecology* 1985; 3(2): 85–94.
68. Besedovsky H. O., A. del Rey: "Interactions between immunological cells and the hypothalamus pituitary-adrenal axis: an example of neuroendocrine immunoregulation." *Recenti Prog Med* 1988; July-Aug. 79 (7–8): 300–304.
69. ______, ______: "Interleukin-1 and glucose homeostasis: an example of the biological relevance of immune-neuroendocrine interactions." *Horm Res* 1989; 31(1–2): 94–99. *Il-1, a cytokine mainly produced by monocytes-macrophages, plays a crucial role in immunological and inflammatory processes. It can also affect neuroendocrine mechanisms and has the capacity to affect glucose homeostasis. Il-1 seems to adjust the "set point" for glucose regulation to a lower level.*
70. ______, ______: "Metabolic and endocrine actions of interleukin-1. Effects on insulin resistant animals." *Ann NY Acad Sci* 1990; 594: 214–221.

71. ______, ______, E. Sorkin: "Neuroendocrine immunoregulation." In: N. Fabris, E. Garaci, J. Hadden, N. A. Mitchison (editors): *Immunoregulation* 1983: 315–339; Plenum Publishing, New York.
71a. Black, D. W., A. Rathe, R. B. Goldstein: "Environmental illness: a controlled study of 26 subjects with '20th Century Disease.'" *JAMA* 1990; 264: 3166–3170.
72. Bliznakov, E. G., G. L. Hunt: *The Miracle Nutrient Coenzyme Q10.* 1987; Bantam Books, Inc., New York.
73. *Blonz, E. R.: "Is there an epidemic of chronic candidiasis in our midst?" (commentary) *JAMA* 1986; 256(12): 3138.
74. Bloom B. S. (ed): *Taxonomy of Educational Objectives* (Handbook I: Cognitive Domain). 1956; David McKay, New York.
75. *BNA Staff Correspondent, Conferences and Seminars, Breckinridge, CO: "Speakers differ on future on immune disregulation claims." *Toxics Law Reporter* 1987; April 1: 1227–1228.
76. *______: "Medical difficulties seen in finding cause of cancer clusters." *Toxics Law Reporter* 1987; April 1: 1228–1229.
77. *______: "Attorney offers analysis of litigation of claims based on fear of risk of cancer." *Toxics Law Reporter* 1987; April 1: 1229–1231.
78. *Bohlen P.: "Chemophobia reappraised" (letter) *Bull Entomol Soc Am,* Summer 1988; 2–3.
79. *Bokina A. I., N. D. Eksler, A. D. Semenenko, et al: "Investigation of the mechanism of action of atmospheric pollutants on the central nervous system and comparative evaluation of methods of study." *Env Hlth Persp* 1976; 13: 37.
80. Bolla-Wilson, K., R. J. Wilson, M. L. Bleecker: "Conditioning of physical symptoms after neurotoxic exposure." *J of Occ Med* 1988; 30(9): 684–686. After neurotoxic exposure, some patients experience recurrence of symptoms when exposed to environmental substances (e.g. perfume, gasoline, and cigarette smoke). Authors propose a classic conditioning model to explain the phenomenon. Essentially this study is limited to two individuals and none of the patients showed abnormal physical or laboratory findings. (See 174a.)
81. Boltansky H., J. Dyer, S. Esworthy, M. Kalinger: "IgE-immunotoxins. I. IgE-intact ricin." *Immunopharmacology* 1987; Sept. 14(1): 35–45.
82. ______, J. Slater, R. Youle, C. Isersky, M. Kaliner: "IgE-immunotoxins. II. IgE ricin A-chain." *Immunopharmacology* 1987; Sept. 14(1): 47–62.
83. Bond, J. A., R. K. Wolff, J. R. Harkema, J. L. Mauderly, R. F. Henderson, W. C. Griffith, R. O. McClellan: "Distribution of DNA adducts in the respiratory tract of rats exposed to diesel exhaust." *Toxicol Appl Pharmacol* 1988; Nov 96(2): 336–346. "These data suggest that DNA adducts levels in discrete location of the respiratory tract may be good measures of the "effective dose" of carcinogenic compounds."
84. Bonneville Power Administration: *Indoor Air Quality.* 3.1–3.13.
85. Boris M., G. Boris, S. Weindorf: "Association of otitis media with exposure to gas fuels." *Clinical Ecology* 1985; 3(4): 195–198.
86. ______, et al: "Antigen induced asthma attentuated by neutralization therapy." *Clinical Ecology* 1985; 3(2): 59–62.
87. Borm, P. J., B. de Barbanson: "Bias in biologic monitoring caused by concomitant medication." *J of Occ Med* 1988; March 30(3): 214–223.
88. Botham, P. A., P. M. Hext, N. J. Rattray, S. T. Walsh, D. R. Woodcock: "Sensitization of guinea pigs by inhalation exposure to low molecular weight chemicals." *Toxicol Let* 1988; 41(2): 159–173.

89. ______, N. J. Rattray, D. R. Woodcock, S. T. Walsh, P. M. Hext: "The induction of respiratory allergy in guinea-pigs following intradermal injection of trimellitic anhydride: a comparison with the response to 2,4-dinitrochlorobenzene." *Toxicol Let* 47 1989; 25–39. TMA–injected animals responded to inhalation challenge (bronchoconstriction). DNCB–injected animals were respiratory unresponsive but contact sensitized.
90. *Boushey, H.A., M. J. Holtzman, J. R. Sheller, J. A. Nadel: "Bronchial hyperreactivity." *Am Rev Respir Dis* 1980; 121: 389–413.
91. Bower, J.: *The Healthy House: How to Buy One; How to Cure a "Sick" One; How to Build One.* Lyle Stuart/Carol Communications, Secaucus NJ.
92. Boxer, M. B., L. C. Grammer, K. E. Harris, D. E. Reach, R. Patterson: "Six-year clinical and immunologic follow-up of workers exposed to trimellitic anhydride." *J of Allergy Clin Immunol* 1987; 80(2): 147–152.
93. Boyles, Jr., J. H.: "Chemical sensitivity: diagnosis and treatment." *Otolaryngol Clin North Am* 1985; Nov. 18(4): 787–795.
94. Brackbill, R. M., N. Mailish, T. Fischbach: "Risk of neuropsychiatric disability among painters in the United States." *Scand J of Work Env Hlth* 1990; Jun 16(3): 182–188. "Painters had significant excess of neuropsychiatric disability . . . construction painters had excess of neuropsychiatric disability in contrast to spray painters."
95. Brain, J. D., B. D. Beck, A. J. Warren: *Variations in susceptibility to inhaled pollutants* 1988; Johns Hopkins University Press.
96. Bridbord K., P. E. Brubaker, B. Gay, Jr., J. G. French: "Exposure to halogenated hydrocarbons in the indoor environment." *Env Hlth Persp* 1975; 11: 215–220. Aside from standard information provided overall, this article points to the composition of propellants of inhalers commonly used by asthma patients. One of the standard propellants still in use today is Freon 114.
97. Briley, M.: "MRI: A new look inside the human body." *Arthritis Today* 1990; Nov.-Dec.: 26–29.
98. *Brodsky, C. M.: "Allergic to everything: a medical subculture." *Psychosomatics* 1983; 24(8): 731–742.

This medical subculture (Clinical Ecology) does not talk about cures; the health-care professionals neither promise nor give hope of eliminating the offending condition, and the patients do not seem to expect it. Like people with diabetes or with long-standing inflammatory bowel disease, they accept the inevitable. In contrast, however, patients seem content with their condition and the reassurance that their symptoms have a physical cause.

In a review of eight patients, Brodsky found withdrawal from work, a lifestyle engineered to avoid exposure to putative noxious substances, and an identity as a disabled person. Brodsky believes that support groups "support the patients' perceptions of themselves as sick and afflicted, and, in turn, support their nonrecovery."

In conclusion, the author states, "We can regard it as likely that the emergence of this ideology may be a result, at least in part, of the failure of psychiatry to provide explanations and regimens that provide the benefits described above (the patient's recovery)." (See 174a.)

99. *______: "Psychological factors contributing to somatoform diseases attributed to the work-place. The case of intoxication." *J of Occ Med* 1983; 25: 459–464.

Profile of 70 people who believed they had been injured but had no organic basis for their complaints.

100. *______: "Multiple chemical sensitivities and other 'environmental illnesses': a psychiatrist's view." In: M. R. Cullen (editor), *Workers with Multiple Chemical Sensitivities,* State of the Art Reviews, Oct.-Dec. 1987; 2(4): 695–704; Hanley and Belfus, Philadelphia. Provides his recommendations for supportive treatment for SCD patients: acknowledging that symptoms are real and frightening, providing thorough physical examination and laboratory evaluation and, through discussion of results, counsel against harmful treatments and discourage avoidances that limit social functioning. Dr Brodsky also notes that "some of the avoidances have the qualities of phobic responses and therefore (doctors) should not press the patient to be counterphobic." He does not discuss what to do about worker compensation or disability.

101. ______, M. A. Green, E. S. Ogrod: "Environmental illness: Does it exist?" *Patient Care,* Nov. 15, 1989; 41–59. Authors ask, "What evidence is there for clinical ecologists' contention that our toxic environment is to blame?" Two issues are not faced here. First, the conclusion of the authors that the etiology is psychiatric is no more provable (perhaps less so) than the medical opinion that environmental illness is caused by toxics. Second, the authors have an obvious problem with clinical ecologists. The prejudice that they are better scientists than the clinical ecologists is arrogance. That arrogance clouds their own scientific objectivity. What occurs through the suggested management of environmental illness by playing psychiatrist to the patient who thinks he has environmental illness is a lie to begin with. Third, the doctor who pretends to treat a patient for a disease while playing psychiatrist may ultimately do more damage than was done prior to the patient's first visit to the doctor's office, particularly if the doctor is not a practicing psychiatrist.

102. *Brody, J. E. : "Clinical ecology: uncertain quantity." *The New York Times* 1985; Jan. 2: 11–12.

103. Broughton A., J. D. Thrasher: "Antibodies and altered cell mediated immunity in formaldehyde exposed humans." *Comments Toxicology,* 1988, 2(3): 155–174.

104. ______, J. Thrasher, Z. Gard: "Immunological evaluation of four arc welders exposed to fumes from ignited polyurethane (isocyanate) foam: antibodies and immune profiles." *Am J of Ind Med* 1988; 13: 463–472.

105. *Brown, H. S., D. R. Bishop, C. A. Rowan: "The role of skin absorption as a route of exposure for volatile organic compounds (VOCs) in drinking water." *Am J Public Health* 1984; 74: 479–484.

106. Brown, M.: *The Toxic Cloud.* 1987; Harper & Row, New York. Poisoning of outdoor air in the United States.

107. *Bryan, W. T. K., M. P. Bryan: "The application of in vitro cytotoxic reactions to clinical diagnosis of food allergy." *Laryngoscope* 1967; 70: 810–815.

108. *Buckley, P.: "Supportive psychotherapy—a neglected treatment." *Psych Ann* 1986; 16: 515–521. Advocates supportive psychotherapy.

108a. Bujnowski, K.: "About the SPECT." *CFIDS Chronicle* 1990; Spring-Summer: 58.

109. Buratti, M., O. Pellegrino, G. Caravelli, D. Xaiz, C. Valla: "Application of high-pressue liquid chromatography in the analysis of urinary metabolites of aromatic solvents." *Med Lav* 1989; May-June 80(3): 254–263. Method "permits simultaneous determination of metabolites of ethylbenzene, styrene, toluene, xylene isomers, benzene, phenol and cresol isomers in diluted urine samples."

110. Burbacher, T. M., P. M. Rodier, B. Weiss: "Methylmercury developmental neurotoxicity: a comparison of effect in humans and animals." *Neurotoxicol Teratol* 1990; May-June 12(3): 191–202.
111. *Burge, P. S. , M. Finnegan, N. Horsfield, D. Emery, P. Austwick, P. S. Davies, C. A. C. Pickering: "Occupational asthma in a factory with a contaminated humidifier." Source unknown. pp. 248–253. Described a case of 35 printers with work related asthma symptoms related to humidifier antigens as evidenced by positive prick tests and symptomatic improvement after cleaning of humidifiers without any change in other work practices. The importance of this example is that the initial assessment would probably have been that the printing materials were responsible for the illness. It emphasizes the need for precise diagnosis as a guide to resolution of illnesses thought to be due to "chemicals."
112. Burger, E. J., R. G. Tardiff, J. A. Bellanti (Eds): *Environmental Chemical Exposures and Immune System Integrity*. 1987; Princeton Scientific Publishing Co., Princeton NJ.
113. *Burr, M. L., T. G. Merritt: "Food tolerance: a community survey." *Br Nutr* 1983; 42: 217–219. The authors found no association between food intolerance and allergic histories; inverse correlation between food intolerance and IgE was described.
114. Burse, V. W., S. L. Head, M. P. Korver, P. C. McClure, J. F. Donahue, L. L. Needham: "Determination of selected organochlorine pesticides and polychlorinated biphenyls in human serum." *J of Anal Toxicol* 1990; May-June 14(3): 137–142.
115. *Burstein, A.: "Treatment of post-traumatic stress disorder with imipramine." *Psychosomatics* 1984; 24: 681. An uncontrolled study reporting beneficial effects of imipramine on the symptoms of post-traumatic stress disorder. The Impact of Events Scale (IES) was used. The author urges well-controlled, double-blind studies of the pharmacologic treatment of PTSD. Measures of PTSD include intensification of symptoms on exposure to events that symbolize or resemble the strategic event, avoidance of activities that arouse recollections of the traumatic event and memory impairment and difficulty concentrating.
116. *Butcher, B. T., C. E. O'Neill, M. A. Reed, J. E. Salvaggio, H. Weill: "Development and loss of toluene diisocyanate reactivity: immunological, pharmacologic and provocative challenge studies." *J of Allergy Clin Immunol* 1982; 70: 231–235. A fascinating, well documented report of asthma related to radishes which developed concurrently with asthma to toluene diisocyanate, and gradually resolved with removal from TDI exposure. The authors indicate that this is the "first report of unrelated food reactivity developing concurrently with occupational asthma." They note that radishes contain allyl and benzyl isothiocyanate, but that these substances are also present in cabbage, brussels sprouts, garlic and cress, which the patient could eat without difficulty.
117. Byers, V., A. Levin, D. Ozonoff, R. Baldwin: "Association between clinical symptoms and lymphocyte abnormalities in a population with chronic domestic exposure to industrial solvent-contaminated domestic water supply and a high incidence of leukaemia." *Cancer Immunology Immunotherapy* 1988; 27: 77–81.
118. Caffrey, E., G. Sladen, P. Isaacs, K. Clark: "Thrombocytopenia caused by cow's milk." *Lancet* Aug. 8, 1981; 316.

119. *Cain W. S.: "Contribution of the trigeminal nerve to perceived odor magnitude." *Ann NY Acad Sci* 1974; 237: 28–34. A study by an expert in the field of olfaction and psychophysical responses which addresses the role of the trigeminal nerve in the perceived magnitude of olfactory stimulation (odors), and to adaptation to odors. The author concludes that the "common chemical sense can be seen to intrude on the subtle world of olfaction." Provides an important avenue of investigation into chemical sensitivity disorders since odors are so often the triggers of symptoms.

120. Caine, D. B., A. Eisen, E. McGeer, P. Spencer: "Alzheimer's disease, Parkinson's disease, and motoneurone disease: abiotrophic interaction between aging and environment." *Lancet* Nov. 8, 1986; 2(8515): 1067–1070.

The hypothesis is that Alzheimer's disease, Parkinson's disease and motoneurone disease are due to environmental damage to specific regions of the central nervous system and that the damage remains subclinical for several decades but makes those affected especially prone to the consequences of age-related neuronal attrition.

121. Calabrese, E.: *Pollutants and High Risk Groups: The Biological Basis of Increased Human Susceptibility to Environmental and Occupational Pollutants.* 1978, John Wiley and Sons, New York.

122. California Air Resource Board: *Draft report on formaldehyde as a toxic air contaminant.* 1990.

123. *California Medical Association Scientific Board Task Force on Chemical Ecology: "Clinical ecology—a critical appraisal." *West J of Med* 1986; 144: 239–245. A presentation of the conclusions about clinical ecology as reached by a task force composed of allergists, immunologists, neuroscientists and pathologists as well as occupational, epidemiological, pediatric and psychiatric physicians. In the opinion of this committee, "clinical ecology does not constitute a valid medical discipline," "scientific and clinical evidence to support the diagnosis of 'environmental illness' and 'cerebral allergy' or the concept of massive environmental allergy is lacking," and clinical ecology lacks "a single, standardized definition among medical practitioners." The conclusions are reproduced in detail here: The task force collected material as for any subject review and included all information supplied by individual clinical ecologists and by their professional organizations.

No convincing evidence was found that patients treated by clinical ecologists have unique, recognizable syndromes, that the diagnostic tests employed are efficacious and reliable or that the treatments used are effective. Even though clinical ecology has existed for approximately 50 years, only a few studies have been conducted that are scientifically sound. Most have such serious methodological flaws as to make their conclusions unacceptable. Those few studies that used scientifically sound methods have provided evidence that the effectiveness of certain treatment methods used by clinical ecologists is based principally on placebo response.

Undoubtedly, some patients suffer from illnesses that cannot be readily diagnosed and for which only supportive treatments exist. It may even be true that some or all of the hypotheses and treatments proposed by clinical ecologists are valid but we found no evidence to support them. These hypotheses and treatments should be subjected to modern, scientific methods of evaluation. We think that this can be done provided genuine interest exists.

The task force is concerned that unproved diagnostic tests are being widely used by clinical ecologists in what may be incorrect or inappropriate applications. Decisions made on the basis of these tests can lead to misdiagnosis, resulting in patients being denied other supportive treatments and becoming psychologically dependent, believing themselves seriously and chronically impaired. This possibility underscores the need for more adequate scientific studies to prove or disprove the value of clinical ecology tests and treatments. To consider the current practice of clinical ecology experimental is misleading, however. It can only be considered experimental when its practitioners adhere to scientifically sound research protocols and inform their patients about the investigative nature of their practice.

124. California Senate Office of Research: "Pesticides at Home: Uncertain Risks and Inadequate Regulations." California State Senate. (Date unknown.)
125. *Campbell, D., R. E. Sanderson, S. G. Laverty: "Characteristics of a conditioned response in human subjects during extinction trials following a single traumatic conditioning trial." *J of Abnorm Soc Psychol* 1964; 68(6): 627.
126. *Campbell, G. H.: "In defense of clinical ecologists" (letter). *Emergency Medicine* Sept. 30, 1986: 11–12.
127. *Campbell, J. R. (UPI): "Everyday chemicals make victims sick." *The State,* Columbia SC, Aug. 25, 1983. Newspaper article concerning a book entitled *How to Live with the New 20th Century Illness—A Resource Guide for Living Chemically Free,* written by Linda Weiss.
128. *Caplinger, K. J.: "'Allergic to Everything': 20th century syndrome" (letter). *JAMA* 1985; 253(6): 842.
129. Carmichael P., et al: "Sudden death in explosives workers." *Arch Env Hlth* 1963; 7: 50–65.
130. Carson, R.: *Silent Spring.* 1962; Houghton Mifflin Co., Boston.
131. *Carter, K. C.: "Germ theory, hysteria, and Freud's early work in psychopathology." *Med Hist* 1980; 24: 259–274. Historical perspective.
132. *Casale, T. B., M. Kaliner: "Allergic reactions in the respiratory tract." In: John Bienenstock, editor, *Immunology of the Lung and Upper Respiratory Tract;* 1984; McGraw-Hill, New York. A review by noted NIH investigators in the field of allergy which provides an overview of the major features of the human allergic response. The authors point to a broadening view of allergic illness, and urge that the reader be aware that "immediate-type hypersensitivity mechanisms and mast cells as well as basophils may be extensively involved in other types of inflammation than those classically associated with allergy such as asthma."
133. *Castleman, B. I., G. E. Ziem: "Corporate influence on threshold limit values." *Am J of Ind Med* 1988; 13: 531–559.
134. CBS News Transcript: *60 Minutes:* "Is There Poison in Your Mouth?" 1990; Dec. 16, 23(14): 2–11. Deals with the amalgam issue.
135. Chandler, M. J., C. R. Zeiss, C. L. Leach, N. S. Hatoum, et al: "Levels and specificity of antibody in bronchoalveolar lavage and serum in an animal model of trimellitic anhydride–induced lung injury." *J of Allergy Clin Immunol* 1987; 80(2): 223–229. *The authors conclude that specific antibodies may play a major role in the lung injury induced by TMA.*
136. *Chan-Yeung, M., S. Lam: "State of art: occupational asthma." *Am Rev Resp Dis* 1986; 133: 686–703. A state of the art review by one of the foremost investigators in the field of occupational asthma. Provides a list of the many

substances known to cause occupational asthma. Dr. Chan-Yeung also summarizes the evidence that atopy is not a risk factor for asthma due to low molecular weight substances, and that a substantial number of people with occupational asthma will develop persistent illness despite removal from the work environment.

137. *Check, W.: "Eat, drink and be merry—or argue about food 'allergy'." *JAMA* 1983; 250: 701–711.

138. *Chow, C. K.: "Nutritional influences on cellular antioxidant defense systems." *Am J of Clin Nutr* 1979; 32: 1066.

138a. Chu, D.: "Immunotherapy with Chinese medicinal herbs. 1. immune restoration of local xenogeneic graft-versus-host reaction in cancer patients by fractionalized astragalus membranaceus in vitro." *J of Clin Lab Immunol* 1988; 25: 119–123.

138b. ______: "Immunotherapy with Chinese medicinal herbs. 2. reversal of cyclophosphamide-induced immune suppression by administration of fractionated astragalus membranaceus in vivo." *J of Clin Lab Immunol* 1988; 25: 125–129.

139. Clayman, C. B. (Ed): *The American Medical Association Encyclopedia of Medicine*. 1989; Dorling Kindersley Limited and the American Medical Association, Random House, New York.

140. *Clinical Toxicology of Commercial Products*, 5 ed. 1984; Gosselin, Smith, and Hodge.

141. *Cochran, D. G.: "Our chemophobic society." *Bull Entomol Soc Am* 1983; Fall: 128–133 (newsletter).

142. Cohen, F. E., P. A. Kosen, I. D. Kuntz, L. B. Epstein, T. L. Ciardelli, K. A. Smith: "Structure-activity studies of interleukin-2." *Science* 1986; Oct. 17 234(4774): 349–352.

143. Cohn, J. R., E. A. Emmett: "The excretion of trace metals in human sweat." *Ann Clin Lab Sci*, 1978; 8(4): 270–275.

144. *Coleman, B. C. (AP): "Complaints concerning total allergy rise." *Midland Daily News* 1985; Feb. 23. Newspaper article describing the controversy concerning the existence of total allergy syndrome.

145. *Condie, L. W.: "Toxicological problems associated with chlorine dioxide." *J of Am Water Works Assoc* 1986; June: 73–78.

146. Cone, J. E.: "Health hazards of solvents." *State Art Rev Occup Med* 1986; Jan.–March 1(1): 69–87.

147. ______: "Public health—theory and practice in occupational medicine programs." *Toxicol Ind Hlth* 1989; July 5(4): 49–55, 79–84.

148. *______, R. Harrison, R. Reiter: "Patients with multiple chemical sensitivities: Clinical diagnosis subsets among an occupational health clinic population." In: M. R. Cullen (editor), *Workers with Multiple Chemical Sensitivities*, State of the Art Reviews, Oct.–Dec. 1987; 2(4): 721–738: Hanley and Belfus, Philadelphia. Reiterates the multi-system complaints of people with chemical sensitivity disorders.

149. Conners, T. A.: "Effects of drugs on structure, biosynthesis, and catabolism of nucleic acids, proteins, carbohydrates, and lipids." In: S. M. Bacq, R. Capek, R. Paoletti, J. Renson: *Fundamentals of Biomedical Pharmacology*. 1971; Pergamon Press, Oxford.

150. Connolly, D.: "Toxics: Too risky to insure? Yes, no, maybe so." *Toxics Law Reporter* 1988; 3(23): 715–723.

151. *Cornish, H. H., J. Adefuin: "Ethanol potentiation of halogenated aliphatic solvent toxicity." *Am J of Ind Hygiene* 1966; 27: 57.

152. Corwin, A.: "A chemist looks at health and disease." Proceedings of the Society for Clinical Ecology, 12th Advanced Seminar, Key Biscayne, Florida, 1978.
153. Cory-Slechta, D. A., B. Weiss, C. Cox: "Tissue distribution of Pb in adult vs. old rats: a pilot study." *Toxicology* 1989; Dec. 1 59(2): 139–150. Exposed old rats exhibited comparatively lower brain weight than old controls; exposed old rats showed Pb-induced elevations of zinc protoporphyrin compared to adult Pb rats; exposed old rats blood lead values increased over exposure while adult rats declined; exposed old rats had more brain lead concentration and liver Pb levels, but bone Pb levels were higher in adult rats. "Tissue Pb distribution may be markedly altered when exposure occurs during the later stages of life."
154. *Cotterill, J. A.: "Total allergy syndrome" (letter). *Lancet* 1982; March 3: 628–629.
155. Council on Environmental Quality, Executive Office of the President: *Env Trends.* July 1981; U.S. Government Printing Office, 0-297-877: QL 2, Washington, D.C.
156. Courpas, M.: *Indoor Air Pollution: Cause for Concern?* 1988; Congressional Research Service, Washington, DC, 88-745ENR.
157. *Cowart, V. S.: "Health fraud's toll: Lost hopes, misspent billions. Medical News and Perspectives," *JAMA* 1988; 259(22): 3229–3230. A report on the National Health Fraud Conference. An estimation that medical "quackery" costs Americans $25 billion per year. Victims are characterized as 1) unsuspecting, 2) chronically ill with desperation overriding common sense, 3) "susceptible to magic," and 4) people with antagonistic attitudes. *The real tragedy is that people with clearly treatable conditions are put on bogus treatments.*
158. Cowley, G., R. Crandall: "Bad water, faulty genes; closing in on the causes of Parkinson's disease." *Newsweek,* 1990; Sept. 3: 73. Nearly all of the dozen or so studies published in the past five years have linked Parkinson's disease to chemical exposure.
159. *Crayton, J. W., T. Stone, G. Stein: "Epilepsy precipitated by food sensitivity; report of a case with double-blind placebo-controlled assessment." *Clin Encephalogy* 1981; 12: 192.
160. Cronstein, B. N., F. R. Rose, C. Pugliese: "Adenosine, a cytoprotective autocoid: effects of adenosine on neutrophil plasma membrane viscosity and chemoattractant receptor display." *Biochem Biophys Acta* 1989; 987(2): 176–180.
161. *Crook, W. G.: "The coming revolution in medicine." *J of Tenn Med Assoc* 1983; 76(3).
162. *Cross, C. E., B. Halliwell, A. Allen: "Antioxidant protection: a function of tracheobronchial and gastrointestinal mucous." *Lancet* 1984; 1: 1328.
163. Cullen, M., M. G. Charniak, L. Rosenstock: "Occupational medicine, No. 2." *New England Journal of Medicine,* March 8, 1990; 322(10): 675–683.
164. *Cullen, M. R. : "The worker with multiple chemical sensitivities: an overview." In: M. R. Cullen (editor), *Workers with Multiple Chemical Sensitivities,* State of the Art Reviews, Oct.–Dec. 1987; 2(4): 655–662; Hanley and Belfus, Philadelphia. In assembling this review, the editor acknowledged that "the level of knowledge was slight, the tenacity of opinions great and that those with differing views had long since ceased serious dialogue or debate." The purpose of the review was their hope to "hasten the only viable approach we know to such a clinical problem—serious, open-minded, scientific inquiry."
165. *______: "Multiple chemical sensitivities: summary and directions for future investigators." In: M. R. Cullen (editor), *Workers with Multiple Chemical Sen-*

sitivities, State of the Art Reviews, Oct.–Dec. 1987; 2(4): 801–804; Hanley and Belfus, Philadelphia.

The health problems of workers who react to low levels of environmental pollutants and chemicals . . . has posed a serious dilemma for health providers from a wide area of disciplines. The inability of these professionals to provide satisfactory care from the patient's perspective has led to the emergence of new and alternative clinical theories and approaches, challenging traditional views. Unfortunately, the success of these alternative approaches has also not been demonstrated, fueling an ever widening and hostile debate in which the patient is held hostage and virtually all clinicians are rendered impotent because of widely known intraprofessional disagreements.

166. ______, L. Rosenstock: "The challenge of teaching occupational and environmental medicine in internal medicine residencies." *Arch Int Med* 1988; Nov. 148(11): 2401–2404. "Few medical residents receive required or elective training in occupational medicine." Analysis is done "in the hope that a proper balance can ultimately be struck between economic and academic imperatives."
167. Czirjak, L., A. Bokk, G. Csontos, G. Loerincz, G. Szegedi: "Clinical findings in 61 patients with progressive systemic schlerosis." *Acta Derm Venerol (Stockh)* 1989; 69(6): 533–536. "Female predominance and sclerodermal involvement of trunk commonly demonstrated. Prior occupational exposure to chemicals was found in 28% of patients."
168. Dadd, D.: *Nontoxic and Natural.* 1984; Jeremy P. Tarcher, Los Angeles.
169. ______: *The Nontoxic Home.* 1986; Jeremy P. Tarcher, Los Angeles.
170. Dager, S. R., J. P. Holland, D. S. Cowley, D. L. Dunner: "Panic disorder precipitated by exposure to organic solvents in the work place." *Am J of Psych* 1987; Aug. 144(8): 1056–1058. Study describes "three cases of idiosyncratic response to occupational solvent exposure, with symptoms characteristic of panic disorder." (See 174a.)
171. Daniell W. E., W. G. Couser, L. Rosenstock: "Occupational solvent exposure and glomerulonephritis. A case report and review of the literature." *JAMA* 1988; April 15 259(15): 2280–2283. "Solvent exposure may play a significant contributing role in the development of GN."
172. Dansereau, C.: "Who is polluting Washington? It's your right to know." *Washington Toxics Coalition Alternatives* 1990: Summer 9(2): 1, 3. Major air pollution sources: Boeing, Longview Fibre Co., Chevron Chemical Co., Weyerhaeuser; major water pollution sources: Weyerhaeuser, ITT Rayonier. Leading air pollution chemicals: methanol, toluene, acetone; major water pollution chemicals: sulfuric acid, ammonium sulfate (solution), ammonia.
173. Daum, S.: "Nitroglycerin and Alkyl Nitrates." In: W. Rom (editor), *Environmental and Occupational Medicine* 1983: 639–648; Little, Brown and Co., Boston.
173a. Davidoff, L. L.: "Models of multiple chemical sensitivities (MCS) syndrome: using empirical data (especially interview data) to focus investigations." Paper presented at the Multiple Chemical Sensitivities Workshop, sponsored by the Association of Occupational and Environmental Clinics, Washington DC, Sept. 21, 1991.
174. ______: "Multiple Chemical Sensitivities." *Amicus Journal* 1989; Winter.
174a. ______: "Multiple chemical sensitivities: research on psychiatric/psychosocial issues." Paper presented at the symposium Multiple Chemical Sensitivities and the Environment II: Diagnosis and Therapy, sponsored by the

divisions of Environment and Occupational Health and Safety at the annual meeting of the American Public Health Association, Atlanta, Georgia, Nov. 13, 1991. The author reveals the lack of scientific vigor in the 13 published studies that purport to examine psychiatric aspects of MCS. Those articles, an "uninterpretable muddle," are Bibliography entries: 71a, 80, 98, 170, 187, 573, 610, 611a, 629, 652, 661, 680, 681.

175. *_____ (editor): *Chemical Sensitivity Connection* (newsletter); Nov. 1988: 8.
176. *Davis, E. S.: "Ecological Illnesses." *Trial* 1986; Oct: 34–40.
177. *_____: "The legal side of ecological illness." *Clinical Ecology* 1986; 4: 77–80. Provides a good description of the practical problems encountered by people with this syndrome. Advises lawyers to avoid getting caught in crossfire between the American Academy of Allergy and Immunology and the American Academy of Environmental Medicine. Finally, he states "there is no substitute for research." A summary article by the editor of the Ecological Illness Law Report, an "independent newsletter providing information to chemical victims and their families." He believes that ecological illnesses are emerging as major public health problems, but that the lack of definitive medical information and government recognition pose "major but not insurmountable obstacles to just compensation for chemical victims and their lawyers."
178. _____: "Chemicals, risk and the public." *Chicago Tribune*, Saturday, April 29, 1989.
179. *Dean, J. H., M. Luster, C. Boorman: "Methods and approaches for assessing immunotoxicity: an overview." *Env Hlth Persp* 1982; 43: 27.
179a. Dean, R. J.: "In defense of tight building syndrome." *For the Defense* 1991; Aug.: 2–6.
180. DeBruin, A.: *Biochemical Toxicology of Environmental Agents*. 1976; Elsevier, North Holland Biomedical Press.
181. DesCotes, J.: *Immunotoxicology of Drugs and Chemicals*. 1986, Elsevier, New York.
182. *DeSilva, P.: "TLVs to protect 'nearly all workers.'" *Appl Indus Hyg* 1986; 1:49–53.
183. Dick, R. B.: "Short duration exposures to organic solvents: the relationship between neurobehavioral test results and other indicators." *Neurotoxicol Teratol* 1988; Jan.-Feb. 10(1): 39–50. Short duration exposures to solvents at low concentrations can induce pre-narcotic effects: mucous membrane irritation, tearing, nasal irritation, headache, nausea—signs of mild toxicity. Higher exposures can induce narcosis: intoxication, incoordination, exhilaration, sleepiness, stupor, and the beginning stages of anesthesia. "Safe exposure levels are difficult to determine because: mild toxic effects are reported subjectively, solvent concentrations cannot be documented, and effects are reversible." The need to set limits is important to "prevent development of more serious cases of chronic solvent neurotoxicity."
184. *Dillard, C. J., R. E. Litov, W. M. Savin, et al: "Effects of exercise, vitamin E and ozone on pulmonary function and lipid peroxidation." *J of Appl Physiol* 1978; 45: 927. An example of research on the effects of a vitamin on the response to air pollutants.
185. Dinman, B. D.: "Arsenic: Chronic human intoxication." *J of Occ Med* 1960; 2: 137.
186. Dossing, M.: "Occupational toxic liver damage." *J of Hepatol* 1986; 3: 131–135. "There are good reasons for suspecting many industrial chemicals as hepatotoxic hazards." There is need to know "if continuous or intermittent

exposure to the various industrial chemicals with or without accompanying alcohol consumption may lead to liver disease. . . . Tests to reveal early hepatotoxic hazards in industry are urgently needed."

187. Doty, R. L., D. A. Deems, R. E. Frye, R. Pelgerg, A. Shapiro: "Olfactory sensitivity, nasal resistance, and autonomic function in patients with multiple chemical sensitivities." *Arch Otolaryngol* 1988; Dec. 114: 1422–1427. "The present results confirm a number of the largely anecdotal reports of somatic and behavioral symptoms of patients with MCS. It is apparent from these observations that individuals suffering from MCS are experiencing alterations in a variety of autonomic functions, including respiration and nasal airway patency. However, why or how such symptoms are triggered remains a mystery." (See 174a.)

188. *Drossman, D. A.: "The problem patient. Evaluation and care of medical patients with psychosocial disturbances." *Ann Int Med* 1978; 88: 366–372.

188a. Dudley, D. L., E. Welke: *How to Survive Being Alive*. Doubleday, New York, 1977.

189. *Duell, P. B., W. E. Morton: "Henock-Schonlein purpura following thiram exposure." *Arch Int Med* 1987; 147: 778–779. A case report of Henoch-Schonlein purpura which occurred coincident to a heavy exposure to the widely used industrial and agricultural agent tetramethylthiuram disulfide.

189a. Duffy, F. H.: "Clinical Value of Topographic Mapping and Quantified Neurophysiology." *Arch Neurol* 1989; 46: 1133–1134. The author's position on qEEG and evoked potentials data is that it functions best as an "organicity detector."

190. *Durlach, J.: "Rapports expérimentaux et cliniques entre magesium et hypersensibilité." *Rev Fr Allerg* 1975; 5: 133–146.

191. *Earley, L. W., O. Von Mering: "Growing old the outpatient way." *Am J of Psych* 1969; 125: 135–139.

192. *Eaton, K. K.: "The incidence of allergy—has it changed?" *Clin Allergy* 1982; 12: 107–110.

193. Ecobichon, D., R. Joy: *Pesticides and Neurological Diseases* 1982; Boca Raton: CRC Press, Inc.

194. *Edgar, R. T., E. Fenyves, W. Rea: "Air pollution analysis used in operating an environmental control unit." *Ann Allergy* 1979; 42: 166–173. Description of air sampling procedures used in Dr. Rea's environmental unit.

195. *Egger, J., et al: "Controlled trial of oligoantigenic treatment in the hyperkinetic syndrome." *Lancet* 1985; March (1): 540–545.

196. *Eisenberg, L.: "What makes persons 'patients' and patients 'well'?" *Am J of Med* 1980; 69: 277.

197. *Elias, J. A., A. I. Levinson: "Hypersensitivity reactions to ethylenediamine in aminophylline[1-3]." *Am Rev Resp Dis* 1981; 123: 550–552. A case report of severe exfoliative erythroderma after intravenous administation of aminophylline with subsequent positive skin patch testing to aminophylline and ethylenediamine, but not theophylline, suggesting a cell-mediated immune reaction.

198. Elliott, E.: "The future of toxic torts: of chemophobia, risk as a compensable injury and hybrid compensation systems." *Houston Law Review* 1988; 25: 781–786.

199. *Ellis, E. F.: "Clinical ecology; myth and reality." (University of) Buffalo ______________ 1986; 17: 24–28.

200. **Emergency Medicine*; April 30, 1986: 630. Summary of Stewart and Raskin's

Can Med Assoc J article. Views Environmental Illness as a new name for an old problem.

201. Environmental Hazard Management Institute: *Household Hazardous Waste Wheel.* P.O. Box 70, Durham NH 03824.
202. Estrin, W. J., S. A. Cavalieri, P. Wald, C. E. Becker, J. R. Jones, J. E. Cone: "Evidence of neurologic dysfunction related to long-term ethylene oxide exposure." *Arch Neurol* 1987; Dec. 44(12): 1283–1286. "Neurologic dysfunction may result from long-term low-dose exposure to ethylene oxide and . . . these effects may occur at exposure levels common in hospital sterilizer operations."
203. Evans, G., S. Colome, D. Shearer: "Psychological reactions to air pollution." *Env Research* 1988; 45: 1–15.

203a. Fackeledy-Larsen, L.: "About the BEAM." *CFIDS Chronicle* 1990; Spring-Summer: 57.

204. Fauci, A.: "The revolution in the approach to allergic and immunologic diseases." *Ann Allergy* 1985; 55: 632–633.
205. Fawcett, I. W., A. J. N. Taylor, J. Pepys: "Asthma due to inhaled chemical agents—epoxy resin systems containing phthalic acid anhydride, trimellitic acid anhydride and triethylene tetramine." *Clin Allergy* 1977; 7: 1–14.
206. *Febrega Jr., H.: "The idea of medicalization: an anthropological perspective." *Persp Biol Med* 1980; 24: 129–142.
207. Fein, G., J. Jaconson, et al: "Prenatal exposure to polychlorinated biphenyls: effects on birth size and gestational age." *J of Ped* 1984; 105: 315–320.
208. *Feldman, R. C., N. L. Ricks, E. L. Baker: "Neuropsychological effects of industrial toxins." *Am J of Ind Med* 1980; 1: 211–227.
209. Feldman, R. G.: "Occupational neurology." *Yale J of Bio Med* 1987; 60: 179–186.

    Clinical manifestations of headache, memory disturbance, and peripheral neuropathy are commonly encountered presentations of the effects of occupational hazards. . . . Occupational and environmental circumstances must be explored when evaluating patients with neurologic disorders.

210. Fenske, R., et al: "Potential exposure and health risks of infants following indoor residential pesticide applications." *Am J of Pub Hlth,* 1990; 80(6): 689–693.
211. Fiedler, N.: "Understanding stress in hazardous waste workers." *Occ Med* 1990; Jan.–March 5(1): 101–108.
212. Fielder, R.J., E. A. Dale, G. S. Sorrie, C. M. Bishop, M. Greenberg, B. H. Hogben, M. J. Van Der Heuvel, M. Topping: *Toxicity Review 8, Part 1, Trimellitic Anhydride (TMA).* 1983; Health and Safety Executive, London, Her Majesty's Stationery Office.
213. Findlay, G. M., A. S. W. deFreitas: "DDT movement from adipocyte to muscle cell during lipid utilization." *Nature* 1971; 229: 63–65.
214. *Fink, J. N., E. F. Banaszak, W. H. Thiede, J. J. Barboriak: "Interstitial pneumonitis due to hypersensitivity to an organism contaminating a heating system." *Ann Int Med* 1971; 74: 80–83. A careful case report of interstititial pneumonitis due to contamination of a furnace humidifier. The authors conclude that a "thorough environmental search should be carried out in all cases of so-called 'idiopathic' interstititial pulmonary disease."
215. *Finn, R., A. G. Gennerty, R. Ahman: "Hydrocarbon exposure and glomerulonephritis." *Clin Nephrol* 1980; 14: 173–175.

216. *Finnegan, M. J., C. A. C. Pickering, P. S. Burge: "The sick building syndrome: prevalence studies." *Brit Med J* 1984; 289: 1573–1575. A provocative prevalence study of symptoms associated with office buildings. Multi-system symptoms are present in an increased prevalence in mechanically ventilated and air conditioned buildings in contrast to "naturally ventilated" ones. Because of the design of the study, the "syndrome must be accepted as a definite entity and cannot be dismissed as hysteria." The authors conclude that "although the symptoms of the sick building syndrome do not represent a disease but rather a reaction to the working environment, the scale of the problem is probably considerable, and the high degree of dissatisfaction seen in the study demands attention from architects, engineers, and the medical community." The authors state that "more research is needed . . . of a longitudinal nature" and that "the facility to alter and measure numerous variables in the working environment and to question the workers repeatedly about their symptomatology should be included in the design of such a study."

217. *Fiore, M. C., H. A. Anderson, R. A. Hong, R. Golubjatnikov, J. Seiser, D. Nordstrom, L. Hanrahan, D. Belluck: "Chronic exposure to aldicarb-contaminated groundwater and human immune function." *Env Research* 1986; 41: 633–645.

218. *Fischer-Homberger E.: "Hyponchondriasis of the eighteenth century—neurosis in the present century." *Bull Hist Med* 1972; 46: 391–401.

219. Flanagan, R. J., M. Ruprah, T. J. Meredith, J. D. Ramsey: "An introduction to the clinical toxicology of volatile substances." *Drug-Saf* Sept.-Oct. 1990; 5(5): 359–383.

Acute poisoning with organic solvents and other volatile compounds now usually follows deliberate inhalation or ingestion of these compounds. . . . The products abused are cheap and readily available despite legislation designed to limit supply. Volatile substance abuse is not illegal and only a minority of abusers are known to progress to heavy alcohol or illicit drug use. . . . Clinically volatile substance abuse is characterised by a rapid onset of intoxication and rapid recovery. Euphoria and disinhibition may be followed by hallucinations, tinnitus, ataxia, confusion, nausea and vomiting. . . . Long term exposure to n-hexane is associated with the development of peripheral neuropathy, while prolonged abuse (notably of toluene or chlorinated solvents) can cause permanent damage to the central nervous sytem, heart, liver, kidney and lungs. . . .

220. Flodin, U., M. Fredriksson, B. Persson: "Multiple myeloma and engine exhausts, fresh wood, and creosote: a case-referrent study." *Am J of Ind Med* 1987; 12(5): 519–529.

Diesel-powered vehicles emit substantially more particles than do gasoline-powered vehicles with contemporary emission control systems. The DEP are submicron in size and readily inhaled. . . . In animal studies, exposure to high levels of DEP overwhelms the normal clearance mechanisms and results in lung burdens of DEP that exceed those predicted from observations at lower exposure concentrations. . . . Material contains more than a thousand individual compounds and is mutagenic.

221. ______, ______, ______, L. Hardell, O. Axelson: "Background radiation, electrical work, and some other exposures associated with acute myeloid leukemia

in a case-referrent study." *Arch Env Hlth* 1986; March-April 41(2): 77–84. "There was association between leukemia morbidity and background radiation, X-ray treatment, and electrical work. Styrene is a risk factor. Other factors less clearly associated."

222. Foo, S. C., J. Jeyaratnam, D. Koh: "Chronic neurobehavioural effects of toluene." *Br J of Ind Med* July 1990; 47(7): 480–484.

Statistically significant differences between workers exposed to toluene and controls in neurobehavioural tests measuring manual dexterity (grooved peg board), visual scaning (trail making, visual reproduction, Benton visual retention, and digit symbol), and verbal memory (digit span) were observed. Further, the performance at each of these tests was related to time weighted average exposure concentrations of air toluene. The workers exposed to toluene had no clinical symptoms or signs. The question arises as to whether these impairments in neurobehavioural tests are reversible or whether they could be a forerunner of more severe damage.

223. *Forman, H. J., E. I. Rotman, A. B. Fisher: "Role of selenium and sulfur-containing amino acids in protection against oxygen toxicity." *Lab Invest* 1983; 49: 148–153.
224. Foster, S., P. Chrostowski: "Inhalation Exposures to Volatile Organic Contaminants in the Shower." 1987. Presented: 80th annual meeting of the American Pollution Control Association June 21–26, 1987.
225. *Franck, C.: "Eye symptoms and signs in buildings with indoor climate problems ('office eye syndrome')." *Acta Ophthal* 1986; 64: 306–311. A study of eye irritation in office workers showing significant associations between symptoms and objective evidence of an unstable precorneal film or epithelial damage using the methods of "break-up time" and Lissamine green staining. Important research questions identified by the author include determining whether the observed changes in eye function are caused by the office environment or if they are a pre-existing condition which makes it more difficult to tolerate the conditions in the office. This is a possible avenue for investigation for CSD problems.
226. Franzblau, A., L. Rosenstock, D. L. Eaton: "Use of inductively coupled plasma-atomic emission spectroscopy (ICP-AES) in screening for trace metal exposures in an industrial population." *Env Research* 1988; June 46(1): 15–24.
227. Friedman, R.: *Sensitive Populations and Environmental Standards* 1981; The Conservation Foundation, Washington, DC.
228. *Galland, L.: "Biochemical abnormalities in patients with multiple chemical sensitivities." In: M. R. Cullen (ed.), "Workers with Multiple Chemical Sensitivities," *State of the Art Reviews,* Oct.–Dec. 1987; 2(4): 713–720; Hanley and Belfus, Philadelphia. Retrospective analysis of data gathered on patients seen in medical consultation in a non-occupational setting. Deficiencies in a variety of vitamins and enzymes were reported in both CSD and control patients.
229. *Galland, L.: "Magnesium and immune function, an overview." *Magnesium* (in press).
230. Gammage, R., S. Kaye (ed.): *Indoor Air and Human Health* 1985; Lewis Publishers, Chelsea MI.
231. Generoso, W. M., K. T. Cain, L. A. Hughes, G. A. Sega, P. W. Braden, D. G. Gosslee, M. D. Shelby: "Ethylene oxide dose and dose-rate effects in the mouse dominant-lethal test." *Env Mutagenesis* 1986; 8:1–7.

232. Gerdes, K., J. Selner: "Bronchospasm Following IV Dextrose." 1980. Presented: American College of Allergy, 36th Scientific Congress, Jan. 19–23, 1980.
233. Gershon, S., F. Shaw: "Psychiatric sequelae of chronic exposure to organophosphorus insecticides." *Lancet* 1961; 1: 1371–1374.
234. Gillner, M.: *Trimellitic anhydride (TMA)—A hazard analysis.* Information Secretariat, Swedish National Chemicals Inspectorate, P.O. Box 1384, S-171, 27 Solna, Sweden, 1989. 45 pp.
235. Givhan, R.D.: "A sniff penalty—one whiff can be too much for those who react to compounds in perfume." *Detroit Free Press,* March 18, 1990.
236. Glaser, R. A., J. E. Arnold, S. A. Shulman: "Comparison of three sampling and analytical methods for measuring m-xylene in expired air of exposed humans." *Am Ind Hyg Assoc J* 1990; March 51(3): 139–150. Comparison of the average and individual mixed to alveolar ratios of m-xylene and carbon dioxide showed that mainstream-mixed sampling was accurate and that sidestream-mixed sampling was not.
237. *Gleeson, J. G.: *Chemically induced immune disregulation closing Pandora's box.* Forensic Medicine Seminar 1984; Oct. 25; 41 pp. Tips for lawyers representing defendants in cases of alleged Chemically-Induced Immune Disregulation (CIID).

If plaintiff is successful in convincing a jury that the body's shield against disease has been lowered, then only a handful of complaints over the plaintiff's lifetime may not be attributable to the chemical exposure. Therefore, the claim of CIID must be considered to be an extremely dangerous one in terms of the damage potential.

Discusses standards for admission of expert testimony. Thinks CIID is like the "mythical story of Pandora, who was entrusted with a box containing all of the ills that could plague mankind and opened it. . . ."
238. Godish, T.: "Indoor air pollution in offices and other non-residential buildings." *J of Env Hlth,* Jan/Feb. 1986; 48(4): 190–195.
239. *Goerth, C. R.: "Trend of home work poses new health, safety challenges." *Occ Hlth Safety* 1984: 31. Cites forecasts that 15–20 million people will be employed at home by the end of the decade.
240. *Golbert, T. M.: "A review of controversial diagnostic and therapeutic techniques employed in allergy." *J of Allergy Clin Immunol* 1975; 56: 170.
241. Goldstein, R. A.: "Efforts by the United States to coordinate the prevention of occupational allergic diseases in the workplace." *J Allergy Clin Immunol* 1986; Nov. 78 (5 Pt 2): 1086–1088.

The investigator who studies OADs must realize that results may impact social, ethical, and moral issues that create economic dilemmas. This is different from most research endeavors, which create warm appreciation for research findings. Finally, the researcher may be asked to support, defend, or deny a position that argues or extrapolates beyond the scientific findings. . . . Confusion and distrust occasionally result. Working on OAD requires enormous understanding from the interested parties. Task force recommendations that fail to consider nonmedical and nonscientific needs for industry and labor are not likely to be welcomed or implemented."

242. Goldstein, R. A.: "Immune reactions in a changing environment. USA initiatives." *Int Arch Allergy Appl Immunol* 1989; 88(1–2): 256–258.

Among the disciplines available to assess adverse health consequences of xenobiotics ("strange" substances in our environment), application of modern immunological methods in concert with traditional toxicological studies have to date demonstrated significant progress in drug allergy, food allergy, environmentally induced lung disease and autoimmunity. These successes have come from the collaboration of immunologists, allergologists, pulmonologists, pharmacologists and toxicologists. In fact a newer discipline of immunotoxicology has emerged in order to deal with these complex issues. The National Institutes of Health, through a series of workshops and research initiatives, and in collaboration with other US government agencies, including the Environmental Protection Agency, the National Institute of Environmental Health Sciences, and the National Academy of Sciences, is attempting to foster research aimed at enhancing progress in the field of immunotoxicology. The overall aim is to encourage the use of modern immunologic approaches to the study of the alleged harmful effects of xenobiotics on the immune system. Success will permit the development of improved diagnostic tools followed by initiatives concerned with prevention. Results are expected to have an impact on social, legal, and economic issues within society.

243. Golos, N., et al: *Coping with Your Allergies* 1979; Simon and Schuster, New York.
244. *Goode, W. J.: "Encroachment, charlatanism and the emerging profession: psychology, sociology and medicine." *Am Soc Rev* 1960; 25: 902–914.
245. *Goodman, J. W., S. Fong, G. K. Lewis, et al: *Immunol Rev* 1978; 39: 35–59.
246. Grammer, L. C., K. E. Harris, M. A. Shaughnessy, P. Sparks, G. H. Ayers, L. C. Altman, R. Patterson: "Clinical and immunologic evaluation of 37 workers exposed to gaseous formaldehyde." *J of Allergy Clin Immunol* 1990; Aug. 86(2): 177–181.

Because there has never been a case of defined immunologically mediated respiratory or occular disease as a result of exposure to gaseous formaldehyde, this study used clinical and immunologic criteria developed for immunologic respiratory diseases that result from inhalational exposure to trimellitic anhydride. None of the workers had IgE or IgG antibody to F-human serum albumin or an immunologically mediated respiratory or occular disease caused by F; however, some of the workers appeared to experience irritant symptoms caused by workplace exposure to F or other irritant chemicals.

247. ______, R. Patterson: "Occupational immunologic lung disease." *Ann Allergy* 1987; 58(3): 151–159. Asthma and hypersensitivity pneumonitis occur in wide variety of occupations and from wide variety of antigens. Education for prevention and early treatment is needed.
248. Graneek, B. J., S. R. Durham, A. J. Newman-Taylor: "Late asthmatic reactions and changes in histamine responsiveness provoked by occupational agents." *Bull Eur Physiopathol Resp* 1987; 23(6): 577–581.
249. Grasso, P.: "Neurotoxic and neurobehavioral effects of organic solvents on the nervous system." *Occupational Medicine,* State of the Art Reviews, July–Sept. 1988; 3(3): 525–537; Hanley and Belfus, Philadelphia.

250. *Gray, P. B.: "Dioxin damage suit ties up courthouse and angers judiciary." *Wall Street Journal* 1987; Jan. 13: 1. Newspaper article describing a three-year toxic tort trial, *Kemner vs. Monsanto,* to determine whether citizens of Sturgeon, Mo., were harmed from a rail-car spill.
251. Green, M. A.: "Questions and answers: Allergic to everything: 20th century syndrome." *JAMA* 1985; 253(6): 842.
252. Greenfield, E. J.: *House Dangerous: Indoor Pollution in Your Home and Office and What You Can Do About It* 1987; Vintage Books, NY.
253. *Grieco, M.: "Controversial practices in allergy." *JAMA* 1982; 247(22): 3106–3111. A summary of studies which fail to establish effectiveness of 1) intracutaneous or low-level modified RAST titration as a guide to immunotherapy, and 2) provocative subcutaneous or sublingual testing or the leukocyto-toxicity assay for the diagnosis of food allergy.
254. Guillemin, R., M. Cohn, T. Melnechuk (editors): *Neural Modulation of Immunity* 1983; Raven Press, New York.
255. Gundy S.: "Cytogenetical studies on a large control population and on persons occupationally exposed to radiation and/or to chemicals." *Ann Ist Super Sanita* 1989; 25(4): 549–555.

All people are exposed to mutagens environmentally, occupationally, therapeutically or due to life style. 163 occupationally exposed to different kinds of mutagens. Chromosomal aberrations: 2 to 6 times higher in persons occupationally exposed to ionizing radiation; 2 to 4 times higher in persons occupationally exposed to chemical mutagens such as vinyl chloride and organic solvents such as benzene and toluene; 5 to 6 times higher in persons exposed to organophosphorus insecticides. Neither chromosomal aberration frequencies nor sister chromatid exchanges differed significantly between smokers and non smokers in control and exposed persons.

256. Gurka, G., R. Rocklin: Immunologic responses during allergen-specific immunotherapy for respiratory allergy. *Ann Allergy* 1988; 61: 239–243.
257. *Gyntelberg, F., et al: "Acquired intolerance to organic solvents and results of vestibular testing." *Am J of Ind Med* 1986; 9: 363–370.
258. Hackney, J., W. Linn, S. Karuza, R. Buckley, D. Law, D. Bates, M. Hazucha, L. Pengelly, F. Silverman: "Effects of ozone exposure in Canadians and Southern Californians. Evidence for adaptation?" *Arch Env Hlth* 1977; 32(2): 110–116.
259. ______, ______, J. Mohler, C. Collier: "Adaptation to short-term respiratory effects of ozone in men exposed repeatedly." *J of Appl Physiol* 1977; 43(1): 82–85.
260. Hadnagy, W., N. H. Sumayer: "Genotoxicity of particulate emission from gasoline-powered engines evaluated by short-term bioassays." *Exp Pathol* 1989; 37(1–4): 43–50.

Atmospheric pollutants, expecially airborne particulates, contain a large number of genotoxic substances capable of inducing human health effects via inhalation. One important source of air pollutants are exhaust particles from automobile traffic. This concerns mainly diesel exhaust for which genotoxic properties are evident. With respect to particle emissions produced by gasoline-powered cars little information on a genotoxic potential is available. In this study, 3 particulate emission extracts from different gasoline-powered cars driven with leaded or unleaded gasoline were investigated for cytotoxic and genotoxic activities. . . . All tested extracts were found to induce a broad spectrum of cytotoxic and genotoxic effects suggesting that gasoline exhausts are under high suspicion of contributing to health in human populations via air pollution.

261. Hafferty, W.: "Whose files are they anyway? Unlocking your health records." *Modern Maturity* April-May, 1991; 34(2): 68–70.
261a. Hallett, M.: "Treatment of peripheral neuropathies." *J of Neurol Neurosurg Psych* 1985; 48: 1193–1207.
262. *Hane, M. O., J. Axelson, C. Blume, et al: "Psychological function changes among house painters." *Scand J of Work Env Hlth* 1977; 3: 91–99.
263. *Hanninen, H.: "Psychological picture of manifest and latent carbon disulfide poisoning." *Br J of Ind Med* 1971; 28: 374–381.
264. *______, L. Eskelinen, K. Husman, et al: "Behavioral effects of long-term exposure to a mixture of organic solvents." *Scand J of Work Env Hlth* 1976; 4: 240–251.
265. Harkonen, H., A. Lehtniemi, A. Aitio: "Styrene exposure and the liver." *Scand J of Work Env Hlth* 1984; 10: 59–61.
266. Harrington, J. M., H. Whitby, C. N. Gray, F. J. Reid, T. C. Aw, J. A. Waterhouse: "Renal disease and occupational exposure to organic solvents; a case referrent approach." *Br J Ind Med* 1989; Sept. 46(9): 643–650. "No relation was found between exposure to 10 different solvents and renal cancer or glomerulonephritis."
267. Harrow, A. J.: *A Taxonomy of the Psychomotor Domain.* 1972; David McKay, New York.
268. Hattis, D., L. Erdreich, M. Ballew: "Human variability in susceptibility to toxic chemicals: A preliminary analysis of pharmacokinetic data from normal volunteers." *Risk Analysis* 1987; 7: 415–426.
269. Haustein, U. F., V. Ziegler: "Scleroderma and scleroderma-like diseases caused by environmental pollutants." *Derm Beruf Umwelt* 1986; May-June 34(3): 61–67. Inducing substances:

plastics (vinyl chloride, epoxy resins), solvents (chlorinated, aromatic, and aliphatic hydrocarbons), drugs (bleomycin, pentazocine), cocaine (abuse), and contaminated rapeseed oil. Paraffin and silicon can act as adjuvants and induce a progressive systemic sclerosis, the latter after long term exposure.

270. Hayes, R. B., T. Thomas, D. T. Silverman, P. Vineis, W. J. Blot, T. J. Mason, L. W. Pickle, P. Correa, E. T. Fontham, J. B. Schoenberg: "Lung cancer in motor exhaust-related occupations." *Am J of Ind Med* 1989; 16(6): 685–695."The 50% excess risk for lung cancer associated with employment in motor exhaust-related occupations could not be explained by greater use of cigarettes or by other occupational exposures among these workers."
271. Herbert, F. A., R. Orford: "Pulmonary hemorrhage and edema due to inhalation of resins containing tri-mellitic anhydride." *Chest* 1970; 76(5): 546–551.
272. *Herbert, V., W. T. Jarvis, G. P. Monaco: "Commentary: Obstacles to nutrition education." *Health Values: Achieving High Level Wellness* 1983; 7(2): 38–41. Warns of the dangers of the "gurus of nutrition misinformation." Believes that states should restrict the role of "alternative practitioners" since many are trained in "diploma mills" and their patients use them in place of orthodox medicine.

273. Herzberg, V. L., K. A. Smith: "T cell growth without serum." *J of Immunol* 1987; Aug. 15 139(4): 998–1004. "The realization that serum is only necessary for the earliest stage of T cell activation will now enable studies designed to identify the critical individual serum components and to define their mechanism of action."
274. *Hessl, S. M. : "Management of patients with multiple chemical sensitivities at occupational health clinics." In M. R. Cullen (editor), *Workers with Multiple Chemical Sensitivities,* State of the Art Reviews, Oct.–Dec. 1987; 2(4): 779–790; Hanley and Belfus, Philadelphia.
275. Heyer N., N. S. Weiss, P. Demers, L. Rosenstock: "Cohort mortality study of Seattle fire fighters: 1945–1983." *Am J of Ind Med* 1990; 17(4): 493–504. "In this analysis a trend of increasing risk with increasing exposure was observed for diseases of the circulatory system."
276. Hirzy, J., R. Morison: "Carpet/4-Phenylcyclohexane Toxicity: The EPA Headquarters Case." Presented at the annual meeting of the Society for Risk Analysis, October 1989, San Francisco.
277. Hirzy, J. W.: "Dialogue—The Other Voice from EPA: The Role of the Headquarters Professional Union." *Env Law Reporter* 1990; 20 ELR 10057–10060.
278. Hodgson, M. J., A. E. Heyl, D. H. Van Thiel: "Liver disease associated with exposure to 1,1,1-trichloroethane." *Arch Int Med* 1989; Aug. 149(8): 179–188. "1,1,1-trichloroethane should be reconsidered as an agent with potential hepatotoxicity in man."
279. *Hoffman, R. E., et al: "Health effects of long term exposure to 2, 3, 7, 8-tetrachlorodibenzo-p-dioxin." *JAMA* 1986; 255: 3031.
280. *Holmes, G. P., et al: "Chronic fatigue syndrome: a working case definition." *Ann Int Med* 1988; 108: 387–389. A proposal for a working definition to improve the comparability and reproducibility of clinical research and epidemiological studies, and to provide a rational basis for evaluating patients who have chronic fatigue of undetermined cause. The working definition was formulated by an informal working group of public health epidemiologists, academic researchers and clinicians who developed a consensus on the salient clinical characteristics of what was initially called Chronic Ebstein-Barre Virus Syndrome. The authors wisely chose to avoid giving a name to the syndrome which would imply a specific causal agent.
281. Hotz, P., J. Pilliod, D. Soederstroem, F. Rey, M. A. Boillat, H. Savolainen: "Relation between renal function tests and a retrospective organic solvent exposure score." *Br J of Ind Med* 1989; Nov. 46(11): 815–819. "Results suggest that relations do exist for the N-acetylbeta-D-glucosaminidase (NAG) activity, erythrocyturia, and, perhaps, albuminuria but not for the protein creatinine ratio or for leucocyturia."
282. *"How to read clinical journals: III. To learn about a diagnostic test." *Can Med Assoc J* 1981; 124: 869–872. Proposes six guides for reading articles about the clinical course and prognosis of diseases:
    1. Was an inception cohort assembled?
    2. Was the referral pattern described? (Four biases are possible: centripetal bias, poularity bias, referral filter bias and diagnosis access bias.)
    3. Was complete follow-up achieved? (Should be greater than 80 percent.)
    4. Were objective outcome criteria developed and used?
    5. Was the outcome assessment "blind"?
    6. Was adjustment for extraneous prognostic factors carried out?

    Articles not meeting these criteria should be discarded.

283. *"How to read clinical journals: IV. To determine etiology or causation." *Can Med Assoc J* 1981; 124: 985–990.
1. Were basic methods that were used weak or strong? Methods ranked from strongest to weakest include: randomized clinical trials, cohort studies, case-control studies and case studies.
2. Apply the diagnostic tests for causation by:
a. Is there evidence from true experiments in humans?
b. Is the association strong?
c. Is the association consistent from study to study?
d. Is the temporal relationship correct?
e. Is there a dose response gradient?
f. Does the association make epidemiologic sense?
g. Does the association make biologic sense?
h. Is the association specific?
i. Is the association analogous to a previously proven causal association. That is, the criteria for a clinical decision to act include a certainty about causation a consideration of the consequences of all alternative courses of action.

284. *"How to Read Clinical Journals: V. To Distinguish useful or even harmful therapy." *Can Med Assoc J* 1981; 124: 1156–1162. Outlines criteria for validity and applicability of intervention studies as:
1. Was the assignment of patients to treatments really randomized?
2. Were all clinically relevant outcomes reported?
3. Were the study patients recognizably similar to your own?
4. Were both statistical and clinical significance considered?
5. Is the therapeutic maneuver feasible in your practice?
6. Were all patients who entered the study accounted for at its conclusion?
The authors note that

study results and interpretations . . . may meet with considerable resistance when they discredit the only clinical approach currently available for managing a condition; clinicians still may elect to do something, even if it has no demonstrable benefit, rather than do nothing. Finally study results may be rejected, regardless of their merit, if they threaten the prestige or livelihood of their audience.

285. *Humphreys, S. L.: "An application of risk: pesticides in toxic tort litigation." *Toxics Law Reporter* 1987; Nov. 18: 696–704. Examines recent cases in pesticide litigation, focuses on emerging legal issues and problems associated with cases involving residential and occupational exposure to pesticides. Cites *Ferebee vs. Chevron*: "A cause-effect relationship need not be clearly established . . . before a doctor can testify that, in his opinion, such a relationship exists."

286. Hunter, D.: *The Diseases of Occupations.* 1978; Hodder and Stoughton, London.

287. Ikatsu, H., T. Nakajima, T. Okino, N. Murayama: "Health care of workers engaged in waste water treatment. 1) The exposure conditions to organic solvents in workers engaged in waste water treatment." *Sangyo Igaku* 1989; Sept. 31(5): 355–362. "Working conditions and health care for workers engaged in waste water treatment facilities" should be improved "to prevent workers from becoming intoxicated by organic solvents."

288. "Indoor Air Quality: Sick Building Syndrome" (author unidentified). *Medical/ Scientific Update,* 1986; Nov.-Dec. 5(10): 1–5. National Jewish Center for Immunology and Respiratory Medicine, Denver, Colorado. Identifies six symptoms: nasal, eye and mucous membrane irritation, lethargy or fatigue, dry skin, and headaches. Symptoms occur in repeated pattern. Etiologies: allergic, infectious, exposure to single chemical, and low level exposures.

289. Infurna, R., B. Weiss: "Neonatal behavioral toxicity in rats following prenatal exposure to methanol." *Teratology* 1986; June 33(3): 259–265. "Data suggest that prenatal MEOH exposure induces behavioral abnormalities early in life that are accompanied by overt toxicity."

290. Iregren, A.: "Effects on human performance from acute and chronic exposure to organic solvents: a short review." *Toxicology* 1988; May 49 (2–3): 349–358.

291. Ishikawa, S.: "Eye injury by organic phosphorus insecticides—preliminary report." *Jap J of Ophthalmol,* 1970; 15: 60–68.

292. ______, M. Miyata: "Development of myopia following chronic organophosphate pesticide intoxication: an epidemiological and experimental study." In W. H. Merigan, B. Weiss (editors), *Neurotoxicity of the Visual System.* 1980; Raven Press, New York.

292a. Itil, T. M., C. D. Patterson, N. Polvan, A. Bigelow, B. Bergey: "Clinical and CNS effects of oral and I.V. Thyrotropin-releasing hormone in depressed patients." *Dis Nerv Syst* 1975; 36(9): 529–536.

293. *IUES/WHO Working Group: "Use and abuse of laboratory tests in clinical immunology: critical considerations of eight widely used diagnostic procedures." *Clin Exp Immunol* 1981; 46: 662.

294. Jacobson, J., S. Jacobson: "New methodologies for assessing the effects of prenatal toxic exposure on cognitivie functioning in humans." In M. Evans (editor), *Toxic Contaminants and Ecosystem Health: A Great Lakes Focus* 1988; John Wiley and Sons, New York.

295. ______, ______, H. Humphrey: "Effects of in utero exposure to polychlorinated biphenyls and related contaminants on cognitivie functioning in young children." *J of Ped* 1990; 116: 38–45.

296. Jensen, L. K., H. Klausen, C. Elsnab: "Organic brain damage in garage workers after long-term exposure to diesel exhaust fumes." *Ugeskr-Laeger* 1989; Sept. 4, 151(36): 2255–2258.

Diesel motors are employed to an increasing extent for occupational transport and fumes from diesel driven vehicles constitute an increasing problem as regards atmospheric pollution but, in particular, they constitute a considerable risk to health for the workers exposed to diesel exhaust fumes in their daily work.

Study shows: 14 garage workers (2–29 years exposure). Symptoms: headache, vertigo, fatigue, irritation of mucous membranes, nausea, abdominal discomfort or diarrhea. Seven (more than 5 year exposure) complained of memory failure, difficulty concentrating, irritability, increased sleep requirement, psychological changes or reduced libido. Of the 7, 6 were given neuropsychological examination showing slight organic brain damage.

Diesel exhaust fumes contain many toxic substances: carbon monoxide, nitrous gases, sulphur oxides, aldehydes, and hydrocarbons.

297. *Jewett, D. L., M. R. Greenberg: "Placebo responses in intradermal provocation testing with food extracts" (abstract). *J of Allergy Clin Immunol* 1985; 75: 205.

298. Johnson, A., W. Rea: "Review of 200 Cases in the Environmental Control Unit, Dallas." Presented at the Seventh International Symposium on Man and His Environment in Health and Disease; Feb. 25–26, 1989, Dallas, Texas.
299. Joneja, J. V., L. Bielory: *Understanding Allergy, Sensitivity and Immunity, a Comprehensible Guide.* 1990, Rutgers University Press, New Brunswick.
300. *Jones, D. P.: "Pesticides stir fears, suits over ill effects." *Schenectady (NY) Gazette*, July 2, 1987. Newspaper article examining the controversy involving pesticide applications. A proponent of tightening regulations concerning lawn-spraying, Paul F. Gosselin, supervising inspector for the Massachusetts Pesticide Board, states, "We don't know all there is to know about the health effects of pesticides, so before all the reviews are done at the federal level, what we need to do is reduce exposure."
301. Jones, S. J., V. L. Yu, P. Rudge, A. Kriss, C. Gilois, N. Hirani, R. Nijhawan P. Norman, R. Will: "Central and peripheral SEP defects in neurologically symptomatic and asymptomatic subjects with low vitamin B12." *J of Neurol Sci* 1987; Dec. 82 (1–3): 55–65.
302. *Juhlin, L., et al: "Blood glutathione peroxidase levels in skin diseases: Effects of selenium and Vitamin E treatment." *Acta Derm-Venerol (Stockh)* 1982; 62: 211–214.
303. Kabiersch, A., A. del Rey, C. G. Honegger, H. O. Bosedovsky: "Interleukin-1 induces changes in norepinephrine metabolism in the brain." *Brain Behav Immun* 1988; Sept. 2(3): 267–274.
304. *Kailin, E., R. Collier: "Relieving therapy for antigen exposure" (letter). *JAMA* 1971; 217: 78.
305. Kaliner, M.: "Immediate hypersensitivity." *J of Allergy Clin Immunol* 1989; Dec. 84 (6 Pt 2): 1028–1031.
306. Kalliokoski, P.: "Solvent containing processes and work practices: environmental observations." *Prog Clin Biol Res* 1986; 220(3): 21–30. "Organic solvents still comprise a significant occupational health hazard." In Finland, proper enclosures and ventilation have made a difference in occupational exposure, but there are other factors to consider. There is "possible existence of solvent misuse. This may not develop into the level of solvent sniffing, but into a milder addiction. Workers may adopt habits that cause unnecessary exposure."
307. *Kalsner, S., R. Richards: "Coronary arteries of cardiac patients are hyperreactive and contain stores of amines: A mechanism for coronary spasm." *Science* 1984; March 30: 1435–1437.
308. Kammuller, M., N. Bloksma, W. Seinen: "Chemical-induced autoimmune reactions and Spanish toxic oil syndrome. Focus on hydantoins and related compounds." *Clin Toxicol* 1988; 26(3–4): 157–174.
309. Kare, M.: "Direct pathway to the brain." *Science* 1968; 163: 952–953.
310. *Katon, W., R. K. Ries, A. Kleinman: "The prevalence of somatization in the primary care." *Compr Psychiatry* 1984; 25(2): 208.
311. *Katz, D. H.: "The allergic phenotype. Manifestations of allergic breakthrough and imbalance in normal damping of IgE antibody production." *Immunol Rev* 1978; 1: 77–108.
312. *Kay, M. M. B.: "Aging of cell membrane molecules leads to appearance of an aging antigen and removal of senescent cells." *Gerontology* 1985; 42: 821.
313. Keefe, T., L. Mounce, et al: "Chronic neurological sequelae of acute organophosphate pesticide poisoning." *Arch Env Hlth* 43: 38–45.
314. Keefe, T. J., E. P. Savage, H. W. Wheeler: "3rd National study of hospitalized

pesticide poisonings in the United States, 1977–1982," 1989; Fort Collins, COM, Colorado State University.

315. *Kellner, R.: "Functional somatic symptoms and hypochondriasis, a survey of empirical studies." *Arch Gen Psych* 1985; 42: 821.
316. *______: *Somatization and Hypochondriasis.* 1986; New York, Praeger Scientific.
317. Kerr, F., J. Pozuelo: "Suppression of physical dependence and induction of hypersensitivity to morphine by stereotopic hypothalamic lesions in addicted rats." *Mayo Clinic Proceedings* 1971; 46: 653–665.
318. *Kessler, L. G., P. D. Cleary, J. D. Burke: "Psychiatric disorders in primary care: results of a follow-up study." *Arch Gen Psych* 1985; 42: 583.
319. Kime, Z. R.: *Sunlight* 1980; World Health Publications, Penrun CA.
320. King, D.: "Psychological and behavioral effects of food and chemical exposure in sensitive individuals." *Nutrition and Health* 1984; 3: 137–151.
321. *King, D. S.: "Can allergic exposure provoke psychological symptoms: a double-blind test." *Bio Psych* 1981; 16: 3–17.
322. *King, W. P., R. G. Fadal, W. A. Ward, R. J. Trevino, W. B. Pierce, J. A. Stewart, J. H. Boyles, Jr.: "Provocation-neutralization: a two-part study. Part II. Subcutaneous neutralization therapy: a multi-center study." *Otolaryngol Head Neck Surg* 1988; 99(3): 272–277.
323. *______, W. A. Rubin, R. G. Fadal, W. A. Ward, R. J. Trevino, W. B. Pierce, J. A. Stewart, J. H. Boyles, Jr.: "Provocation-neutralization: a two-part study. Part I. The intracutaneous provocative food test: a multi-center comparison study." *Otolaryngol Head Neck Surg* 1988; 99(3): 263–271.
324. *Kinnell, H. G.: "Total allergy syndrome" (letter). *Lancet* 1982; March 3; 628–629.
325. *Kirk-Othmer Encyclopedia of Chemical Technology,* third ed., Vol. 18, 1982; John Wiley and Sons, New York.
326. *Kitchner, I., R. Greenstein: "Low dose lithium carbonate in the treatment of post-traumatic stress disorder—Brief communication." *Milit Med* 1985; 150: 378.
327. Kitzhaber, J.: "A healthier approach to health care." In *Issues in Science and Technology,* 1990–91; Winter: 59–65. National Academy of Sciences, National Academy of Engineering, Institute of Medicine. The "Oregon Plan" seeks to extend coverage by prioritizing services on the basis of cost-effectiveness.
328. Klees, J. E., A. Lash, R. M. Bowler, M. Shore, C. E. Becker: "Neuropsychologic impairment in a cohort of hospital workers chronically exposed to ethylene oxide." *J of Toxicol Clin Toxicol* 1990; 28(1): 21–28. "CNS dysfunction and cognitive impairment may result from chronic ethylene oxide exposure in hospital central supply units."
329. *Klein, G. L., R. W. Ziering, Girsh, et al: "The allergic-irritability syndrome: four case reports and a position statement from the Neuroallergy Committee of the American College of Allergy." 1985; 55: 22–24. (Unidentified source.)
330. *Knave, B., B. Anshelm-Olsson, et al: "Long-term exposure to jet fuel. II. A cross-sectional epidemiologic investigation on occupationally exposed industrial workers exposed to various solvents." *Scan J of Work Env Hlth* 1978; 4: 19–45.
331. Kniker, W.: "Deciding the future for practice of allergy and immunology." *Ann Allergy* 1985; 55(2): 106–113.
332. *Kolb, L. C.: "Treatment of chronic post-traumatic stress disorder." *Curr Psych Ther* 1986; 23: 119.

333. *Koller, L. D.: "Effect of chemical sensitivity on the immune system." *Immunol Allergy Pract* 1985; 7: 405–417.
334. Kolstad, H. A., L. P. Brandt, K. Rasmussen: "Chlorinated solvents and fetal damage. Spontaneous abortions, low birth weight and malformations among women employed in the dry-cleaning industry." *Ugeskr-Laeger* 1990; Aug. 27 152(35): 2481–2482. Exposure to perchlorethylene, a chlorinated solvent, may cause reproductive failure. Among 886 women: 12 spontaneous abortions, one malformation, 10 low birth weight.
335. *Komisaruk, B. R., C. Beyer: "Responses of diencephalic neurons to olfactory bulb stimulation, odor and arousal." *Brain Research* 1972; 36: 153.
336. Kraljic, J., I. Zrilic, J. Saric: "Changes in the blood composition in workers exposed to solvents containing benzene." *Arch Hig Rada Toksokol* 1989; Dec. 40(4): 367–371. Results "show significant drop in number of leukocytes in workers exposed for a long time." After exposure ceased, number of leukocytes increased.
337. Krathwohl, D. R., B. S. Bloom, B. B. Masia: *Taxonomy of Educational Objectives (Handbook II: Affective Domain).* 1956; David McKay, New York.
338. Kraut, A., et al: "Neurotoxic effects of solvent exposure on sewage treatment workers." *Arch Env Hlth,* 1988; July-Aug. 43(4).
339. Kreiss, K.: "The epidemiology of building-related complaints and illness." In J. Cone, M. Hodgson (editors), "Problem Buildings: Building-Associated Illness and the Sick Building Syndrome." *Occupational Medicine,* State of the Art Reviews Oct.-Dec. 1989; 4(4): 575–592; Hanley and Belfus, Philadelphia.
340. Kroker, G., R. Marshal, T. Randolph: "Acrylic denture intolerance in multiple food and chemical sensitivity." *Clinical Ecology* 1982; 1(1): 48–52.
341. *Kumar, P., R. Marier, S. H. Leech: "Hypersensitivity pneumonitis due to contamination of a car air conditioner." *New England Journal of Medicine* 1981; 305: 1531–1532. A case report of mold contaminating a car air conditioner. Again emphasizes the need for clinical detective work.
342. Kurtz, P.: "Behavioral and biochemical effects of malathion." Study No. 51-051-73-76. Aberdeen Proving Grounds MD: U.S. Army Environmental Hygiene Agency.
343. Kusters, E., R. Lauwerys: "Biological monitoring of exposure to monochlorobenzene." *Int Arch Occ Env Hlth* 1990; 62(4): 329–331. In a study of 44 male subjects. "On the average workers excreted 3 times more 4-chlorocatechol than 4-chlorophenol. . . . No tendency for metabolite concentration to increase during workweek."
344. *LaDou, J. (editor): "The Microelectronics Industry." In *Occupational Medicine,* State of the Art Reviews, Jan. 1985; Hanley and Belfus, Philadelphia.
345. LaMarte, F., J. Merchant, T. Casale: "Acute systemic reactions to carbonless carbon paper associated with histamine release." *JAMA* 1988; 260(2): 242–243.
345a. Lamielle, M.: Statement before the Subcommittee on Health and Safety, U.S. House of Representatives, July 24, 1991.
346. ______: *The workplace environment: the good . . . the bad . . the sometimes impossible. Worklife* (a publication of the President's Committee on the Employment of People with Disabilities), Summer 1989.
347. Landrigan, P. J.: "Prevention of toxic environmental illness in the twenty-first century." *Env Hlth Persp* June 1990; 86: 197–199.

Previous introductions of new technologies have frequently resulted in unanticipated occupational and environmental illness. Prevention of such illness in the twenty-first century requires stringent application of two fundamental principles of public health: evaluation of new technologies before their introduction, and surveillance of exposed persons after the introduction of new technologies. Failure to establish these basic preventive mechanisms in advance will inevitably result in the development of new toxic diseases in the twenty-first century.

348. *Laseter, J. L., I. R. DeLeon, W. J. Rea, J. R. Butler: "Chlorinated hydrocarbon pesticides in environmentally sensitive patients." *Clinical Ecology* 1983; 2: 3–12.
349. *Last, J. M.: "Epidemiology and health information." In Last, J. M.: *Public Health and Preventive Medicine.* 1983; Appelton-Century-Crofts, Norwalk, Connecticut, pp. 9–74. Basic definitions of epidemiology.
350. Lavelle, M.: "Sometimes the U.S. just says 'No'." *Nat Law J* 1989; July 24, 11(46): 35–37. Non-acquiescence is simply opting not to follow the law of district and circuit courts. This throws a "wild card into the process of justice for any person who relies on Uncle Sam for benefits. . . ."
351. Leach, C. L., N. S. Hatoum, H. V. Ratajczak, C. R. Zeiss, P. J. Garvin: "Evidence of immunologic control of lung injury by trimellitic anhydride." *Am Rev Resp Dis* 1988; 137(1): 186–190. Sensitized serum and single TMA challenge as necessary and sufficient conditions for TMA induced lesions.
352. ______, ______, ______, ______, J. C. Roger, P. J. Garvin: "The pathologic and immunologic response to inhaled trimellitic anhydride in rats." *Toxicol Appl Pharmacol* 1987; 87(1): 67–80.
353. ______, ______, R. L. Sherwood, C. R. Zeiss, P. J. Garvin: "Pulmonary cellular and antibody response to trimellitic anhydride inhalation." *Inhalation Toxicology* 1989; 1(1): 37–47. Responses included capillary hemorrhage and severe inflammation.
354. ______, ______, C. R. Zeiss, P. J. Garvin: "Immunologic tolerance in rats during 13 weeks of inhalation exposure to trimellitic anhydride." *Fund Appl Toxicol* 1989; 12(3): 519–529.
355. *Lebowitz, M. D.: "Occupational exposures in relation to symptomatology and lung function in a community population." *Env Research* 1977; 14: 59–67. A community population study by a respected epidemiologist to determine whether workers encountered in a general population study show symptom rates and lung function impairment rates commensurate with their occupational exposure. It was found that many individuals had multiple exposures for varying lengths of time, and that those with exposures to smoke, auto exhaust and other compounds had higher rates of symptomatology and lung function impairment, and that these were often dose related. The authors conclude that there is benefit to studying those in the general population who have occupational exposures.
356. Ledbetter, A. D., C. L. Leach, N. S. Hatoum, J. C. Roger: "The generation and detection of particulate aerosols of trimellitic anhydride and trimellitic acid for inhalation exposures." *Am Ind Hyg Assoc J* 1987; 48(1): 35–38.
357. *Lee, R. E.: "Environmental hypersensitivity: would we really accept the results of sound research?" *Can Med Assoc J* 1986; 134: 1333–46.
358. *Legro, W.: "Under siege." *Organic Gardening* 1988; April: 58–60, 65–67. Describes the problems of farmers with what Dr. Alan Levin of San Francisco calls "CAIDS" (Chemically Acquired Immune Deficiency Syndrome). Levin asserts that a farmer suffers damage to both his nervous system and his immune system by repeated exposures to pesticides, insecticides, herbicides and fungicides.

359. Lemanske, Jr., R. F., M. Kaliner: "Late-phase IgE-mediated reactions. *J of Clin Immunol* 1988; Jan. 8(1): 1–13.

360. Letz, G. L. Wugofski, J. E. Cone, R. Patterson, K. E. Harris, L. C. Grammer: "Trimellitic anhydride exposure in a 55-gallon drum manufacturing plant: clinical, immunologic, and industrial hygiene evaluation." *Am J of Ind Med* 1987; 12(4): 407–417. "Material safety data sheet did not list TMA as ingredient. The measurement of PEFR may be useful in identifying TMA-exposed workers with late respiratory systemic syndrome."

361. *Levin, A., et al: "Immune complex mediated vascular inflammation in patients with food and chemical illness" (abstract). *Ann Allergy* 1981; 47: 138.

362. *Levin, A. S., V. S. Byers: "Environmental illness: a disorder of immune regulation." In: M. R. Cullen, editor, *Workers with Multiple Chemical Sensitivities*, State of the Art Reviews, Oct.–Dec. 1987; 2(4): 669–682; Hanley and Belfus, Philadelphia. A presentation by one of the proponents of the hypothesis that CSD is a disorder of immunoregulation. Summarizes data on T-cell helper/suppressor ratios in several populations.

362a. Levin, H.: "The evaluation of building materials and furnishings for a new office building." Submitted for publication in *Practical Control of Indoor Air Problems, Proceedings of IAQ '87*, sponsored by ASHRAE, June 1987.

363. *Levine, L. I.: "Treatment of '20th Century Disease'" (letter). *Can Med Assoc J* 1986; 134: 875.

364. *Levine, S. A.: "Oxidants/anti-oxidants and chemical hypersensitivities." *J of Biosocial Res* 1983; 4. Part 1: pp. 51–54; Part 2: pp. 102–105.

365. *______, J. H. Reinhardt: "Biochemical-pathology initiated by free radicals, oxidant chemicals and therapeutic drugs in the etiology of chemical hypersensitivity disease." *J of Orthomol Psych* 1983; 12: 166–183.

366. *Lewis, B. M.: "Workers with multiple chemical sensitivities: psychosocial intervention." In M. R. Cullen (editor), *Workers with Multiple Chemical Sensitivities*, State of the Art Reviews, Oct.–Dec. 1987; 2(4): 791–800; Hanley and Belfus, Philadelphia.

In the problem of MCS three elements emerge that involve the need for psychosocial assessment and intervention, including the occurrence of environmental exposures in the workplace, the recurrence of symptoms subsequently and the restriction in life style affecting patients and family members. Utilizing case material, the author discusses the implications of each of these diagnostic areas.

367. *Lewis T. R.: "Identification of sensitive subjects not adequately protected by TLVs." *Appl Indus Hyg* 1986; 1: 66–69.

368. *Leydecker, M. (GNS): "Chemicals imprison helpless woman." *The Pensacola (FL) Journal*, May 25, 1981. Newspaper article describing one woman's experience with "20th century disease."

369. Lezak, M. D.: *Neuropsychological Assessment* (2nd edition). 1983; Oxford University Press, New York.

370. Lieber, C. S.: "Microsomal ethanol-oxidizing system." *Enzyme* 1987; 37(1–2): 45–56. Sidelight: "acutely, ethanol consumption inhibits the metabolism of other drugs through competition for an at least partially shared microsomal detoxification pathway."

371. *Likoff, R., C. Znockes, et al: "Vitamin E and aspirin depress prostaglandin in protection of chickens against Escherichia coli infection." *Am J of Clin Nutr* 1981; 34: 245. Another study of the effects of drugs and vitamins on biologic function.

372. *Lindermann, C. G., C. M. Zitrin, D. F. Klein: "Thyroid dysfunction in phobic patients." *Psychosomatics* 1984; 25: 603–606.
373. *Lindstrom, K.: "Psychological performances of workers exposed to various solvents." *Scand J of Work Env Hlth* 1973; 2: 129–139.
374. *_____, H. Harkonen, S. Hernberg: "Disturbances in psychological functions of workers occupationally exposed to styrene." *Scand J of Work Env Hlth* 1976; 2: 129–139.
375. *Liska, B., W. Stadelman: "Accelerated removal of pesticides from domestic animals." *Residue Rev* 1969; 29: 51.
376. Liu, F. T., F. R. Bargatze, D. H. Katz: "Induction of immunologic tolerance to the trimellate haptenic group in mice: model for a therapeutic approach to trimellitic anhydride-induced hypersensitivity syndromes in humans." *J of Allergy Clin Immunol* 1980; 66(4): 322–326.
377. Lockey, R.: "Fatalities from immunotherapy and skin testing." *J of Allergy Clin Immunol* 1987; 79(4): 660–677.
378. Lolin, Y.: "Chronic neurologic toxicity associated with exposure to volatile substances." *Hum Toxicol* 1989; July 8(4): 293–300. "Main disorders associated with volatile substance abuse are peripheral neuropathy, cerebellar disease, chronic encephalopathy and dementia."
379. *Lowell, F. C.: "Some untested diagnostic and therapeutic procedures in clinical allergy" (editorial). *J of Allergy Clin Immunol* 1975; 56: 168–169.
380. *Lum, L. C.: "Total allergy" (letter). *Brit Med J* 1982; 284: 1044–45.
381. Lundholm, M., R. Rylander: "Occupational symptoms among compost workers." *J of Occ Med* 1980; 22: 256–257. "Exposure to sewage sludge and composted household garbage may cause acute symptoms including: fever, chills, eye infections, and diarrhea accompanied by increase in total immunoglobin levels and fibrogen degradation products in the urine from gram-negative bacteria and endotoxins."
382. *Luster, M., R. Faith, G. Clark: "Laboratory studies on the immune effects of halogenated aromatics." *Ann NY Acad Sci* 1979; 320: 473–486.
383. *_____, _____, _____: "Assessment of immunologic alteration caused by halogenated aromatic hydrocarbons." *Ann NY Acad Sci* 1979; 320: 572–578.
384. _____, D. Wierda, G. J. Rosenthal: "Environmentally related disorders of the hematologic and immune systems." *Med Clin North Am* 1990; March 74(2): 425–440. "Possibility that chemical induced damage to the immune system may be associated with potential pathological conditions."
385. Lux, W. E., J. F. Kurtzke: "Is Parkinson's disease acquired? Evidence from a geographic comparison with multiple sclerosis." *Neurology*, March 1987; 37(3): 467–471.

In the coterminous United States, MS mortality rates demonstrate a north-south gradient, which is confirmed by more sophisticated—and more expensive—prevalence studies. Mortality rates from idiopathic Parkinson's disease show a similar north-south gradient, and they correlate significantly with the MS mortality and prevalence data. This demonstration that Parkinson's disease may be place-related provides support for the hypothesis that Parkinson's disease, like MS, is an acquired, environmental illness.

385a. Lyles, W. B.: "Sick building syndrome." *Southern Med J* 1991; Jan. 84(1): 65–71.

386. *McCay, P. B., D. D. Gibson, K. L. Fong, K. R. Hornbrook: "Effect of glutathione peroxidase activity on lipid peroxidation in biological membranes." *Biochem Biophys Acta* 1976; 431: 459–469.
387. McClellan, R. O.: "Health effects of exposure to diesel exhaust particles." *Annu Rev Pharmacol Toxicol* 1987; 27: 279–300.

Diesel powered vehicles emit substantially more particles than do gasoline-powered vehicles with contemporary emission control systems. The DEP are submicron in size and readily inhaled. Approximately one-fourth of the particle mass inhaled by people is deposited in the pulmonary region, some of which is retained with a half-life of several hundred days. . . . Some studies . . . suggest exposure to DE enhances the effect of the known carcinogens.

388. *McClory, R.: "The yeast of our problems." *Chicago's Free Weekly Reader* 1988; Jan. 22:1, 16–24.

It is precisely this depressing sense of being sick all over that lead EI (Environmental Illness) sufferers to gravitate to clinical ecologists and to one another—that, and the bewildered expressions on the faces of many of the doctors by whom they have been treated. The ecologists offer an integrated explanation for their illness and a measure of cautious hope. Fellow sufferers offer support along with their own war stories. "When at any moment on any day you can be zapped by practically anything you come in contact with, you get desperate," says Lynn Lawson. "You simply have to get some answers."

389. McCrory, W., C. Becker, C. Cunningham-Rundles, R. Klein, J. Mouradian, L. Reisman: "Immune complex glomerulopathy in a child with food hypersensitivity." *Kidney International* 1986; 30(4): 592–598.
390. McDonald, A. D., J. C. McDonald, B. Armstrong, N. M. Cherry, R. Cote, J. Lavoie, A. D. Nolin, D. Robert: "Fetal death and work in pregnancy." *Br J of Ind Med* 1988; March 45(3): 148–157.
391. *McGovern, J. J.: "Correlation of clinical food allergy symptoms with serial pharmacological and immunological changes in the patient's plasma" (abstract). *Ann Allergy* 1980; 44: 57.
392. *______: "The role of naturally-occurring haptens in allergy" (abstract). *Ann Allergy* 1981; 47: 123.
393. *______, J. A. Lazaroni, M. F. Hicks, et al: "Food and chemical sensitivity: clinical and immunologic correlates." *Arch Otolaryngol* 1983; 109: 292–297.
394. *______, ______, P. Saifer, et al: "Clinical evaluation of the major plasma and cellular measures of immunity." *J of Orthomol Psych* 1983; 12: 60.
395. McGrath, K. G., D. Roach, C. R. Zeiss, R. Patterson: "Four-year evaluation of workers exposed to trimellitic anhydride—a brief report." *J of Occ Med* 1984; 26(9): 671–675.
396. *McKenna, P. J.: "Disorders with overvalued ideas." *Br J of Psych* 1984; 145: 579–585.
397. *McLellan, R. K.: "Biological interventions in the treatment of patients with multiple chemical sensitivities." In M. R. Cullen (editor), *Workers with Multiple Chemical Sensitivities,* State of the Art Reviews, Oct.–Dec. 1987; 2(4): 791-800; Hanley and Belfus, Philadelphia.

Emphasizing physiologic interventions, the author points out that such biologic approaches should be applied in the context of a more holistic therapeutic stra-

tegem. The author offers eclectic medical management techniques developed on the front line, fully recognizing that rarely are "cures" possible and that some approaches have theoretical scientific merit whereas others have evolved empirically.

398. *Maclennan, J. G. "Candida and 20th century disease" (letter). *Can Med Assoc J* 134: 1112–1113.
399. *Mage, D. T., R. B. Gammage: "Evaluation of changes in indoor air quality occurring over the past several decades." In R. B. Gammage, S. B. Kay, V. A. Jacobs (editors), *Indoor Air and Human Health* 1985: 5–36; Lewis Publishers, Chelsea MI. An excellent, concise summary of the changes in indoor air that have occurred inside residences and office buildings. The authors note that we are "in the era of synthetic organic materials." There is a "plethora of volatile organic compounds in the indoor environment" resulting from emissions from plastics, paints, sprays, pesticides, automotive interior products, personal and household items, furnishings and building materials." In forecasting future trends, the authors note that "next to nothing is known about human reactions to the simultaneous exposure to several organic compounds. Considering the biological activity of many VOC, this lack of knowledge is cause for concern. Future high priority research will be conducted to evaluate health effects, source locations and emission strengths of VOC. The authors note the increasing trend toward spending time indoors, the increasing proportion of people working indoors and the sizable increases forecast in the number of people working at home.
400. *Maiback, H.: "The excited skin syndrome (alias the angry back)." In K. Ring, G. Burg (editors), *New Trends in Allergy* 1981: 208–221; Springer-Verlag, New York.
401. Makower, Joel: *Office Hazards* 1981; Tilden Press, Washington DC. Identifies hazards common to the office setting.
402. *Mandell, M., A. Conte: "The role of allergy in arthritis, rheumatism and polysymptomatic cerebral, visceral and somatic disorders: a double-blind study." *J of Int Acad Prev Med* 1982; July 5–6.
403. Marjot, R., A. A. McLeod: "Chronic non-neurological toxicity from volatile substance abuse." *Hum Toxicol* 1989; July 8(4): 301–306. "Toluene and chlorinated hydrocarbons 1,1,1-trichloroethane and trichloroethylene can cause permanent damage to the kidney, liver, heart, and lung in certain volatile substance abusers."
404. *Marks, J. G., J. J. Trautlein, C. W. Zwillich, L. M. Demers: "Contact urticaria and airway obstruction from carbonless paper." *JAMA* 1984; 252: 1038–1040. An intriguing case report of a blinded challenge to carbonless copy paper which resulted in multiple symptoms including fatigue, headache, nausea, itching and mucosal burning. Flow volume loops demonstrated upper airway obstruction and plasma samples demonstrated decrease of PGE2, and elevations of PGF2alpha, thromboxane B2 and 6-keto-PGF1alpha. More carefully performed studies of this type are needed.
405. *Masa, L.: "The infection women don't talk about." *Parade* 1986; Aug. 17:17. Article concerning the problems of yeast infection in women. Alludes to the candida hypersensitivity hypothesis.
406. Marshall, E.: "The rise and decline of Temik." *Science* 1985; 229: 1370.
407. *______: "Woburn case may spark explosion of lawsuits." *Science* 1986; 234: 418–420. News article about the Woburn lawsuit alleging childhood leukemia resulting from TCE-contaminated wells.

408. *______, Title 15, "Pesticide Applicator's Law," Subtitle 02. Authority: Agriculture Article, $$2–103 and 5–204, Annotated Code of Maryland.
409. *Maryland Department of Agriculture, Title 15, "Pesticide Use Control," Subtitle 05. "Use and sale of pesticides, certification of pesticide applicators and pest control consultants and licensing of pesticide businesses." Authority: Agriculture Article, $$2–103 and 5–204, Annotated Code of Maryland.
410. Maryland State Department of Education: "Indoor Air Quality: Maryland Public Schools." 1987.
411. Massachusetts, Commonwealth of: *Indoor Air Pollution in Massachusetts: Final Report* 1989; Published by Michael J. Connolly, Secretary of State.
412. Massad, E., P. H. Saldiva, C. D. Saldiva, M. P. Caldeira, L. M. Cardoso, A. M. deMorais, D. F. Calheiros, R. da Silva, G. M. Boehm: "Toxicity of prolonged exposure to ethanol and gasoline autoengine exhaust gases." *Env Res,* 1986; Aug. 40(2): 479–486. "Comparative chronic inhalation study: results demonstrated that the chronic toxicity of the gasoline-fueled engine is significantly higher than that of the ethanol engine."
413. Massioui, F. E., F. Lille, N. Leservre, P. Hazemann, R. Garnier, S. Dally: "Sensory and cognitive event related potentials in workers chronically exposed to solvents." *J of Toxicol Clin Toxicol* 1990; 28(2): 203–219. "Findings support presence of minor dysfunction of the nervous system."
414. *Mathison, D. A., D. D. Stevenson, R. A. Simon: "Asthma and the home environment." *Ann Int Med* 1982; 97: 128–129. An editorial from the Divison of Allergy and Immunology at the respected Scripps Clinic and Research Foundation. Aeroirritants aggravate asthma in patients of all ages. Perhaps the greatest nemesis of asthmatic patients is tobacco smoke, so much so that many patients consider themselves allergic to smoke despite the fact that IgE reactivity to smoke per se does not account for the reaction. Other aeroirritants in the home may include fumes from cooking and heating appliances, dusts, fumes from chemical cleaning (especially oven cleaning) and gardening aids, fresh newsprint, smoke from fireplaces, aromatic terpines from evergreen Christmas trees, hairsprays and other aerosols.

For the asthmatic patient who has a history of exacerbaton of symptoms coincident to exposures to aeroallergens within the home and who is confirmed to have IgE antibodies to these by cutaneous tests, it is reasonable to recommend preventive measures to be taken to reduce the exposures.

Because most studies suggest that measures to reduce aeroallergens and aeroirritants in the home environment result in improvement of asthma, such measures need be considered in the management of the asthmatic patient. We assume these measures help reduce the smoldering irritation, edema and inflammation of the tracheobronchial tree that perpetuate asthma and the person's reactivity to other factors that contribute to his asthma.

415. *Matsumura, Y.: "The effects of ozone, nitrogen dioxide and sulfur dioxide on the experimentally induced allergic respiratory disorder in guinea pigs. I. The effect on sensitization with albumin through the airway. II. The effects of ozone on the absorption and the retenton of antigen in the lung. III. The effect of the occurrence of dyspneic attacks." *Am Rev Resp Dis* 1970; 102: 420–427; 102: 438–443; 102: 444–447.
416. *May, C.: "Food allergy: lessons from the past." *J of Allergy Clin Immunol* 1982; 69: 255–259.

417. Mendell, M. J., A. H. Smith: "Consistent Pattern of Elevated Syptoms in Air-conditioned Office Buildings: A Reanalysis of Epidemiologic Studies." *Am J of Pub Hlth* 1990; 1193–1199.
418. *Mendelson, G.: "'Compensation Neurosis': an invalid diagnosis." *Med J Aus* 1985; 142: 561.
419. *Mercurio, S. D., G. F. Combs: "Selenium-dependent glutathione peroxidase inhibitors increase toxicity of prooxidant compounds in chicks." *J of Nutr* 1986; 116: 1720–1726.
420. Merigan, W. H., B. Weiss (editors): *Neurotoxicity of the Visual System*. 1980; Raven Press, New York.
421. Metcalf, R. L., et al: "Laboratory model ecosystem studies of the degradation and fate of radiolabeled tri-, tera-, and pentachlorobiphenyl compared with DDT." *Arch Env Contam* 1971; 3: 151–163.
422. Metz, S.: "Anti-inflammatory agents as inhibitors of prostaglandin synthesis in man." *Med Clin North Am* 1981; 65(4): 713–753.
423. Miller, C.: "Mass psychogenic illness or chemically-induced hypersusceptibility?" Presented at the H.E.W. Symposium on the Diagnosis and Amelioration of Mass Psychogenic Illness, Chicago IL, May 30–June 1, 1979.
423a. Miller, C. S.: "Possible models for multiple chemical sensitivity." Paper presented at the Association of Occupational and Environmental Clinics, Washington DC, Sept. 20–21, 1991.
424. *Miller, J.: "A double-blind study of food extract injection therapy: a preliminary report." *Ann Allergy* 1978; 38: 37–50. A double-blind crossover study addressing the question of whether food extract injection reduced symptoms precipitated by foods. A correlation existed between decreased symptoms and the neutralizing dose. In three instances, subsequent placebo injections also were associated with decreased symptoms. The investigators conclude that this is a holdover phenomenon. The problem with this interpretation as initially presented by the California Medical Association Task Force is that "the interpretation of the investigator indicates that regardless of outcome, patients who received the neutralizing dose would improve (and therefore,) this study cannot be accepted as sound evidence. Further studies using this design strategy would appear to have merit, however." Statistically inappropriate data analysis.
425. *______: "Treatment of active herpes virus infections with influenza virus vaccine." *Ann Allergy* 1979; 42: 295–305. Study was not blinded, patients not randomly assigned.
426. *Miller, J. B.: "Hidden food ingredients, chemical food additives and incomplete food labels." *Ann Allergy* 1978; 41: 93–98. A discussion based on data from 1978.
427. *Miller, M.: "The untouchables." *Guideposts* 1982; April: 2–7.
428. *Miller, M. H.: "Accident Neurosis." *Brit Med J* 1961; 919–925, 992–998.
428a. Mishkin, M., T. Appenzeller: "The Anatomy of Memory," *Scientific American* Special Report, 1987.
429. Moeller, C., L. Odfvist, B. Larsby, R. Tham, T. Ledin, L. Bergholtz: "Otoneurological findings in workers exposed to styrene." *Scand J of Work Env Hlth* 1990 June; 16(3): 189–194. Eighteen workers' long term exposure (6–15 years). Disturbances in central auditory pathways (7 workers), abnormal central processing of impulses from different sensory equilibrium organs, larger sway area in posturography, poorer ability to suppress vestibular nystagmus in visual suppression test. Central nervous system disturbances from low level

styrene exposure may not be detected in psychometric testing but it may be apparent in otoneurological tests.

430. ______, L. M. Odkvist, J. Thell, B. Larsby, D. Hyden, L. M. Bergholtz, R. Tham: "Otoneurological findings in psycho-organic syndrome caused by industrial solvent exposure." *Acta Otolaryngol (Stockh)* 1989; Jan.–Feb. 107 (1–2): 5–12. "Test battery used strongly indicated CNS lesions due to industrial solvents."

431. Molhave, L.: "Dose-response relation of volatile organic compounds in the sick building syndrome." *Clinical Ecology* 1986/87; IV(2): 52–56.

432. *______, B. Bach, O. F. Pedersen: "Human reactions during controlled exposures to low concentrations of organic gases and vapours known as normal indoor air pollutants." In B. Berglund, T. Lindvall, J. Sundell (editors), *Indoor Air: Proceedings of the 3rd International Conference on Indoor Air Quality and Climate. Sensory and Hyperreactivity reactions to sick buildings.* 1984: 431–436. Swedish Council for Building Research, Stockholm, Sweden. A landmark study, the first in the world to systematically evaluate human responses to VOC mixtures. In response to controlled exposure to 5 mg/m^3 and 25 mg/m^3 of a mixture of 22 VOCs, symptoms of mucosal irritation were present and greater than clean air exposure. The level of each individual VOC alone would not have caused the symptoms. No adaptation was observed. This study suggests that low level exposure to VOCs can in fact be associated with symptoms.

433. *______, B. Bach, O. F. Pedersen: "Human reactions to low concentrations of volatile organic compounds." *Env Intl* 1986; pages unknown. Another paper describing Molhave's landmark study. "The reports on feelings of dry mucous membranes were strongly correlated with exposure, and correlated further with the questionnaire reports of irritation symptoms and deteriorated air quality but not to reports of odor intensity. The subjective evaluations about odor intensity and odor quality, therefore, seem to refer to different aspects of indoor air quality.

434. *Monro, J., J. Brostoff, C. Carini: "Migraine is a food-allergic disease." *Lancet* 1984; Sept.(2): 719–721.

435. *Montalbano, J.: "Bitter living through chemistry." *U of I Chicagoan* 1986; June 7: 16.

436. *Moore, J.: "The immunotoxicology phenomenon." *Drug and Chemical Toxicology* 1979; 5: 67.

437. *Mooser, S. B.: "The epidemiology of multiple chemical sensitivities (MCS)." In M. R. Cullen (editor), *Workers with Multiple Chemical Sensitivites,* State of the Art Reviews, Oct.–Dec. 1987; 2(4): 663–668; Hanley and Belfus, Philadelphia. Cites the absence of a uniform definition and common criteria making estimates of prevalence impossible. Cites need for further research.

438. Morgan, D., C. C. Roan: "The metabolism of DDT in man." *Toxicology* 1974; 5: 39–97.

439. Morgan, M. S., J. E. Camp: "Upper respiratory irritation from controlled exposure to vapor from carbonless copy forms." *J of Occ Med* 1986; 28: 415–419.

440. Morris, P. D., T. D. Koepsell, J. R. Daling, J. W. Taylor, J. L. Lyon, G. M. Swanson, M. Child, N. S. Weiss: "Toxic substance exposure and multiple myeloma: a case-control study." *J of Natl Cancer Inst* 1986; June 76(6): 987–994. Risk occurs with exposures to pesticide, painting materials, carbon monoxide, and borderline for metals and organically high polymers (plastics and elastomers). "No significant associations exist for exposure to fertilizer, dyes

and inks, alkalies, acids, other caustic substances, chemical asphyxiants, aliphatic hydrocarbons, chlorinated hydrocarbons, aromatic hydrocarbons, aldehydes and keytones, ethers, esters, oils, dusts, or asbestos."

441. Morrow, L., C. Thomas, et al: "PET and neurobehavioral evidence of tetrabromoethane encephalopathy." *J of Neuropsych* 1990; Fall 2(1): 341–345. Case report. Although, "organic solvents have been implicated in a variety of central nervous system (CNS) disturbances . . . the existence of solvent-induced encephalopathy remains controversial." PET scan to assess regional cerebral metabolic activity demonstrated variations (significant reduction in regional uptake); topographic EEG demonstrated asymmetry; neurobehavioral assessment demonstrated deficits in a number of functional areas. The MMPI showed "significant elevations on virtually every scale, with the largest elevations noted on the scales measuring depression, somatic concerns, anxiety, confusion, and disturbances in thought. In this case a negative CT and neurologic exam has led to a diagnosis of major depression with no organic involvement. Such misdiagnoses may lead to considerable hardship for persons who are labeled 'psychiatric' cases and denied work-related compensation or appropriate treatment."

442. Morrow, L. A., C. M. Ryan, G. Goldstein, M. J. Hodgson: "A distinct pattern of personality disturbance following exposure to mixtures of organic solvents." *J of Occ Med* 1989; Sept. 31(9): 743–746. Striking similarities to post–traumatic stress disorder.

443. ______, ______, M. J. Hodgson, N. Robin: "Alterations in cognitive and psychological functioning after organic solvent exposure." *J of Occ Med* 1990; May 32(5): 444–450. "Exposure to organic solvents has been linked repeatedly to alterations in both personality and cognitive functioning." Tested 32 workers with exposures to mixed organic solvents against blue collar workers with no history of exposure. "Significant differences in all cognitive domains other than general intelligence: learning and memory, visuospatial, attention and mental flexibility, psychomotor speed. In addition . . . clinically significant levels of depression, anxiety, somatic concerns, and disturbances in thinking were noted."

444. *Moses, M., R. Lilis, K. D. Crow, et al: "Health status of workers with past exposure to 2, 3, 7, 8-tetrachlorodibenzo-p-dioxin in the manufacture of 2, 4, 5-trichlorophenoxyacetic acid: comparison of findings with and without chloracne." *Am J of Ind Med* 1984; 5: 161.

445. *Muranaka, M., S. Suzuki, K. Koizumi, S. Takafuji, T. Miyamoto, R. Ikemori, H. Tokiwa: "Adjuvant activity of diesel-exhaust particulates for the production of IgE antibody in mice." *J of Allergy Clin Immunol* 1986; 77: 616. Provocative study which addresses the hypothesis that the increased prevalence of allergic rhinitis in Japan is due to the increase in air pollution due to diesel cars. Intraperitoneal injection of antigen mixed with diesel exhaust particles was associated with an increased primary IgE response and a persistent IgE antibody response when compared to injection of antigen alone.

446. Mustafa, M., D. Tierney: "Biochemical and metabolic changes in the lung with oxygen, ozone and nitrogen dioxide toxicity." *Am Rev Resp Dis* 1978; 118: 1061–1090.

447. Namba, T., C. Nolte, J. Jackrel, D. Grob: "Poisoning due to organophosphate insecticides." *Am J of Med* 1971; 50: 475–492.

448. National Academy of Sciences: *Drinking Water and Health.* Vol. I. National Academy Press, 1977.

449. ______, Institute of Medicine: "The Role of the Primary Care Physician in Occupational and Environmental Medicine." 1988.

450. National Archives and Records Administration, Office of the Federal Register: Code of Federal Regulations Title 20, Parts 1 to 399: "Employees' Benefits." Revised April 1, 1988. Contains the law regarding administration of the Office of Workers' Compensation Programs (federal government workers' compensation program).

451. National Center for Environmental Health Strategies: "Indoor Pollutants, Hèalth Risks and Involuntary Exposure to Fragrances." *The Delicate Balance*, March 27, 1990; p. 5. In an NIOSH study of 2,983 chemicals in the fragrance and cosmetic industry, 884 were identified as toxic. Of the 884, 314 cause biological mutations, 218 cause reproductive problems, 778 cause acute toxicity, 146 cause tumors, 376 cause skin and eye irritation.

452. National Federation of Federal Employees Local 2050 and American Federation of Government Employees Local 3331: "Indoor air quality and work environment study, EPA Headquarters buildings." Nov. 20, 1989.

453. *National Institute for Occupational Safety and Health: "Guidance for Indoor Air Quality Investigations." 1987; Cincinnati NIOSH. Guidance based on extensive experience evaluating indoor air quality complaints.

453a. National Research Council: *Biologic Markers in Immunotoxicology*. 1992; National Academy Press, Washington DC. In 1989 the American College of Physicians published a position statement on chemical sensitivity in an article titled "Clinical Ecology" by Abba Terr. This article has been used to discourage research and discriminate against CS patients. The National Research Council makes this statement (page 135) regarding Terr's conclusions: "Terr's conclusions are a poorly supported opinion expressed by one who has evaluated patients on behalf of a workers' compensation appeals board."

453b. ______: *Multiple Chemical Sensitivities Addendum to Biologic Markers in Immunotoxicology*. 1992; National Academy Press, Washington DC.

454. ______: *Toxicity Testing Strategies to Determine Needs and Priorities*. 1984; National Academy Press, Washington DC. Of the ingredients in fragrances, 84 percent have minimal or no toxicity or neurobehavioral toxicity data. The other 16 percent contain agents which can cause cancer, birth defects, central nervous system disorders, allergic reactions, chemical and multiple chemical sensitivity, and other effects.

455. National Safe Workplace Institute: *Beyond Neglect: The Problem of Occupational Disease in the U.S.—Labor Day '90 Report*. 1990; National Safe Workplace Institute, Chicago, Illinois.

456. National Toxicology Program. Symposium summary: "Immunological hypersensitivity resulting from environmental or occupational exposure to chemicals: A state of the art workshop summary." *Fund Appl Toxicol* 1982, 2: 327–330.

457. *Nelson, J. C.: "Treatment of patients with minor psychosomatic disorders." *Social Casework* 1969; 50: 581.

458. Nelson, N.: "Perspectives on diesel emissions health research." In J. Lewtas (editor), *Toxicological Effect on Emission from Diesel Engines*; 1982: 371–375; Elsevier Biomedical, New York.

459. Nero, A.: "Controlling indoor air pollution." *Scientific American* 1988; 258(5): 42–48.

460. New Jersey Department of Health, Division of Occupational and Environmental Health: *Surveillance of Occupational Illnesses, Injuries, and Hazards in New Jersey*. July 1988.

461. *New Scientist: "You are what you eat—or are you?" *Forum* 1984; Oct. 11: 34–36.
462. Newman-Taylor, A. J., K. M. Venables, S. R. Durham, B. J. Graneek, M. D. Topping: "Acid anhydrides and asthma." *Int Arch Allergy Appl Immunol* 1987; 83(3/4): 435–439. "Persistence of airway hyperresponsiveness in asthmatic patients after avoidance of exposure may indicate a permanent hyperresponsiveness caused by the asthma inducing exposure."
463. *Nikiforuk, G., M. Nikiforuk: Platforms: evidence for the 'hypersensitivity syndrome." *Can Med Assoc J* 1986; 134: 1343–1344. An angry rebuttal to Stewart and Raskin's paper which says that these authors "relegated a group of 18 patients 'purportedly suffering from 20th century disease' to two compartments of the psychiatric wastebasket: one for victims of depression and the other for those with somatiform disorder." The authors state that this "assails the use of vernacular science, i.e. labelling people on the basis of dubious, non-specific criteria." The authors cite a variety of studies in the area of immunotoxicology and make a plea for "a more positive dialogue . . . to marshall talent and resources to answer a basic simple question: Is hypersensitivity on the increase in the population."
464. *Noffsinger, L. (AP): "Some flee from pesticide spraying." *AP Domestic News* 1981; July 13.
465. "Occupational asthma from a low-molecular weight organic chemical" (author unidentified). *JAMA* 1980; 244(15): 1667–1668. Studied workers occupationally exposed to trimellitic anhydride. "Four respiratory syndromes: coughing or rhinorrhea; asthma or rhinitis; late respiratory systemic syndrome (LRSS). . . pulmonary disease anemia (PDA). . . . Coughing syndrome was a simple irritant effect, but the others were caused by immunologic sensitization."
466. Odkvist, L., et al: "Solvent-induced central nervous system disturbances appearing in hearing and vestibulo-oculomotor tests." *Clinical Ecology* 1985; 3(3): 149–153.
467. *O'Donnell, C., L. Friedman: "Allergic to life." *The Daily Herald*, Suburban Living Section 1986; Nov. 20: 1, 3.
468. *______, ______: "Doctor gets patient's blessings, not medic." *The Daily Herald*, Suburban Living Section 1986; Nov. 20: 3.
469. *______, ______: "Here's where to write or call." *The Daily Herald*, Suburban Living Section 1986; Nov. 20: 3.
469a. Onischenko, T. G.: "Cognitive rehabilitation." *CFIDS Chronicle* 1991; 1(2): 7–28. There are remarkable CFS-CS parallels: (1) the description here of "CFS dementia" and cognitive impairment common in the CS patient and (2) "multiple spotty lesions" shown in MRIs of CFIDS patients and patterns common to MRIs of CS patients which might be described in like manner. Though this article focuses only on CFS, researchers should compare these two groups with respect to brain impairment structurally, metabolically, electrically, and cognitively.
470. *Paglia, D. E., W. N. Valentine: "Studies on the quantitative and qualitative characterization of erythrocyte glutathione peroxidase." *J of Lab Clin Med* 1967; 70: 158–169.
471. Palassis, J., J. C. Posner, E. Slick, K. Schulte: "Air sampling and analysis of trimellitic anhydride." *Am Ind Hyg Assoc J* 1981; 42(11): 785–789.
472. Pan, Y., A. Johnson, W. Rea: "Aliphatic hydrocarbon solvents in chemically sensitive patients." *Clinical Ecology* 1987–88; 5(2): 126–131.

473. Parker, S. E.: "Use and abuse of volatile substances in industry." *Hum Toxicol* 1989; July 8(4): 271–275. Supports "occurrence for substance abuse (particularly organic solvents) in industry, but extent of practice is unknown. Proposed Control of Substances Hazardous to Health Regulations (COSHH) will bring greater emphasis on assessment of risk."
474. Parrish, G., W. Chrostek, R. Hartle: "Health hazard evaluation report no. HETA 82-355-1375, R and S Manufacturing Co., Columbia, Pennsylvania." *Govt Reports Announcements and Index (GRA&I)*, 1985, Issue 11.
475. Patel, J. M., E. R. Block: "Acrolein-induced injury to vascular endothelial cells." *In Vitro Toxicol* 1990; 3(3): 269–279. Acrolein is a reactive metabolite of a variety of environmental chemicals. It is implicated in vascular permeability. "Acrolein reacts with cellular glutathione and protein sulfhydryl, fluidizes membranes, and increases membrane leakiness. These changes were only partially reversible."
476. Patterson, R., W. Addington, A. S. Banner, G. E. Byron, M. Franco, F.A. Herbert, M. B. Nicotra, J. J. Pruzansky, M. Rivera, M. Roberts, D. Yawn, C. R. Zeiss: "Antihapten antibodies in workers exposed to trimellitic anhydride fumes: a potential immunopathogenic mechanism for the trimellitic anhydride pulmonary disease–anemia syndrome. *Am Rev Resp Dis*, Vol. 120, 1979; 1259–1267. "The pathogenesis of the TMA pulmonary disease and anemia syndrome may be a complex interaction between the chemical toxicity of TMA fumes, an immune reaction against TM haptenized proteins, degree of TMA fume exposure of the individual worker."
477. Patterson, R., K. E. Harris: "Responses of human airways to inhaled chemicals." N *Engl Reg Allergy Proc* 1985; 6(3): 238–240.

Sensitization to TMA can take several forms—IgE-mediated asthma and rhinitis, a late reaction in the lung which resembles hypersensitivity pneumonitis, and an irritated airways syndrome. Antibody studies show that TMA can combine with bodily constituents to form new antigenic determinants (NADs) *which are probably the most immunogenic form of the compound.*

478. ______, K. E. Harris, W. Stopford, G. Van der Heiden, et al: "Irritant symptoms and immunologic responses to multiple chemicals: importance of clinical and immunologic correlations." *Int Arch Allergy Appl Immunol* 1988; 85(4): 467–471.
479. ______, K. M. Nugent, K. E. Harris, M. E. Eberle: "Immunologic hemorrhagic pneumonia caused by isocyanates." *Am Rev Resp Dis* 1990; 141(1): 226–230. Immunologic hemorrhagic pneumonia from paint sprayed on warm metal surfaces.
480. *______, V. Pateras, L. C. Grammer, K. E. Harris: "Human antibodies against formaldehyde—human serum albumin conjugates or human serum albumin in individuals exposed to formaldehyde." *Int Arch Allergy Appl Immun* 1986; 79: 53.
481. ______, M. Roberts, K. E. Harris, D. Levitz, C. R. Zeiss: "Pulmonary and systemic immune responses of rhesus monkeys to intrabronchial administration of trimellitic anhydride." *Clin Immuno Immunopoathol* 15, 1980; 357–366.
482. ______, ______, C. R. Zeiss, J. J. Pruzansky: "Human antibodies against trimellityl proteins: comparison of specificities of IgA and IgE classes." *Int Arch Allergy Appl Immunol* 1981; 66(3): 332–340.
483–4. ______, I. M. Suszko, C. R. Zeiss, J. J. Pruzansky: "Characterization of

hapten-human serum albumins and their complexes with specific human antisera." *J of Clin Immunol* 1981; 1(3): 181–185.

485. ______, C. R. Zeiss, J. J. Pruzansky: "Immunology and immunopathology of trimellitic anhydride pulmonary reactions." *J of Allergy Clin Immunol* 1982; 70(1): 19–23.

486. Payan, D., J. McGillis, E. Goetzl: "Neuroimmunology." *Adv Immunol* 1986; 39: 299–323.

487. Pedretti, L. W., B. Zoltan: *Occupational Therapy Practice Skills for Physical Dysfunction,* 3rd Ed. 1990; C. V. Mosby, St. Louis.

488. Pekari, K., M. L. Riekkola, A. Aitio: "Simultaneous determination of benzene and toluene in the blood using head-space gas chromatography." *J of Chromatog* 1989; July 21 491(2): 309–320. An application of the method in monitoring exposed workers.

489. *Perona, G., et al: "In vivo and in vitro variations of human erythrocyte glutathione peroxidase activity as result of cells aging, selenium availablility and peroxide activation." *Br J of Haematol* 1978; 39: 399–408.

490. Persaud, T. V.: "The pregnant woman in the work place: potential embryonic risks." *Anat Anz* 1990; 170(3–4); 295–300. Risk factors identified: "industrial solvents, air pollution, water pollution, noise, anesthetic agents, and video display terminals."

491. *Pevsner, J., P. B. Sklar, S. H. Snyder: "Odorant-binding protein: localization to nasal glands and secretions." *Proc Natl Acad Sci* 1986; 83(13): 4942–4946.

492. Philpott, W., et al: *Brain Allergies: The Psycho-Nutrient Connection* 1980; Keats, New Canaan CO.

493. Pien, L. C., C. R. Zeiss, C. L. Leach, N. S. Hatoum, et al: "Antibody response to trimellityl hemoglobin in trimellitic anhydride-induced lung injury." *J of Allergy Clin Immunol* 1988; 82(6): 1098–1103.

493a. Pleil, J. D.: "Determination of organic emissions from new carpeting." *App Occ Env Hyg* 1990; Oct. 5(10): 693–699.

494. *Podell, R. N.: "Intracutaneous and sublingual provocation and neutralization." *Clinical Ecology* 1983; 11: 13–20.

495. Pope, B. L.: "Immunopharmacology: a new frontier." *Can J of Physiol Pharmacol* 1989; June 67 (6): 537–545.

496. *Porter, W. P., R. Hinsdell, A. Fairbrother, et al: "Toxicant-disease-environment interaction associated with suppression of immune system, growth and reproduction." *Science* 1984; 224: 1014.

497. *Prah, J. D., V. A. Benignus: "Trigeminal sensitivity to contact chemical stimulation: A new method and some results." *Perception and Psychophysics* 1984; 35: 65–68. An important research technique which allows direct examination of nasal trigeminal sensitivity without concomitantly stimulating the olfactory sense. This method could be used to test the hypothesis that individuals with chemical sensitivity disorders have a lowered threshold for trigeminal pain and irritation.

498. Prody, A. C., P. Dreyfus, R. Zimir, H. Zakut, H. Soreq: "De novo amplification within a 'silent' human cholinesterase gene in a family subjected to prolonged exposure to organophosphorous insecticides." *Proc Natl Acad Sci* 1988; 86(2): 690–694.

499. *Pross, H. F., J. H. Day, R. H. Clark, R. E. M. Lees: "Immunologic studies of subjects with asthma exposed to formaldehyde and ureaformaldehyde foam insulation (UFFI)." *J of Allergy Clin Immunol* 1987; 79: 797–810.

500. *Quill, T. E.: "Somatization Disorder. One of medicine's blind spots." *JAMA*

1985; 254: 3075–3079. Discussion of diagnostic criteria for somatization disorder and the importance of a long-term relationship with a primary care provider who will treat the patient and his symptoms seriously and respectfully but who is not compelled to invasively evaluate all symptoms.

501. Quinlan, P., J. M. Macher, L. E. Alevantis, J. E. Cone: "Protocol for the comprehensive evaluation of building-associated illness." *Occ Med* 1989; Oct.–Dec. 4(4): 771–797.

502. Randolph, T.: "Fatigue and weakness of allergic origin (allergic toxemia) to be,differentiated from nervous fatigue or neurasthenia." *Ann Allergy* 1945: 3: 418–430.

503. _____: *Environmental Medicine: Beginnings and Bibliographies of Clinical Ecology*. 1987; Clinical Ecology Publications, Fort Collins CO.

504. _____, R. Moss: *An Alterantive Approach to Allergies.* 1980; Lippincott and Crowell, New York.

505. *Randolph, T. G.: "Allergic-type reactions to industrial solvents and liquid fuels." *J of Lab Clin Med* 1954; 44: 910. The author observes that 1) many patients in Northwestern Indiana "remained chronically ill with specifically undiagnosed allergic-type manifestations"; 2) fumes are particularly irritating to allergic individuals; and 3) there is "no easy way to detect this subtle syndrome." Precipitating causes of allergic-type manifestations included fresh newsprint and rubbing alcohol. This is a clinical description without presentation of data.

506. *_____: "Allergic-type reactions to mosquito abatement fogs and mists." *J of Lab Clin Med* 1954; 44: 910. Descriptive abstract of multi-system symptoms reportedly associated with insecticide mists ranging from burning of the eyes to coughing to a stuporous depression to muscle aching.

507. *_____: "Sensory aspects of cerebral allergy." *J of Lab Clin Med* 1954; 44: 910. Descriptive abstract alluding to experimental exposures of "specifically sensitized individuals" to allergenic foods and drugs. The author believes that manifestations of cerebral allergy to include hyperesthesia, paresthesia, and anesthesia with anosmia, ageusia, transient numbness, analgesia, blindness, deafness and these symptoms have improperly been labelled "hysteria."

508. *_____: "Allergic-type reactions to motor exhausts." *J of Lab Clin Med* 1954; 44: 912. Report of symptoms associated with inhalation of auto exhaust including rhinitis, coughing, nausea, and abdominal cramps or cerebral reactions including "going to sleep at the wheel" and "drunkenness" in the absence of alcohol. Again, no controlled exposures are included in this clinical abstract report.

509. *_____: "Allergic-type reactions to chemical additives of food and drugs." *J of Lab Clin Med* 1954; 44: 913. The author states his clinical impression that misdiagnosis of food or drug allergy may be made in individuals with reactions to additives; he emphasizes presence of constitutional and cerebral symptoms.

510. *_____: "Allergic-type reactions to indoor utility gas and oil fumes." *J of Lab Clin Med* 1954; 44: 913. Abstract reporting 50 patients having symptoms consisting of "respiratory symptoms, chronic fatigue, myalgia, arthralgia, headache, generalized edema and cerebral manifestations varying from slowness of thought to stupor or mania." Again, no controlled exposure to assess symptoms.

511. _____: "Allergic-type reactions to synthetic drugs and cosmetics." *J of Lab Clin Med* 1954; 44: 914. Brief clinical description of a wide range of acute symptoms interpreted as indicating intolerance of "synthetic" drugs. Drugs

include sulfonamides, aspirin, synthetic vitamins, antihistamines, etc. Warns against a "chronic addictive" response which is a side effect of a medication repeatedly taken to control the primary response.

512. *_____: "Sodium bicarbonate in the treatment of allergic conditions." *J of Lab Clin Med* 1954; 44: 914. Refers to the "Acid-Anoxia-Endocrine Theory of Allergy" and advocates IV sodium bicarbonate to relieve acute and chronic allergic manifestations. Not a controlled trial.

513. *_____: "Depressions caused by home exposure to gas and combustion products of gas, oil and coal." *J of Lab Clin Med* 1955; 46: 942. Descriptive abstract showing association between exposures to utility gas and to combustion products of gas, oil and coal with a multi-system response with prominent depression. Not a controlled study.

514. *_____: *Human Ecology and Susceptibility to the Chemical Environment.* 1981. Charles C. Thomas, Springfield IL.

515. *_____: "Emergence of the specialty of clinical ecology." *Clinical Ecology* 1982–83; 1: 84–90.

516. *_____: "Graphic representation of clinical ecology." *Clinical Ecology* 1983; 2: 27–33.

517. *_____: "The development of ecologically focused medical care." *Clinical Ecology* 1985; 3: 6–16.

518. Rapoport, J. L.: "The biology of obsessions and compulsions." *Scientific American* 1989; March 260(3): 82–89.

519. *Raskin, N. H.: "Chemical headaches." *Ann Rev Med* 1981; 32: 63–71.

520. Rasmussen, K., S. Sabroe: "Neuropsychological symptoms among metal workers exposed to halogenated hydrocarbons." *Scand J of Soc Med* 1986; 14(3): 161–168. "Highly significant associations between exposure to halogenated hydrocarbons and symptoms of psychological dysfunction. A dose-response-like relation could be demonstrated."

521. Rea, W.: "Chemical hypersensitivity and the allergic response." *Ear Nose and Throat Journal* 1988; 67(1): 50–56.

522. _____, et al: "Toxic volatile organic hydrocarbons in chemically sensitive patients." *Clinical Ecology* 1987; 5(2): 70–74.

523. *Rea, W. J.: "Environmentally triggered thrombophlebitis." *Ann Allergy* 1976; 37: 101–109. Clinical description by one of the leading clinical ecologists.

524. *_____: "Environmentally triggered small vessel vasculitis." *Ann Allergy* 1977; 38: 245–251. Clinical description by one of the leading clinical ecologists.

525. *_____: "Environmentally triggered cardiac disease." *Ann Allergy* 1978; 40: 243–251. A report of twelve patients with "multi-symptomatology related to smooth muscle sensitization" and arrhythmias of unknown etiology with no evidence of arteriosclerosis on catheterization.

526. *_____: "Diagnosing food and chemical sensitivity." *Continuing Education* 1979; Sept. 47–59.

527. *_____: "The environmental aspects of ear, nose and throat disease: Part I." *J.C.E.O.R.L. and Allergy Digest* 1979; 41: 41–54.

528. *_____: "The environmental aspects of ear, nose and throat disease: Part II." *J.C.E.O.R.L. and Allergy Digest* 1979; 41: 54–56.

529. *_____: *Environmentally triggered disorders* 1982; Basal, Switzerland, Sandorama IV: 27–31.

530. *_____: "Ecologic orientation in thoracic and cardiovascular surgery." Chapter 73, pages 650–660 in *Clinical Ecology.*

531. *______: "The environmental aspects of cardiovascular disease" (source unknown). A summary paper with no specific data which includes a description of some of Rea's fundamental hypotheses including technological lag, total body load, masking or adaptation, bipolarity and biochemical individuality.

"The weight of the individual's environmental burden upon the body's homeostatic mechanisms appears to be an overwhelmingly important factor in the breakdown of resistance." (Note: the problem with this hypothesis is that in most instances it is not possible to measure an individual's environmental burden, and the measures of "breakdown of resistance" are not generally accepted.)

"Oedema, localized or general, seems to be the initial pathological event observed in most individuals sensitive to environmental incitants." (Note: the problem with this observation is that edema is a non-specific inflammatory response to a variety of stimuli. The presence of edema does not point to environmental triggers.)

Cardiovascular effects which Rea believes result from environmentally triggered diseases include nontraumatic phlebitis, nonarteriosclerotic arrhythmias, vasculitis, Raynaud's disease, mysotis, fibrositis, myalgias, and possible heart attacks and strokes. (Note: the problem with this list is that while there are specific reports of specific agents in specific instances being associated with these problems, the article does not provide these specific examples, and specific guidelines by which an individual practitioner could make these diagnoses in individual patients are lacking.)

532. *______: "Environmentally triggered large-vessel vasculitis." In F. Johnson and J. T. Spencer, Jr. (editors), *Allergy: Immunology and Medical Treatment.* Year Book Medical Publishers, Chicago: 185–187.

533. *______: "Reduction of chlorinated hydrocarbon pesticides with environmental control unit treatment." Chicago, 18th Advanced Seminar, American Academy of Environmental Medicine, 12 pages.

534. ______: "Relationship of food and chemical sensitivities to acute respiratory failure." *Clinical Ecology* (issue data unavailable).

535. ______, I. R. Bell, C. W. Suits, R. W. Smiley: "Food and chemical susceptibility after environmental chemical overexposure; case histories." *Ann Allergy* 1978; 41: 101–110.

536. *______, J. R. Butler, J. L. Laseter, I. R. DeLeon: "Pesticides and brain-function changes in a controlled environment." *Clinical Ecology* 1984; 2: 145–150.

537. ______, et al: "T & B lymphocyte parameters measured in chemically sensitive patients and controls." *Clinical Ecology* 1986; 4(1): 11–14.

538. *______, M. J. Mitchell: "Chemical sensitivity and the environmental." *Immunology and Allergy Practice* 1982; 4(5): 21–31, 157–67.

539. *______, D. W. Peters, R. E. Smiley, et al: "Recurrent environmentally triggered thrombophlebitis: a five-year follow-up." *Ann Allergy* 1981; 47: 338–344. Clinical description by one of the leading clinical ecologists. Describes study in which environmental modification allegedly prevented recurrent thrombophlebitis.

540. *______, R. N. Podell, M. L. T. Williams, et al: "Elimination of oral food challenge reaction by injection of food extracts." *Arch Otololaryngol* 1984; 110: 248–252. A presentation of studies on a selected group of patients who could be "neutralized" by the subcutaneous injection of food extracts. One neutralizing dose and two placebo doses were used, but the technician and subject

were informed after each injection was judged to be positive or negative, permitting educated guesses as to the identity of subsequent injections. The applicability of this study to a more general group of reactive subjects is unknown.

541.*______, C. W. Suits: "Cardiovascular disease triggered by foods and chemicals." In J. W. Gerrard: *Food Allergy: New Perspectives*; 99–113; Charles C. Thomas, Springfield IL.

542. Redlich, C. A., S. W. Beckett, J. Sparer, K. W. Barwick, C. A. Riely, H. Miller, S. L. Sigal, S. L. Shalat, M. R. Cullen: "Liver disease associated with occupational exposure to the solvent dimethylformamide." *Ann Int Med* 1988; 108(5): 680–686.

543. *Rees, W.: "Total Allergy" (letter) *Brit Med J* 1982; 284: 1044–1045.

544. Regenstein, Lewis: *How to Survive in America the Poisoned.* 1986; Acropolis Books, Washington DC.

545. Reidenberg, M., et al: "Lupus erythematosus–like disease due to hydrazine." *Am J of Med* 1983; 75: 363–370.

546. Reilly, F. D., R. E. McCafferty, E. V. Cilento: "Hepatic microvascular regulatory mechanisms. X. Effects of alpha-one or -two adrenoceptor blockade on glucoregulation in normotensive endotoxic ras with optimal perfusion and flowrates." *Microcirc Endothelium Lymphatics* 1988; Aug. 4(4): 293–309.

547. *Reinberg, A., E. Sidi, J. Ghata: "Circadian reactivity rhythms of human skin to histamine or allergen and the adrenal cycle." *J of Allergy* 1965; 36: 273–283.

548. Reinhold, R.: "When Life is Toxic." *New York Times Magazine,* Sept. 16, 1990; Section 6, p. 50–70.

549. "Report of the Ad Hoc Committee on Environmental Hypersensitivity Disorders." G. M. Thomson et al. 1985; Ministry of Health, Ontario, Canada (2 volumes).

550. *"Report of the American Industrial Health Council: Cancer, pollution and the workplace." The American Industrial Health Council; 15 pp.

551. *"Report of the Asthma and Allergy Foundation of America: The potential for quackery and questionable treatment in asthma and allergy medicine." Consumer Advisory Service Bulletin No. 1; 11 pp.

We believe that medical quackery involves the promotion and use by a health care provider of any diagnostic or treatment method, or drug based on claims that cannot be supported by what the body of responsible scientific and medical experts consider to be well-designed clinical trials (that is, free from human bias and repeatable.) Fraud involves the intention of any individual or organization to receive payment for health care services or products that have not been clearly shown to accomplish that which is promoted. Good allergy medicine: A personal history, physical examination, allergy testing and other laboratory testing. Good allergy treatment: avoid the substance that causes the allergic reaction. Where avoidance therapy is not practical or is ineffective, a wide selection of drugs is available to help relieve symptoms. Questionable practices include:

1. *Cytotoxicity Testing,*
2. *Provocation and Neutralization, and*
3. *Urine Autoinjection*

These practices substitute ineffective methods for practical medical technique and can rob an unsuspecting individual of precious time, money and the hope of relief.

552. *"Report of the Food Allergy Committee of the American College of Allergists on the clinical evaluation of the sublingual provocative testing method for diagnosis of food allergy." *Ann Allergy* 1974; 38: 185–191.
553. *"Report of the Food Allergy Committee of the American College of Allergists on the sublingual method of provocative testing for allergy," April 12, 1973. *Ann Allergy* 1973; 31: 382–385.
554. *"Report of the 36th Annual Congress of the American College of Allergists." *Convention Reporter* 10(8), June 1980 (newsletter).
555. *"Report of the U.S. Dept. of Health and Human Services: Sublingual provocative and neutralization therapy for food allergies." Assessment Report Series, HRST, 1981; 1(9); 6 p. Sublingual provocative testing and neutralization therapy for food allergy are widely used but lack scientific evidence of effectiveness. These therapies should be considered experimental at this time.
556. *Rest, K. M.: "Problems of special groups." In J. M. Last: *Public Health and Preventive Medicine*; 1986; Appleton-Century-Crofts, East Norwalk CT.
557. *Reynolds, R. D., C. L. Natta: "Depressed plasma pyridoxal phosphate concentrations in adult asthmatics." *Am J of Clin Nutr* 1985; 41: 684–688.
558. *Rich, L. A., J. Palenik: "Right to know in the lawn care industry's front yard." *Chemical Week*, Environment Section 1985; June 26: 15–16. Magazine article discussing the $2.3 billion chemical lawn care industry's opposition to right-to-know laws for lawn spraying. David Dietz, director of the Pesticide Public Policy Foundation of Salem OR, states "You can't legislate and you can't regulate on a general basis to protect the most hypersensitive person."
559. *Rinkel, H. J.: "Inhalant allergy: I. The wheeling response of the skin to serial dilution testing." *Ann Allergy* 1949; 7: 625–630.
560. Rinsky, R. A., A. B. Smith, R. Hornung, et al: "Benzene and Leukemia: An epidemiologic risk assessment." *New England Journal of Medicine* 1987; 316: 1044–1050.
561. *Ripperer, V.: "Total allergy syndrome" (letter). *Lancet* 1982; March 13: 628–629.
562. Rivera, M., M. B. Nicotra, G. E. Byron, R. Patterson, et al: "Trimellitic anhydride toxicity: a cause of acute multisystem failure." *Arch Int Med* 1981; 141(8): 1071–1074. Following TMA exposure patient experienced respiratory failure, anemia, gastrointestinal bleeding. Multisystem failure should signal occupational hazards search in differential diagnosis.
563. *Robertson, A. S., P. S. Burge, A. Hedge, J. Sims, F. S. Fill, M. Finnegan, C. A. Pickering, G. Dalton: "Comparison of health problems related to work and environmental measurements in two office buildings with different ventilation systems." *Brit Med J* 1985; 291: 373–376. A cross-sectional study of "building sickness" in two buildings. In the air conditioned building as opposed to the naturally ventilated building, there were increases in symptoms of rhinitis, nasal blockage and sore throat, lethargy, and headache. Enviromental assessment showed no difference between the two buildings in temperature, humidity, air velocity, positive and negative ions, carbon monoxide, ozone, and formaldehyde. The factors responsible for the differences in symptoms were therefore not identified.
564. Rodgers, Sherry A.: *The E. I. Syndrome: A Rx for the Environmental Illness.* 1986; Prestige Publishers, Syracuse NY.
565. ______: *Tired or Toxic?* 1990; Prestige Publishers, Syracuse NY.
566. *Rodin, J.: Somatoipsychics and attribution. *Person Soc Psychol Bull* 1978; 4: 531.

567. *Rogers, M. P., D. Dubey, P. Reich: "The influence of the psyche and the brain on immunity and disease susceptibility: a critical review." *Psychosom Med* 1979; 41: 147–164.
568. Root, D. E., et al: *Diagnosis and treatment of patients presenting subclinical signs and symptoms of exposure to chemicals which accumulate in human tissue.* Proceedings of the National Conference on Hazardous Wastes and Environmental Emergencies, May 14–16, 1987, Hazardous Materials Control Research Institute.
569. Root, D. E., G. T. Lionelli: Excretion of a lipophilic toxicant through the sebaceous glands: a case report. *J of Toxicol Cut and Ocular Toxicol* 1987; 6(1): 13–17.
570. Rosen, G., I. M Anderson, L. Juringe: "Reduction of exposure to solvents and formaldehyde in surface-coating operations in the woodworking industry." *Ann Occ Hyg* 1990; June 34(3): 293–303. Exposure reductions "through training, adjustment of existing equipment, and minor technical measures."
571. *Rosenberg, C.: *The Cholera Years.* 1962: 199–200; University of Chicago Press, Chicago.
572. Rosenberg, L. E., K. G. Haglid: "Long term neurotoxicity of styrene. A quantitative study of glial fibrillary acidic protein (GFA) and S-100." *Br J of Ind Med,* May 1989; 46(5): 316–320.

> *Little information exists about the possible neurotoxicity of styrene. The present study was designed to explore whether long term inhalation exposure (three months) to styrene (90 and 320 ppm) could induce long lasting astroglial alterations in Sprague Dawley rats. . . . It is concluded that exposure to styrene at moderate exposure levels induces regional, long lasting astroglial reactions that serve as an indicator of solvent induced brain damage.*

573. Rosenberg, S. J., M. R. Freedman, K. B. Schmaling, C. Rose: "Personality Styles of Patients Asserting Environmental Illness." *J of Occ Med,* Aug. 1990; 32(8): 678–681. This article delineates the position of the National Jewish Center for Immunology and Respiratory Medicine: environmental illness is psychiatric in etiology. Authors are no more able to prove that "urban air, organic solvents and pesticides, diesel exhaust, building materials, and tap water" are safe than that the etiology of environmental illness is psychiatric. (See 174a.)
574. Rosenstock, L., P. Demers, N. J. Heyer, S. Barnhart: "Respiratory mortality among firefighters." *Br J of Ind Med* 1990; July 47(7): 462–465. "Results indicate that firefighters are probably at increased risk for dying from nonmalignant respiratory disease."
575. Rosenstock, L., A. Hagopian: "Ethical dilemmas in providing health care to workers." *Ann Int Med* 1987; Oct. 107(4): 575–580. "Appropriate responses . . . can be formulated based on accepted ethical and legal principles."
576. Ross, James W.: *Social Security Disability Benefits.* 1984; Ross Publishing, Slippery Rock PA.
577. *Rossi, F. F.: "Modern evidence and the expert witness" (Source unknown). Discusses implications of 1975 Federal Rules of Evidence (702–705). Notes that the "Frye Standard" (the test is whether the theory is sufficiently established to gain general acceptance) is now in dispute. Courts in 15 jurisdictions have rejected Frye (all that is required is a showing of sufficient reliability to satisfy the requirement of relevance).

578. Rossiter, E.: "Pulmonary function in histology technicians compared with women from Michigan: effects of chronic low dose formaldehyde exposure on a national sample of women" (letter). *Br J of Ind Med* 1990 May 47(5): 358–360.
579. Rothschild, P. R.: *Enzyme-Therapy in Immune Complex and Free Radical Contingent Diseases.* 1988; University Labs Press, Honolulu HI.
580. Rotton, J., J. Frey: "Air pollution, weather and violent crimes: concomitant time-series analysis of archival data." *J of Person Soc Psychol* 1985; 49(5): 1207–1220.
581. *Roueche, B.: "Medical mystery: the doctor who was slowly being poisoned." *Med Econ* 1988; Feb. 15: 211–226.
582. Rousseau, D., et al: *Your Home, Your Health and Well-Being.* 1988; Hartley and Marks, Vancouver, British Columbia.
583. *Rozman, K., T. Rozman, H. Greim: "Enhanced fecal elimination of stored hexachlorobenzene from rats and rhesus monkeys by hexadecane or mineral oil." *Toxicology* 1981; 22: 33.
584. *Rundall, T. G.: "Evaluation of health services programs." In J. M. Last: *Public Health and Preventive Medicine;* 1986: 1831–1848; Appleton-Century-Crofts, East Norwalk CT.
585. Rushing, L. G., J. R. Althaus, H. C. Thompson: "Simultaneous determination of trimellitic anhydride and its trimellitic acid impurity by GC/FID." *J of Anal Toxicol* 1982; 6(6): 290–293.
586. Ryan, C. M., L. A. Morrow, E. J. Bromet, D. K. Parkinson: "Assessment of neuropsychological dysfunction in the workplace; normative data from the Pittsburgh Occupational Exposures Test Battery." *J of Clin Exp Neuropsychol* 1987; Dec. 9(6): 665–679.

Neuropsychologists are being increasingly called upon to assess the neurobehavioral status of adults who have been exposed to toxic chemicals or heavy metals. Unfortunately, the evaluation of blue-collar workers has been hampered by the absence of a brief yet comprehensive battery of sensitive neuropsychological tests that have been administered to a large cohort of demographically similar adults with no prior history of occupational exposure. The paper describes the development of the Pittsburgh Occupational Exposures Test Battery.

587. ———, ———, M. Hodgson: "Cacosmia and neurobehavioral dysfunction associated with occupational exposure to mixtures of organic solvents. *Am J of Psych* 1988 Nov. 145(11): 1442–1445. Administration of a battery of tests to solvent exposed and non-exposed blue collar workers. "Found exposed workers impaired across a wide range of cognitive domains. Given the apparent hypersensitivity of limbic structures to a wide range of . . . toxic agents, it would not be at all surprising to find anatomical and physiological evidence of limbic lobe damage in individuals who have experienced chronic occupational exposure to mixtures of organic solvents."
588. ———, ———, D. Parkinson, E. Bromet: "Low level lead exposure and neuropsychological functioning in blue collar males." *Int J of Neurosci* 1987 Sept. 36(1–2): 29–39. "There is little support for the view that older adults with current blood lead levels in the low to moderate range are at risk for developing significant CNS dysfunction, even though they may have had a past history of excessively high blood lead levels."

589. Ryan, J. J., D. J. Williams: *Symposium on chlorinated dioxins and dibenzofurans in the total environment II, 186th National Meeting of the American Society*, Washington, DC, Aug. 28–Sept. 2, 1983.

590. Saifer, P., N. Becker: "Allergy and autoimmune endocrinopathy: APICH syndrome." In J. Brostoff, S. Challacombe (editors), *Food Allergy and Intolerance*; 1987; 781–796; Bailliere Tindall, Philadelphia.

591. Sale, S. R., R. Patterson, C. R. Zeiss, M. Fiore, et al: "Immune response of dogs and rabbits to intrabronchial trimellitic anhydride." *Int Arch Allergy Appl Immunol* 1982; 67(4): 329–334. Death occurred in two dogs with low dose immunization, in two of four with moderate dose immunization, and in neither of two dogs with high dose immunization. Death did not correlate with levels of anti–TM-E antibody or anti–TM125I-DSA antibody binding, or lymphocyte reactivity. Autopsy revealed hemorrhagic pneumonitis in the four dogs.

592. ______, D. E. Roach, C. R. Zeiss, R. Patterson: "Clinical and immunologic correlations in trimellitic anhydride airway syndromes." *J of Allergy Clin Immunol* 1981; 68(3): 188–193.

593. *Salvaggio, J., L. Aukrust: "Mold induced asthma." *J of Allergy Clin Immunol* 1981; 68: 327–346. A postgraduate course presentation summarizing the biochemical and immunochemical characteristics, classification and taxonomy, complexity, cross reactivity, toxicity and clinical relevance of fungi, and therapeutic considerations for mold-induced asthma. The authors note that clinical and anecdotal evidence attests to the fact that many patients with positive skin tests to crude fungal extracts and bronchial asthma improve after empiric immunotherapy with crude extracts. He notes that

> *the practice of medicine will, to be sure, remain primarily an art rather than a science, and physicians will of necessity continue to use clinical judgement and weigh benefit/risk ratios in prescribing a large number of therapeutic procedures in all fields of medicine that have not been proved to be efficacious by controlled studies. Indeed, one could fill several pages with a list of commonly employed therapeutic procedures in all fields of medicine that have not been proved to be efficacious.*

While the authors accept that many practicing allergists will continue to use immunotherapy to treat mold-sensitive asthmatics, they caution that

> *appropriately controlled immunotherapy studies with mold extracts have simply not been carried out. The characterization and standardization of many species of fungal allergens will be necessary prerequisites to the undertaking of such clinical trials, and it is incumbent on those of us who use these procedures to carry out the necessary antigen characterization studies and controlled therapeutic trials.*

594. *Salvaggio, J. E.: "Presidential address—AAAI: Allergy and clinical immunology—2001." *J of Allergy Clin Immunol* 1986; 78(2): 253–268. Describes the expanding field of allergy and the study of non-IgE related disease processes.

595. Samet, J. (Chairman): "American Thoracic Society—Environmental Controls and Lung Disease (Report of the ATS Workshop on Environmental Controls and Lung Disease, Santa Fe NM, March 24–26, 1988)." *Am Rev Resp Dis* 1990; 142: 915–939.

596. *Samet, J. M., M. C. Marbury, J. D. Spengler: "Health effects and sources of indoor air pollution, Parts 1 and 2." *Am Rev Resp Dis* 1987; 136: 1486–1508.

597. Sandberg, D., C. Bernstein, R. McIntosh, R. Carr, J. Strauss: "Severe steroid responsive nephrosis associated with hypersensitivity." *Lancet* 1977; 1(8008): 388–391.
598. Santodononato, J., S. Bosch, W. Maylan, J. Becker, M. Neal: *Monograph on human exposure to chemicals in the workplace: trimellitic anhydride.* Center for Chemical Hazard Assessment, Syracuse Research Corporation, Syracuse, New York, 1985; Report No. SRC-TR-84-1048, 27 pp.
599. Sax, N. I., R. J. Lewis, Sr.: *Dangerous properties of industrial materials.* 7th Ed., Vol. 3. Van Nostrand Reinhold, New York.
600. Schaumberg, H. H., P. S. Spencer: "Recognizing neurotoxic disease." *Neurology* 1987; Feb. 37: 276–278. Makes the following points: (1) neurotoxic chemicals rarely destroy focal CNS/PNS areas; (2) clinical tests present limitations (testing may occur too late, since many neurotoxics are retained for weeks; there are no tests for many neurotoxics); (3) a strong dose-relationship exists between exposure and response; (4) exposure to different levels of a given toxic may result in different clinical pictures; (5) exposure and onset of illness occur concurrently or with brief latency; (6) chemical formula does not predict toxicity; (7) neurotoxic effect may be enhanced by "innocent-bystander" chemicals (those without known neurotoxic effect); (8) neurotoxic disease may be asymptomatic, and

> *Since many neurotoxic conditions result from prolonged, low-level exposure, and the diseases have an insidious onset, the relationship between toxicant and disease may be obscure to the patients. The clinician must probe for a background of occupational, environmental, or iatrogenic exposure.*

601. Schaumburg, I., K. Molsted: "The influence of chemical occupational environmental factors on reproduction in women in various occupations." *Nord Med* 1989; 104(5): 155–157. Possible hazards in occupations with exposures to: "pesticides, solvents, pharmaceutical products, textile colors, antineoplastic plastic drugs, anaesthetic gases, plastfumes, and metals."
602. Schmid, W. In A. Hollaender (editor): *Chemical Mutagens: Principles and Methods for Their Detection.* Vol. 4, 31–53. 1976; Plenum Press, New York.
603. Schmidt-Camelo, E. A.: "Changes in the intellectual function in workers exposed to mixtures of organic solvents." *Arch Invest Med (Mex)* 1989; Jan.–March 20(1): 107–112. "The intellectual functioning was diminished regarding the previous level in the exposed group and the parameters with more differences between the two groups were: attention, immediate memory, visuomotor coordination, and visual constructive ability." Inferior performance occurred in the exposed group not the non-exposed group.
604. *Schnare, D. W., M. Ben, M. G. Shields: "Body burden reductions of PCB's, PBB's and chlorinated pesticides in human subjects." *Ambio* 1984; 13(5–6): 378–380.
605. *______, G. Denk, M. G. Shields, S. Brunton: "Evaluation of a detoxification regimen for fat stored xenobiotics." *Med Hypoth* 1982; 9: 265.
606. ______, P. C. Robinson: "Reduction of hexachlorobenzene and polychlorinated biphenyl human body burden." International Agency for Research on Cancer, Scientific Publications Series 1986; 77: 597–603.
607. Schneider, Z.: "How clean is it? WashPIRG fights for a Clean Air Act worthy of the name." *WashPIRG REPORTS (the Report of the Washington Public Interest Research Group).* 1990; Summer 6(3): 4–6.

608. *Schottenfeld, R. S.: "Asbestos, lead and old lace: psychiatric manifestations of toxic exposures in the workplace." *Medical Times* 1985; 142(2): 198.

609. *______: "Workers with multiple chemical sensitivities: a psychiatric approach to diagnosis and treatment." In M. R. Cullen (editor), *Workers with Multiple Chemical Sensitivities,* State of the Art Reviews, Oct.–Dec. 1987; 2(4): 739–754; Hanley and Belfus, Philadelphia.

Based on a psychiatric approach, the author discusses the evidence suggesting that psychological factors are significant in leading to or perpetuating symptoms and disability in patients with MCS. He also comments on the role of biological vulnerability; social and cultural factors; associated psychiatric disorders; and finally the treatment implications of psychological and psychiatric diagnosis.

610. *______, M. R. Cullen: "Recognition of occupation-induced post-traumatic stress disorders." *J of Occ Med* 1986; 28: 365. This study excluded any individual with relevant physical impairment or diagnosis of organic mental disorders. (See 174a.)

611. *Schwab, J. H.: "Suppression of the immune response by microorganisms." *Bacteriol Rev* 1975; 39: 121–143.

611a. Schusterman D., J. Balmes, J. Cone: "Behavioral sensitization to irritants/odorants after acute overexposures." *J of Occ Med* 1988; 30: 565–7.

612. *Seelig, M. S.: "Mechanisms by which antibiotics increase the incidence and severity of candidiasis and alter the immunological defenses." *Bacteriol Rev* 1966; 30: 442.

613. Selner, J.: "Chemical sensitivity." In: *Current Therapy in Allergy, Immunology and Rheumatology*; 1988: 48–52; B. C. Decker, Philadelphia. This is one piece which has received significant negative reaction from those who recognize chemical sensitivity. This article is somewhat disjointed. It expresses the opinion that there are four categories of chemical exposures each with its own set of rules. The categories are ambient, occupational, domiciliary, and universal reactors (a diagnostic term associated with environmental medicine). The focus of the article is domiciliary and universal reactors. The author dismisses ambient and occupational exposures as known sources of chemical sensitivity (e.g., TMA causes four distinct clinical syndromes; TDI may be the result of pharmacological diisocyanate metabolites; contact dermatitis is chemical sensitivity). His discussion of domiciliary exposures appears under the heading "sick building syndrome," where he extends the definition of domiciliary to cover home and all the occupational exposures other than industrial. (A word choice other than domiciliary would be more appropriate.) He defines sick building syndrome as having the following symptoms: upper airway and eye mucous membrane involvement, dryness of skin, reddening and itching skin, mental fatigue, extreme awareness of odor. It is interesting that he classifies TMA exposure as occupational (industrial) when it also occurs in the home and office settings with the same set of symptoms. In the focus on universal reactors, he defines the group as not having objective signs and symptoms of disease related to a specific chemical. (Use of language is worth noting. In discussing TMA exposures, which are accepted as legitimate chemical sensitivity if exposure occurred in industrial setting, the term for symptoms is syndrome. In discussing universal reactors, the term disease is used.) In the discussion of universal reactors, the author

makes the following statement without having built up to it: "Psychologic interaction has tended to reveal a disturbing incidence of life threatening physical abuse and sexual abuse in early childhood among these patients."

Without logical buildup, such an idea inserted at the end of the piece could be interpreted as irresponsible, unscientific littering of the literature. Many questions should have been asked prior to publication, chief of which might have been, "What is this doing in here?" followed by "Does early childhood abuse invalidate contact dermatitis or occupational TMA exposure induced reactive airway disease?" or "Did right or left handedness of the patient correlate?"

614. *Selner, J. C., H. Staudenmeyer: "The practical approach to the evaluation of suspected environmental exposures: chemical intolerance." *Ann Allergy* 1985; 55: 665–673. A thoughtful proposal for approaches to the evaluation of chemical sensitivity disorders by a respected team of investigators. The authors state a belief that chemical intolerance is a real and growing problem in our society. They recommend controlled challenge testing with masking of odors as an essential part of the diagnosis and proper treatment of problems of chemical intolerance. They emphasize that in their experiences, chemical intolerance is multifaceted in its etiology, with some individuals objectively demonstrating specific sensitivities and others manifesting reactions to placebo challenges. The latter group are thought to have a somatoform disorder.

615. *______, H. Staudenmeyer: "The relationship of the environment and food to allergic and psychiatric illness." *Environmental and Food Allergies*; 102–146. Additional studies from a careful pair of investigators.

616. *Selye, H.: "The general adaptation syndrome and the diseases of adaptation." *J of Allergy* 1946; 17: 231.

617. Seppalainen, A. M., H. Harkonen: "Neurophysiological findings among workers occupationally exposed to styrene." *Scand J of Work Env Hlth* 1976; 2: 140.

618. Serve, M. P., B. M. Llewelyn, K. O. Yu, G. M. McDonald, C. T. Olson, D. W. Hobson: "Metabolism and nephrotoxicity of tetralin in male Fischer 344 rats." *J of Toxicol Env Hlth* 1989; 26(3): 267–275. "Tetralin is a component of fuels, solvents, and varnishes. . . . Rats treated with tetralin demonstrated the classic lesions of hydrocarbon-induced nephropathy."

619. Seuss, Dr. (Theodor Geisel): *The Lorax* 1971; Random House, New York.

620. *Shakman, R. A.: "Nutritional influences on the toxicity of environmental pollutants." *Arch Env Hlth* 1974; 28: 105–113.

621. *Sharma, R. P.: "Immunologic considerations in toxicology," Vols. I and II. 1986; CRC Press, Boca Raton FL.

622. Sharp, D. S., J. Osterloh, C. E. Becker, A. H. Smith, B. L. Holman, J. M. Fisher: "Elevated blood pressure in treated hypertensives with low-level lead accumulation." *Arch Env Hlth* 1989: Jan.-Feb. 44(1): 18–22.

623. Sherman, J.: *Chemical Exposure and Disease* 1988; Van Nostrand Reinhold, New York.

624. *Shim, C., M. H. Williams: "Effect of odors in asthma." *Am J of Med* 1986; 80: 18–22. A survey indicating that 57 of 60 asthmatics report respiratory symptoms on exposure to common odors. Challenge testing with cologne in four patients was associated with 18–58 percent declines below baseline. Pretreatment with metaproterenol and atropine reduced or prevented the decline. The substances which asthmatics indicated worsen their symptoms

fall into the general category of mixtures of volatile organic compounds (VOCs). While the title of the paper may suggest that the route of the effect is through the olfactory nerve, the authors indicate that other mechanisms may be responsible, including via an immunologic reaction, a local neural reflex, or a direct irritant effect. The authors do not address the question of whether prolonged exposure to the cologne would exacerbate the underlying asthma. Their practical advice is that sensitive asthmatic patients should be advised to eliminate odors from their environment as much as possible.

625. Shusterman, D., P. Quinlan, R. Lowengart, J. Cone: "Methylene chloride intoxication in a furniture refinisher. A comparison of exposure estimates utilizing workplace air sampling and blood carboxyhemoglobin measurements." *J of Occ Med* 1990; May 32(5): 451–454. "Methylene chloride (dichloromethane) is an organic solvent that has found wide use as a degreaser, paint remover, aerosol propellant, and a blowing agent for polyurethane foams, and as a solvent in food processing, photographic film production, and plastics manufacturing." It has known unusual metabolic conversion to carbon monoxide in vivo. It has an oncogenic effect in experimental animals. In workplace exposures conditions may prevail where "controls are inadequate to prevent acute toxicity, much less long-term exposure risks." Potential usefulness of COHb monitoring.

626. Siegel, R. K.: *Intoxication.* 1989; Simon and Schuster, New York.

627. Silverstein, M., N. Maizlish, R. Park, B. Silverstein, L. Brodsky, F. Mirer: "Mortality among ferrous foundry workers." *Am J of Ind Med* 1986; 10(1): 27–43.

628. ______, R. Park, M. Marmor, N. Maizlish, F. Mirer: "Mortality among bearing plant workers exposed to metalworking fluids and abrasives." *J of Occ Med* 1988; Sept. 30(9): 706–714.

629. Simon, G. E., W. J. Katon, P. J. Sparks: "Allergic to life: psychological factors in environmental illness." *Am J of Psych* July 1990; 147(7): 901–906. Article "suggests that psychological vulnerability strong influences chemical sensitivity following chemical exposure." (See 174a.)

630. *Sklar, P. B., R. R. Anholt, S. H. Snyder: "The odorant-sensitive adenylate cyclase of olfactory receptor cells." *J of Biol Chem* 1986; 216(33): 15538–15543.

631. Skov, P., O. Valbjorn: "Danish Indoor Climate Study Group: The sick building syndrome in the office environment: The Danish town hall study." *Env Intl* 1987; 13: 339–349.

632. Sly, R. M.: "Mortality from asthma." *J of Allergy Clin Immunol* 1988; 82(5): 705–717.

633. Smith, A. L.: *Microbiology and Pathology,* 9th edition. 1968; C. V. Mosby Company, St. Louis. Addresses chemical and immunologic injuries prior to 1970s.

634. *Smith, G. R., R. A. Monson, D. C. Ray: "Patients with multiple unexplained symptoms. Their characteristics, functional health and health care utilization." *Arch Int Med* 1986; 146: 69–72.

635. *Smith, H. M.: "The ultimate allergy—to the 20th century." *MD* 1983; July: 71–81.

636. Smith, K. A.: "Dissection of the molecular events occurring during T cell cycle progression." *Adv Exp Med Biol* 1987; 213: 125–128.

637. ______: "The bimolecular structure of the interleukin 2 receptor." *Immunol Today* 1988; Feb. 9(2): 36–37.

638. ______: "Interleukin-2: inception, impact, and implications." *Science* 1988; May 27 240(4856): 1169–1176.

639. *Snyder, S. H., P. B. Sklar, J. Pevsner: "Molecular mechanisms of olfaction." *J of Biol Chem* 1988; 263(28): 13971–13974.

640. *Society for Clinical Ecology. Position paper, 1983–1984. Environmental illness results from a hypersensitivity to food, water, chemicals or pollutants which can result in multiple symptoms and be a manifestation of immune system dysregulation.

Immune system dysregulation can develop over a long period of time and triggered by a single serious viral infection, major stress, fungi infection, particularly Candida albicans, *and accumulative exposure to toxic chemicals, even at low levels found in our everyday environment or massive chemical exposure. Immune system dysregulation often remains undiagnosed, however, because many physicians faced with its incredible array of seemingly unrelated symptoms and unfamiliar with the available diagnostic methods, misdiagnose it as stress, psychosomatic disease or the like. The medications commonly prescribed for these problems may suppress the symptoms to some extent but often further aggravate the problem without dealing with the underlying disease process. When the immune system is malfunctioning it causes a broad range of symptoms and reaction to a number of harmless or even beneficial substances entering the body. The malfunction commonly originates with the T cells. When the normal complement of T cells are reduced in number or when their ability to function is impaired, they can no longer adequately control B cell production of antibodies. Without this control the B cells cannot distinguish harmless dust pollen, animal dander or vital and nutritious foods from toxic chemicals or life-threatening bacteria or viruses. The actual healing process from immune system dysregulation is long, slow and punctuated by exasperating short-term setbacks. These setbacks are part of the healing process and invariably follow a roller coaster pattern. The frequency, duration and severity of setbacks gradually diminish until symptoms are mild and occur only occasionally.*

641. Sotaniemi, E. A., S. Sutinen: "Liver injury in subjects occupationally exposed to chemicals in low doses." *Acta Med Scand* 1982; 212: 207–215.

642. *Sparer, J.: "Environmental evaluation of workers with multiple chemical sensitivities: an industrial hygienist's view." In M. R. Cullen (editor), *Workers with Multiple Chemical Sensitivities,* State of the Art Reviews, Oct.–Dec. 1987; 2(4): 705–712; Hanley and Belfus, Philadelphia.

Using the approach of an industrial hygienist, the author discusses the worker's environment and the information that can be obtained from MCS patient and his workplace. Case studies are used to illustrate the collection of data and problem solving.

643. Sparks, P. J., G. E. Simon, W. J. Katon, L. C. Altman, et al: "An outbreak of illness among aerospace workers." *West J of Med,* July 1990; 153(1): 28–33. Another in the series by this group which reverses the standard medical approach of seeking first the physical ramifications of illness and then, if there is nothing there, turning to psychosocial areas. This article is negatively reviewed by William E. Morton, M.D., Dr. P.H., and Adrianne Feldstein, M.D., M.S., in *West J of Med,* Feb. 1991, page 225. Reviewers address above problem as well as others.

644. *Speer, F.: "The allergic tension-fatigue syndrome." *Pediatr Clin N Am* 1954; 1:1029.

645. Speizer, F., et al: "Palpitation rates associated with fluorocarbon in a hospital setting." *New England Journal of Medicine* 1975; 292(12): 624–626.

646. Spengler, J.: Testimony before the Ways and Means Committee, California State Legislature; Feb. 22, 1988.

647.*Spengler, J. D., K. Sexton: "Indoor air pollution: a public health perspective." *Science* 1983; 221: 9–17. A thoughtful article which establishes the basis for concern about indoor air pollution and calls for "an overall strategy to be developed to investigate indoor exposures, health effects, control options, and public policy alternatives."

648. Sprague, D. E., et al: "Chemical Sensitivity and Pesticides." *J of Pest Reform* 1986; Summer: 17–19.

649. ______, M. J. Milam: "Chemical sensitivity and pesticides." *J of Pest Reform* 1986; Summer: 17–19.

It appears that doubts about chemical sensitivity may have been due to insensitive laboratory techniques. Tody it is quite clear that not only does a relationship exist between chemical exposure and clinical symptoms, but that it exists at an exceedingly low level of exposure.

650. *Sprince, H., C. M. Parker, G. G. Smith: "Comparison of protection by l-ascorbic acid, l-cysteine, and adrenergic-blocking agents against acetaldehyde acrolein, and formaldehyde toxicity: implications in smoking." *Agents Actions* 1979; 9: 407–414.

651. Stankus, R., P. Menon, R. Rando, H. Glindmeyer, J. Salvaggio, S. Lehrer: "Cigarette smoke–sensitive asthma: challenge studies." *J of Allergy Clin Immunol* 1988; 82(3 Pt 1): 331–338.

652. Staudenmayer, H., J. C. Selner: "Neuropsychophysiology during relaxation in generalized, universal 'allergic' reactivity to the environment: a comparison study." *J of Psychosom Res* 1990; 34(3): 259–270. (See 174a.)

653. **Stedman's Medical Dictionary*. 1972; Williams and Wilkins, Baltimore.

654. Steenblock, D.: *Chlorella*. 1987; Aging Research Institute, El Toro CA.

655. Steenland, N. K., M. J. Thun, C. W. Ferguson, F. K. Port: "Occupational and other exposures associated with male end-stage renal disease: a case/control study." *Am J of Pub Hlth* 1990; Feb. 80(2): 153–157. Significant risk factors among 325 men ages 30–69: "consumption of phenacetin or acetaminophen, family history of renal disease, regular occupational exposure to solvents or silica. Particular occupational exposures: solvents used as cleaning agents and degreasers, silica exposures in foundries or brick factories or sandblasting."

656. *Stein, M., R. C. Schiavi, M. Camerino: "Influence of brain and behavior on the immune system." *Science* 1976; 191: 435–440.

657. *Steinbergs, C. Z.: "Removal of by-products of chlorine and chlorine dioxide at a hemodialysis center." *J of Am Water Works Assoc.* June 1986: 94–98.

658. Stein-Streilein, J. E.: CRISP Data Base, National Institutes of Health: Study lung hypersensitivity using 2,4,6 trinitro-1-chlorobenzene and dinitrofluorobenzene (similar chemicals to trimellitic anhydride). 1) "Pulmonary interstitial disease induced by haptens." CRISP/90/HL33709-04. Early and late toxic lesions. 2) "Immunological mechanisms in lung defense and disease." CRISP/90/HL01683-03. Pulmonary and systemic immune responses; delayed responses; natural killer cell activity; lung lesions. Etiology of pulmonary interstitial disease with respect to link between cellular immunity and lung pathology.

659. Stellman, J., M. S. Henifin: *Office Work Can Be Dangerous to Your Health* 1989; Fawcett Crest, New York.
660. *Sterling, D. A.: "Volatile organic compounds in indoor air: an overview of sources, concentrations and health effects." In R. B. Gammage, S. B. Kaye, V. Jacobs (editors), *Indoor Air and Human Health*: 387–402; 1985; Lewis Publishers, Chelsea MI. This author emphasizes the need to further identify and isolate the types of compounds consistently found indoors. "Because of the difficulty in assessing health effects to indoor nonoccupational exposures at low concentrations, more objective determinations of potential health effects from exposure to these compounds need to be developed."
661. *Stewart, D., J. Raskin: "Psychiatric assessment of patients with '20th Century Disease' ('total allergy syndrome')." *Can Med Assoc J* 1985; 133: 1001–1006. (See 174a.)
662. Strahilevitz, M., A. Strahilevitz, J. Miller: "Air pollutants and the admission rate of psychiatric patients." *Am J of Psych* 1979; 136(2): 205–207.
663. *Street, J.: "Methods of removal of pesticide residues." *Can Med Assoc J* 1969; 100: 16.
664. *"Sulfites in drugs and foods." *Medical Letter* 1986; 28: 74.
665. Sullivan, Jr., J. B.: "Immunological alterations and chemical exposure." *J of Toxicol Clin Toxicol* 1989; 27(6): 311–314. "Immunotoxicology is defined as an adverse response of the immune system to a chemical or drug which may result in disease such as autoimmunity, immune suppression, allergy or other hypersensitivity states. Occasionally, immune enhancement is the end result."
666. *"Summary Report of the Task Force on Immunology and Disease" (revised edition). In NIH publication No. 80-940: 144. 1980; U.S. Dept. of Health and Human Services, Bethesda MD.
667. Sunnyhill Research Center: "Recommendations for action on pollution and education in Toronto." Small and Associates, publishers. (No other publishing information available.)
668. *Supramaniam, G., J. O. Warner: "Artificial food additive intolerance in patients with angio-edema and urticaria." *Lancet* 1986; 11: 906.
669. Swanson, J.: *The psychological and educational implications of formaldehyde toxicology* (doctoral dissertation). 1984; University of Northern Colorado, Greeley CO.
670. *Taber, R. N.: "A unified theory of chemical hypersensitivity." *J of Orthomol Psych* 13: 1–9.
671. Tabershaw, I., W. Cooper: "Sequelae of acute organic phosphate poisoning." *J of Occ Med* 1966; 8(1): 5–20.
672. *Tabor, M.: "The stress of job loss." *Occ Hlth Safet* 1982; 5:20.
673. Takeuchi, Y.: "Visual disorders due to organic solvent poisoning." *Sangyo Igaku*, July 1988; 30(4): 236–247.

> *Visual ability has increasingly become very important in recent years in industry which has become highly automated with the rapid introduction of computers. On the other hand, visual disorder due to occupational activity pose a serious occupational health problem. . . . Visual disorders due to carbon disulfide, n-hexane, methanol, toluene, trichloroethylene, butanols, methylethyl ketone (MEK), styrene and mixed or unidentified solvents were reviewed together with corneal ulcer, lenticular changes, visual field changes, retinal changes, visual acuity impairment, acquired dyschromatopsia and other visual*

disorders due to these solvents. Visual disorders are often accompanied with impairment of the central and/or peripheral nervous system and can serve as early indicators of their impairment due to organic solvent poisoning. Especially, acquired dyschromatopsia can be an indicator for the early diagnosis of CNS impairment due to organic solvent poisoning.

674. Talan, J.: "Worried sick at work." *American Health* 1991; Jan.–Feb.: 24.
675. *Tarsh, M. J., C. Royston: "A follow-up study of accident neurosis." *Br J of Psych* 1985; 146: 18.
676. Taylor, G., W. Harris: "Cardia toxicity of aerosol propellants. *JAMA* 1970; 214(1): 81–85.
677. Taylor, S. L., R. K. Bush, J. C. Selner, J. A. Nordlee, M. B. Wiener, K. Holden, J. W. Koepke, W. W. Busse: "Sensitivity to sulfited foods among sulfite-sensitive subjects with asthma." *J of Allergy Clin Immunol* 1988; June 81(6): 1159–1167. "The likelihood of a reaction is dependent on the nature of the food, the level of residual sulfite, the sensitivity of the patient, and perhaps on the form of residual sulfite and the mechanism of the sulfite-induced reaction."
678. Tepper, J. S., B. Weiss: "Determinants of behavioral response with ozone exposure." *J of Appl Physiol* 1986; March 60(3): 868–875.
679. Terr, A.: "Clinical ecology in the workplace." *J of Occ Med* 1989; 31(3): 257–261.
680. *Terr, A. I.: "Environmental illness: review of 50 cases." *J of Allergy Clin Immunol* 1985; 75: 169.
681. *______: "Environmental illness: a clinical review of 50 cases." *Arch Int Med* 1986; 146: 145–149. Three assumptions were examined and disproved: 1) Environmentally induced illness is a disease entity with an identifiable set of clinical features; 2) A significant immunologic abnormality that distinguishes patients from normal persons; and 3) Treatment by clinical ecology methods results in improvement in clinical and relevant laboratory test abnormalities. A clinical review widely cited by opponents of clinical ecology. (See 174a.)
682. *______: "Editorial: Clinical ecology." *J of Allergy Clin Immunol* 1987; 79: 423–426. The heterogenous nature of the clinical presentation was highlighted. Terr did not perform blinded challenges to assess the validity of the diagnoses, so he assumed the diagnoses based on provocation-neutralization testing were invalid. Reportedly, only 2 patients improved, 26 were unchanged and 22 worsened. In the absence of a description of the natural history of their problem, it is not possible to say whether the treatment altered the course of the illness.
683. *______: "'Multiple chemical sensitivities': immunologic critique of clinical ecology theories and practice." In M. R. Cullen (editor), *Workers with Multiple Chemical Sensitivities,* State of the Art Reviews, Oct.–Dec. 1987; 2(4): 683–694; Hanley and Belfus, Philadelphia.

    This article is a critical review of the theories and practice of clinical ecology from the point of view of an immunologist, including commentary on articles from the clinical ecology literature and examination of clinical features, pathology, immunopathogenesis, laboratory evidence, diagnostic methods, treatment and course of the disease.

684. Teshigawara, K., H. M. Wang, K. Kato, K. A. Smith: "Interleukin 2 high-affinity receptor expression requires two distinct binding proteins." *J of Exp Med* 1987; Jan. 1 165 (1): 223–238.

685. Thomas, C. L. (editor): *Taber's Cyclopedic Medical Dictionary*, 16th ed. 1989; F. A. Davis Company, Philadelphia.
686. *Thomas, D. C.: "The newest mystery illness." *Redbook Special Medical Report* 1986; April: 120–121, 152–153.
687. Thrasher, J., R. Madison, A. Broughton, Z. Gard: "Building-related illness and antibodies to albumin conjugates of formaldehyde, toluene diisocyanate, and trimellitic anhydride." *Am J of Ind Med* 15(2): 1989, 187–195.
688. ______, A. Wojdani, G. Cheung, G. Heuser: "Evidence for formaldehyde antibodies and altered cellular immunity in subjects exposed to formaldehyde in mobile homes." *Arch Env Hlth* 1987; 42(6): 347–350. "Exposure to HCHO appears to stimulate IgG antibodies to F-HSA and decrease the proportion of peripheral T cells."
689. Thrasher, J. D.: "Chemical Injury" (lecture). July 18, 1989.
690. ______: "Immune activation and autoantibodies in humans with long-term inhalation exposure to formaldehyde." *Arch Env Hlth* 1990; July/Aug.
691. ______, A. Broughton, P. Micevich: "Antibodies and immune profiles of individuals occupationally exposed to formaldehyde: six case reports." *Am J of Ind Med* 1988; 14: 479–488.
692. ______, ______: *The Poisoning of Our Homes and Workplaces* 1989; Seadora, Inc., Santa Ana, CA. Focus is specific to immune system and effects of formaldehyde toxicity, including brief mention of other toxics.
693. Tollerud, D., J. Clark, L. Brown, C. Neuland, D. Mann, L. Pankiw-Trost, W. Blattner, R. Hoover: "The effects of cigarette smoking on T cell subsets." *Am Rev Resp Dis* 1989; 139(6): 1446–1451.
694. Topping, M. D., K. M. Venables, C. M. Luczynska, W. Howe, A. J. Newman-Taylor: "Specificity of the human IgE response to inhaled acid anhydrides." *J of Allergy Clin Immunol* 1986; 77(6): 834–842. In TCPA and TMA sensitization the "antibody combines with the anhydride and the spatially adjacent portion of the HSA molecule, whereas in the patients sensitized to PA, the antibody is specific for the hapten."
695. *"*Toxics Law Reporter*, Verdicts and Settlements: Environmental exposure. Infants' ailments not caused by landfill, court-appointed guardian Ad Litem concludes." *Toxics Law Reporter* 1986; Nov. 5: 615–616. "It is noted that in none of the thirty cases individually or as a group were reports rendered comparing the experiences of the infant plaintiffs as against a control group." In April 1985, Judge Joelson denied the defendants' motion for summary judgment and held that hazardous waste generators can be held liable for property damage or personal injuries, notwithstanding any safeguards undertaken to dispose of the toxic chemicals.
696. *"*Toxics Law Reporter*, Verdicts and Settlements: Environmental exposure. Jury clears aerojet of all claims in suits alleging immune system damage." *Toxics Law Reporter* 1986; Nov. 5: 613–615. Discusses a case of alleged immune system and psychological damage resulting from contamination of groundwater with trichloroethylene (TCE). The levels in the plaintiffs' well-water was TCE 520 ppb, dichloroethylene 80 ppb and tetrachlavethylene 32 ppb. Testimony included: "it was the general belief among industrial hygienists until the late 1970s that spent chlorinated solvents disposed of in the ground would evaporate harmlessly into the air or be rendered harmless by the curative powers of the earth!" The jurors found the risk assessment of Richard Wilson compelling: this level of TCE represented a potential risk of one additional cancer per one million members of the population.

697. Triebig, G.: "Occupational neurotoxicology of organic solvents and solvent mixtures." *Neurotoxicol Teratol* 1989; Nov.–Dec. 11(6): 575–578. "Experiences in occupational medicine in the Federal Republic of Germany do not support the assumption of high neurotoxic risks in solvent-exposed workers."
698. Turiel, I.: Indoor Air Quality and Human Health 1985; Stanford University Press, Stanford CA.
699. *_____, C. D. Hollowell, R. R. Miksch, J. V. Rudy, R. A. Young: "The effects of reduced ventilation on indoor air quality in an office building." *Environment* 1983; 17: 51–64. A study of an office building in San Francisco where employees noted irritant symptoms. In no case did levels of individual pollutants exceed standards, but levels were often higher indoors compared to outdoors.
700. "'Unbelievable' immune system response" (author and date unidentified). National Jewish Center for Immunology and Respiratory Medicine, Denver CO. LungLine Letter, 2–3. Philippa Marrack, Ph.D., and associates discovered that T cells in response to *Staphylococcus aureus* bacteria and certain food poisoning may flood the body with large quantities of chemicals which may cause an individual's feeling sick or even his death.
701. Unger, L. S., F. D. Reilly: "Hepatic microvascular regulatory mechanisms. VII. Effects of endoportally-infused endotoxin on microcirculation and mast cells in rats." *Microcirc Endothelium Lymphatics* 1986; 3(1): 47–74.
702. _____, _____: "Hepatic microvasulcar regulatory mechanisms. IX. Effects of compound 48/80 on endotoxin-induced changes in microcirculation and mast cell integrity." *Microcirc Endothelium Lymphatics* 1986; 3(2): 109–128.
703. *U.S. Center for National Health Statistics: *ICD-9-CM International Classification of Diseases, 9th revision, Clinical Modification*, Vols. 1, 2, and 3. DHHS Pub. No. (PHS)80–1260.
704. U.S. Coast Guard: *Manual I of the Chemical Hazards Response Information System (CHRIS)*. 1985; Washington DC.
705. U.S. Congress: *Neurotoxins [sic]: At Home and the Workplace*, 99th Congress, 2nd Session, Report 99-827, Sept. 16, 1986; U.S. Government Printing Office, Washington DC (71-0060).
706. _____: *Health Effects of Indoor Air Pollution*, 100th Congress, 1st Session, April 24, 1987, Senate Hearing 100-70, printed for use of the Committee on Environment and Public Works, U.S. Government Printing Office, Washington DC (73-934).
706a. _____: *Identifying and Controlling Immunotoxic Substances*. Office of Technology Assessment. April 1991, GPO Stock #OTA-BP-BA-75.
707. _____: *Issues Related to the Use of, and Exposure to, Various Chemicals*, 101st Congress, 1st Session, March 6, 1989, Senate Hearing 101-112, printed for use of the Committee on Environment and Public Works, U.S. Government Printing Office, Washington DC (96-831).
708. _____: H. R. 1530—*The Indoor Air Quality Act of 1989*, 101st Congress, 1st Session, July 20 and Sept. 27, 1989, No. 89, Congressional Hearing, printed for use of the Committee on Science, Space and Technology, U.S. Government Printing Office, Washington DC (26-090).
709. _____: *Neurotoxicity: Identifying and Controlling Poisons of the Nervous System*. Office of Technology Assessment. April 1990, GPO Stock #052-003-01184-1.
710. _____: *Indoor Air Quality Act of 1990*, S. 657, 101st Congress, 2nd Session, Rept. No. 101-304, May 24, 1990.

710a. U.S. Department of Health and Human Services, Public Health Service, Centers for Disease Control, National Institute for Occupational Safety and Health: *Health Hazard Evaluation Report (HETA 82-355-1375), R & S Manufacturing Company, Columbia, Pennsylvania.* TMA study.

711. _____: *NIOSH Current Intelligence Bulletin 48, Organic Solvent Neurotoxicity,* March 31, 1987. DHHS(NIOSH) Publication No. 87-104.

712. U.S. Department of Health and Human Services, Public Helath Service—National Institutes of Health, National Institute of Environmental Health Sciences: *Environmental Health Perspectives.*

Volume	Subject
1	Polychlorinated Biphenyls
2	Review—Perspective Articles
3	Phthalate Esters
4	Review—Perspective Articles
5	Chlorinated Dibenzodioxins and Dibenzofurans
6	Workshop on the Evaluation of Chemical Mutagenicity Data in Relation to Population Risk
7	Low Level Lead Toxicity and the Environmental Impact of Cadmium
8	Review—Perspective Articles
9	Asbestos
10	Mobile Air Emission, Biometeorological Hazards Abstracts on Heavy Metals in the Environment, Conference II
11	Components of Plastics Manufacture
12	Heavy Metals in the Environment
13	US-USSR Environmental Health Conference
14	Human Health Effects of New Approaches to Insect Pest Control
15	Target Organ Toxicity: Liver and Kidney
16	Target Organ Toxicity: Lung
17	WHO/NIEHS Symposium on Plastics Manufacture
18	Target Organ Toxicity: Development
19	Environmental Arsenic and Lead
20	Proceedings of the Second NIEHS Task Force
21	Vinyl Chloride Related Compounds
22	Air Pollution and Human Health Extrapolation from Animal to Man
23	Aspects of Polybrominated Biphenyls
24	Target Organ Toxicity: Gonads PCB's
25	Factors Influencing Metal Toxicity
26	Target Organ Toxicity: Cardiovascular System
27	Higher Plants as Monitors of Environmental Mutagens
28	Cadmium
29	Pollutants and High Risk Groups
30	USA/USSR Cooperative Research
31	Aneuploidy
32	JAPAN/USA Biostatistics: Statistics and the Environment
33	Target Organ Toxicity: Intestines Effects of Increased Coal Utilization NIEHS Science Seminar

Volume	Subject
34	Aquatic Toxicology: Biological Effects of Mineral Fibers and Particulates
35	Experimental Mode for Pulmonary Research
36	Application of Negative Ion Spectrometry
37	Pollen Systems
38	Target Organ Toxicity: Endocrine System
39	Target Organ Toxicity: Blood
40	Role of Metals in Carcinogenicity
41	Polyvinyl Chloride
42	Environmental Epidemiology
43	Target Organ Toxicity: Immune System
44	Target Organ Toxicity: Eye, Ear, and Other Senses
45	Phthalate Esters
46	Drinking Water Disinfectants
47	Mutagenicity and Carcinogenicity of Air Pollutants
48	Health Effects of Toxic Waste
49	N-Substituted Aryl Compounds
50	Tumor Promotion
51	In Vitro Effects of Mineral Dusts
52	Environmental Epidemiology Air Quality Control NIEHS Science Seminar
53	Asbestos
54	Metallothionein and Cadmium Nephrotoxicity
55	Monograph on Pulmonary Toxicology
56	Methods in Pulmonary Toxicology
57	Glycol Ethers: Mechanisms of Cell Injury
58	Carcinogenic Potency Database Formaldehyde
59	PCBs: Japan-U.S. Symposium
60	PCBs: U.S. Symposium
	Finland-U.S. Symposium
61	Monograph on Structure-Activity and Molecular Mechanisms
62	DNA Adducts
	Environmental Epidemiology
63	Health Effects of Acid Precipitation Environmental Risk Assessment
64	Monograph on Free Radicals
65	Metal-Binding Proteins Phthalic Acid Esters
66	Cotton and Grain Dusts
67	Dietary Mutagens
68	SENCAR Mouse: Author and Subject Indices, Volumes 41–60
69	Drinking Water Disinfectants
70	Airborne Pollutants and Respiratory Cancer: Reproductive and Developmental Toxicology
71	Aquatic Toxicology
72	Methyl Isocyanate
73	Ovarian Pathology Nitrogen Oxides
74	Biomarkers in Reproductive and Developmental Toxicology
75	NIEHS 20th Anniversary
76	Basic Research in Risk Assessment

77 Male Reproductive System
78 Lead–Blood Pressure Relationships: Author and Subject Indices, Volumes 61–73
79 Health Effects of Acid Aerosols
80 Monograph on Regulation of Differentiation in Eukaryotic Cell Systems
81 Scientific Advances in Environmental Health
82 Benzene Metabolism, Toxicity and Carcinogenesis
83 Monograph on Groundwater Quality
84 Calcium Messenger Service
85 Chemicals and Lung Toxicity Upper Respiratory System
86 Butadiene Environmental Health in the 21st Century
87 Biostatistics in Human Cancer Structure-Activity
88 Risk Factors and Mechanisms in Carcinogenesis
89 Advances in Lead Research
90 Methods for Environmental Quantitative Risk Assessment

713. ______: *Issues and Challenges in Environmental Health.* NIH Publication No. 87-861. (Not dated.)
714. ______: *Research Programs.* Jan. 1989; NIH Publication N. 89-2225.
715. U.S. Department of Health and Human Services, Social Security Administration: *Program Operation Manual System, Transmittal No. 12* (SSA Pub. No. 68-0424500), Feb. 1988.
716. ______: *What you have to know about SSI.* Jan. 1989; SSA Pub. No. 01-11011.
717. ______: *Supplemental Security Income.* July 1990; SSA Pub. No. 05-11000.
718. U.S. Department of Health, Education, and Welfare (now Health and Human Services), Public Health Service, Center for Disease Control, National Institute for Occupational Safety and Health: *NIOSH Current Intelligence Bulletin 21, Trimellitic Anhydride (TMA).* Feb. 3, 1978. DHEW (NIOSH) Publication No. 78-121. Human Toxicity: pulmonary edema, sensitization (rhinitis and/or asthma), TMA flu (delayed onset cough, wheezing, labored breathing), irritant effect (running nose, occasional nosebleeds, cough, labored breathing, occasional wheezing), immunologic sensitization.
    According to Asst. Surgeon General, J. Donald Miller, M.D., "trimellitic anhydride . . . can cause pulmonary edema, immunological sensitizations, and asthma symptoms." Warning: "NIOSH recommends that trimellitic anhydride be handled in the workplace as an extremely toxic substance."
719. U.S. Department of Housing and Urban Development, Office of the Assistant Secretary for Housing—Federal Housing Commissioner: "Manufactured Home Construction and Safety Standards; Final Rule." *Federal Register,* Aug. 9, 1984; 31999-32001. "The Department realizes that there are people who will react adversely to extremely low levels of formaldehyde and who are unusually sensitive to formaldehyde's irritant effects."
720. U.S. Department of Labor, Occupational Safety and Health Administration: *Industrial Exposure and Control Technologies for OSHA Regulated Hazardous Substances,* March 1989; 11(11) Substances K–Z.

> *NIOSH recommends that trimellitic anhydride be handled as an extremely toxic agent in the workplace. Exposure may result in: noncardiac pulmonary edema, . . . immunological sensitization, and irritation. . . . Three distinct syndromes: . . . rhinitis and/or asthma, . . . TMA flu, . . . irritant effect.*

The inhalation of TMA appears to be a significant stimulus of systemic immune response.

721. U.S. Environmental Protection Agency: *Dioxins.* 1980. EPA-600/2-80-197.
722. _____: *Formaldehyde and other aldehydes,* National Press, 1981.
723. _____: *Broad scan analysis of the FY82 national human adipose tissue survey specimens.* Dec. 1986, EPA-560/5-86-035.
724. _____: *DCPA fact sheet.* 1988; Washington DC.
724a. _____: *Indoor air quality and work environment study: EPA Headquarters Buildings, Volume IV—Multivariate Statistical Analysis of Health, Comfort, and Odor Perceptions as Related to Personal and Workplace Characteristics;* June 1991.
725. _____: *Pesticides fact handbook.* 1988.
726. _____: *Current Federal Indoor Air Quality Activities.* Aug. 1989; Washington DC; ANR-445.
727. _____, Atmospheric Research and Exposure Assessment Laboratory: *Nonoccupational pesticide exposure study (NOPES), Order ©PB 90-152 224/AS.* April 1990; EPA 600/SE-90/003.
728. _____, Center for Environmental Research, Project Summary: *Indoor air quality in public buildings,* vol. II. L. Sheldon, H. Zelon, J. Sickles, C. Eaton, T. Hartwell, and L. Wallace. Sept. 1988; (EPA/600/S6-88/009b).
729. _____, Consumer Product Safety Commission: *The inside story, a guide to indoor air quality.* Sept. 1988; Washington DC. EPA/400/1-88/004.
730. _____, Office of Air and Radiation: *Indoor air facts 3, ventilation and air quality in offices.* Feb. 1988; Washington DC.
731. _____, Office of Air and Radiation: *Indoor air facts 4, sick buildings.* July 1988; Washington DC.
732. _____, Office of Air and Radiation: *Indoor air facts 5, environmental tobacco smoke.* June 1989; Washington DC.
733. _____, Office of Air and Radiation: *Indoor air facts 6, Report to Congress on Indoor Air Quality.* Aug. 1989.
734. _____, Office of Air and Radiation: *Indoor air facts 7, Residential air cleaners.* Feb. 1990.
735. _____, Office of Air Quality Planning and Standards: *Assessment of health risks to garment workers and certain home residents from exposure to formaldehyde.* April 1987.
736. _____, Office of Drinking Water: *Aldicarb (sulfoxide and sulfone) health advisory.* 1987.
737. *_____, Office of Health and Environmental Assessment: *EPA Indoor Air Quality Implementation Plan (plus appendices).* June 1987. Washington DC. EPA/600/8-87/016.

EPA's indoor air program is geared toward identificaton, characterization, and ranking of indoor air problems and assessment and implementation of appropriate implementation strategies. EPA's research and analytical activities will pursue both a source-specific and generic approach to indoor air pollution. From a source-specific standpoint, the Agency will identify high risk pollutant sources and characterize the exposures and health risks of various populations to those sources. At the same time, the Agency will also pursue broad, cross-cutting strategies aimed at assessing the total exposure of people to indoor air pollutants and developing mitigation strategies which can address multiple pollutants simultaneously through improved building design and management techniques.

EPA will assess appropriate federal actions to mitigate health and environmental risks associated with indoor air quality problems. EPA will also take actions under existing statutes to reduce significant health risks, will refer problems to other federal agencies with appropriate regulatory authorities, or will request separate regulatory authority from Congress, if appropriate.

EPA's indoor air program will also emphasize information dissemination strategies to communicate information to a wide variety of audiences with roles to play in indoor air pollution. Ultimately, the Agency hopes to increase the capabilities of state and local governments, the private sector and individuals to identify and solve immediate health problems associated with pollutants in indoor environments and to reduce overall health risks.

738. ______, Office of Pesticide Programs: *Aldicarb fact sheet* 1988.
739. ______, Office of Pesticide Programs, *Aldicarb special review technical support document* 1988.
740. ______, Office of Policy, Planning and Evaluation: *Comparing risks and setting environmental priorities: overview of three regional projects* 1989.
741. ______, Office of Research and Development: *The total exposure assessment methodology (TEAM) study: summary and analysis,* vol. 1. June 1987; EPA/600/6-87/002a.
742. ______, Office of Toxic Substances: *The Toxics Release Inventory National Perspective,* 1987. June 1989; U.S. Government Printing Office, Washington DC.
743. ______, Office of Water Regulations and Standards: *Risk assessment for 2378–TCDD and 2378–TCDF contaminated receiving waters from U.S. chlorine-bleaching pulp and paper mills.* 1990; Aug., Washington DC.
744. U.S. Public Health Service, Agency for Toxic Substances and Disease Registry in Atlanta, Georgia: *Toxicological profiles set one, two, three, and four.* 1990. Each individual profile discusses the health effects of that chemical and provides a comprehensive bibliography of the current research.

Profile Set One: aldrin, dieldrin, benzene, benzo(a)pyrene, beryllium, chloroform, chrysene, dibenzo(a,h)anthracene, di(2-ethylhexyl)phthalate, lead, nickel, polychlorinated biphenyls, vinyl chloride, arsenic, benzo(a)anthracene, benzo(b)fluoranthene, cadmium, chromium, cyanide, 1,4-dichlorobenzene, heptachlor/heptachlor epoxide, methylene chloride, n-nitrosodiphenylamine, 2,3, 7,8-tetrachlorodibenzo-p-dioxin, tetrachloroethylene, trichloroethylene.

Profile Set Two: benzidine, bis(chloromethyl)ether, carbon tetrachloride, chloroethane, 3,3-dichlorobenzidine, 1,1-dichloroethene, 2,4- & 2,6-dinitrotoluene, isophorone, n-nitrosodimethylamine, pentachlorophenol, selenium, toluene, zinc, bis(2-chloroethyl)ether), bromodichloromethane, chlordane, p,p-DDT, DDE, DDD, 1,2-dichloromethane, 1,2-dichloropropane, hexachlorocyclohexane, mercury, n-nitrosodi-n-propylamine, phenol, 1,1,2,2-tetrachloroethane, 1,1,2-trichloroethane.

Profile Set Three: acrolien, ammonia, bromoform/chlorodibromomethane, chloromethane, creosote, 1,2-diphenylhydrazine, cis, trans 1,2-dischloroethene, ethylbenzene, hexachlorobenzene, nitrobenzene, plutonium, radium, radon, silver thorium, toxaphene, 1,1,1-trichloroethane, uranium, acrylonitrile, asbestos, chlorobenzene, copper, di-n-butylphthalate, total xylenes,

1,1-dichloroethane, endrin/endrine aldehyde, ethylene oxide, naphthalene/2-methylnaphthalene, 14 polycyclic aromatic hydrocarbons, 2,4,5-trichlorophenol.

Profile Set Four: aluminum, barium, boron, 1,3-butadiene, carbon disulfite, cresols, 1,2-dibromoethane, 1,3-dichloropropene, fluorides, manganese, methyl parathion, nitrophenol, styrene, tin, vandium, antimony, 2,3-benzofuran, bromomethane, 2-butanone, cobalt, dibromochloropropane, 2,4-dichlorophenol, endosulfan, a-hezanone, methyl mercaptan, mustard gas, pyridine, thallium, 1,2,3-trichloropropane, vinyl acetate.

745. *U.S. Surgeon General: *Report on Health Promotion and Disease Prevention 1979.* "There is virtually no major chronic disease to which environmental factors do not contribute, directly or indirectly."

746. *VanderWalt, H. S.: "Total allergy syndrome" (letter). *Lancet* 1982; March 13: 628–629.

747. *Van Metre, Jr., T. E.: "Critique of controversial and unproven procedures for diagnosis and therapy of allergic disorders," *Pediatr Clin N Am* 1983; 30(5): 807–817.

748. _____, N. Adkinson, Jr.: "Immunotherapy for aeroallergen disease." In E. Middleton, Jr., C. Reed, E. Ellis, N. Adkinson, Jr., J. Yunginger (editors), *Allergy Principles and Practice*, 3rd edition; 1988; 2: 1327–1343; C. V. Mosby Co., St. Louis.

749. *_____, N. F. Adkinson, Jr., L. M. Lichtenstein, et al: "A controlled study of the effectiveness of the Rinkel method of immunotherapy for ragweek pollen hay fever." *J of Allergy Clin Immunol* 1980; 65: 288–297. A controlled study which failed to demonstrate the efficacy of the Rinkel method.

750. Venables, K. M.: "Low molecular weight chemicals, hypersensitivity, and direct toxicity: the acid anhydrides." *Br J of Ind Med* 1989; 46(4); 222–232.

Direct toxicity effects of acid anhydrides on humans included: skin, eye, nose, and throat irritations; pulmonary effects such as bronchitis, emphysema, hempotysis, and congestion; and general symptoms including anemia, malaise, headache, fever, and dizziness.

Hypersensitivity effects included: asthma, urticaria, contact dermatitis, fever, chills, malaise, anorexia, weight loss, myalgia, late respiratory systemic syndrome, hemoptysis, and hemolysis. Allergic asthma was found to be the major form of hypersensitivity effect. Most asthma caused by acid anhydrides appeared to be immunologically mediated.

751. *Vos, J. G.: "Immune suppression as related to toxicology." CRC *Toxicology.* 1977; 5: 67.

752. Vree, T. B., et al: "Excretion of amphetamines in human sweat." *Arch Int Pharmacodyn* 1972; 199: 311–317.

753. Wallace, L.: "The TEAM study: personal exposures to toxic substances in air, drinking water and breath of 400 residents of New Jersey, North Carolina and North Dakota." *Env Research* 1987; 43: 290–307.

754. *Wallace, L. A.: "Part five. Overview." In R. B. Gammage, S. B. Kaye, V. A. Jacobs (editors), *Indoor Air and Human Health*; 1985; 331–333; Lewis Publishers, Chelsea MI. A summary from recent studies: 1) Indoor median concentrations of volatile organics are consistently greater, by factors of 2 to 5, than outdoor medians; 2) at higher concentrations the indoor-outdoor ratio increases, often beyond factors of 10; 3) concentrations are extremely variable, covering three to four orders of magnitude, indicating the presence of

intense indoor sources; and 4) these sources are many, including paints, adhesives, cleansers, cosmetics and other consumer products and building materials, but also common activities, such as visiting the dry cleaning shop or even taking a hot shower.

755. *______: "Organic chemicals in indoor air: a review of human exposure studies and indoor air quality studies." In R. B. Gammage, S. B. Kaye, V. A. Jacobs (editors), *Indoor Air and Human Health*; 1985; 28: 361–379; Lewis Publishers, Chelsea MI. Presents the rationale for, and some results from, the TEAM study.

Rationale: Many of our most common and useful chemicals are volatile organics. Unfortunately, some of them cause mutations in bacteria and or cancer in animals or man. Several federal agencies have authority to regulate such chemicals. However, before such regulation is undertaken, information on the sources, health effects and human exposure to each chemical must be collected.

Since there are many thousands of chemicals in use, it is necessary to narrow the possible universe from thousands to scores of chemicals. Such efforts are under way in a number of programs.

Results: Every one of 40 organics studied (in 9 studies worldwide) had higher levels indoors than outdoors.

Sources include building materials, furnishings, dry-cleaned clothes, cigarettes, gasoline, cleansers, moth crystals, hot showers, printed materials, etc.

Eleven chemicals were present in more than half of the TEAM study samples: benzene, styrene, ethylbenzene, o-xylene, m + p-xylene, 1,1,1-trichloromethane, trichloroethylene, tetrachloroethylene, m + p-dichlorobenzene, chloroform and carbon tetrachloride. Of these, nine have mutagenic, carcinogenic or co-carcinogenic properties.

756. *______: "The sick building syndrome: a review." Paper 88-110.6 in Proceedings of the 1988 Annual Meeting of the Air Pollution Control Association, Pittsburgh PA.

757. *______, E. D. Pellizzair, T. D. Hartwell, C. M. Sparacino, L. S. Sheldon, H. Zelon: "Results from the first three seasons of the TEAM study: personal exposures, indoor-outdoor relationships, and breath levels of toxic air pollutants measured for 355 persons in New Jersey." Presented at the 78th Annual Meeting of the Air Pollution Control Association, June 1985. A report of the TEAM (Total Exposure Assessment Methodology) Study which was designed to develop and demonstrate methods to measure human exposure to toxic substances in air, food and drinking water, and to measure biological fluids (breath, blood, urine) for the same compounds to determine body burden.

758. *Wallingfor, K.: *NIOSH Industry Air Quality Investigation in Office Buildings.* 1987; NIOSH; Cincinnati OH.

759. Wang, H. M., K. A. Smith: "The interleukin 2 receptor. Functional consequences of its bimolecular structure." *J of Exp Med* 1987; Oct. 1 166(4): 1055–1069.

760. *Ward, A. M., et al: "Immunological mechanisms in the pathogenesis of vinyl chloride disease." *Brit Med J* 1976; 1: 936.

761. Warner, M.: "Diagnosing sick buildings." *Anal Chem* 1990 April 15 62(8): 499A-501A.

762. Wasch, H. H., W. J. Estrin, P. Yip, R. Bowler, J. E. Cone: "Prolongation of the P-300 latency associated with hydrogen sulfide exposure." *Arch Neurol* 1989; Aug. 46(8): 902–904. "Each patient had persistent neurological symptoms, neuropsychological deficits, and abnormally prolonged P-300 latencies."

763. Washington State Interagency Indoor Air Quality Task Force: *Indoor Air Quality Report,* June 1990.
764. Wasner, C., et al: "The use of unproven remedies." *Scientific American* 1980; 23(1): 759–760.
765. *Wasowics, L. (UPI): "'Drunken' child suffers from allergy, doctors say." *UPA Domestic News* 1983; Sept. 28.
766. Wass, U., L. Belin: "An in vitro method for predicting sensitizing properties of inhaled chemicals." *Scand J of Work Env Hlth* 1990; June 16(3): 208–214.
767. *"Water filters." *Consumer Reports* 1983: 68 Feb.
768. *Webster, J. R.: "Medical 'experts' in litigation" (letter). *Ann Int Med* 1988; 108: 637–638. Highlights the problem of misuse or distortion of basic medical concepts by "so-called 'experts' who reflexively and inductively support plaintiffs' claims to their own personal financial benefit."
769. Weiner, M. A.: *Maximum Immunity.* 1987; Pocket Books, New York.
770. *Weinrich, D., B. J. Undem: "Immunological transmission of synaptic transmission in isolated guinea pig autonomic ganglia." *J of Clin Invest* 1987; 79: 1529–1532.
771. Weinstein, Allan M.: *Asthma.* 1987; Fawcett Crest, New York. Thorough treatment of subject of asthma for general reader.
772. *Weiss, B.: "Behavioral toxicology and environmental health science: opportunity and challenge for psychology." *Ann Psychol* 1983: 38: 1174–1187.
773. ______: "Toxic chemical disasters and the implications of Bhopal for technology transfer." *Milbank Q* 1986; 64(2): 216–240.
774. ______: "Environmental contaminants and behavior disorders." *Dev Pharmacol Ther* 1987; 10(5): 346–353. "Incipient toxicity often takes the form of subjective complaints that are later followed by overt impairments."
775. ______: "Implications of behavioral teratology for assessing the risks posed by environmental and therapeutic chemicals." *Prog Brain Res* 1988; 73: 39–49.
776. ______: "Quantitative perspectives on behavioral toxicology." *Toxicol Let* 1988; Oct. 43(1–3): 285–293.
777. *Weiss, L., M. Weiss: *How to Lie with the New 20th Century Illness. A Resource Guide for Living Chemically-Free.* Human Ecology Action League, Franklin MI. 74pp.
778. Weiskopf, M.: "Hypersensitivity to chemicals called rising health problem—some cannot adapt to low doses of toxics, study says." *Washington Post,* Feb. 10, 1990.
779. Welch, L.: "The role of occupational health clinics in surveillance of occupational disease." *Am J of Pub Hlth* 1989; Dec. 79 Suppl.: 58–60.
780. *Welliver, R. C.: "Allergy and the syndrome of chronic Epstein-Barr Virus infection" (editorial). *J of Allergy Clin Immunol* 1986; 78(2): 278–281.
781. Weschler, C. J., H. C. Shields, D. Rainer: "Concentrations of volatile organic compounds at a building with health and comfort complaints." *Am Ind Hyg Assoc J* 1990; May 51(5): 261–268.
782. *White, R. F.: "The role of neurologic testing in the evaluation of toxic CNS disorders." *Seminars in Occupational Medicine* 1986; 1: 191–196.
783. Whorton, D., S. R. Larson, N. J. Gordon, R. W. Morgan: "Investigation and work-up of tight building syndrome." *J of Occ Med* 1987; Feb. 29(2): 142–147.
784. Whyatt, R.: "Intolerable risk: the physiological susceptibilty of children to pesticides." *J of Pest Reform* 1989; 9(3): 5–9.
785. *Wide, L., H. Bennich, S. G. O. Johannsson: "Diagnosis of allergy by an in vitro test for allergen antibodies." *Lancet* 1967; 2: 1105–1108.

785a. Wilson, C.: "Adding Insult to Injury." *Our Toxic Times* 1992; 3(5): 2–3.
786. *Wojdani, A., J. D. Thrasher, G. Heuserr, G. P. Cheung: "Humoral and cellular immunity and IgE antibodies in humans chronically exposed to low concentrations of formaldehyde." *Arch Env Hlth* 1987, Nov.-Dec. 42(6): 347.
787. Wolff, M., H. Anderson, K. Rosenman, I. Selikoff: "Equilibrium of polybrominated biphenyl (PBB) residues in serum and fat of Michigan residents." *Bull Env Contam Toxicol* 1979; 21(6): 775–781.
788. ______, ______, I. Selikoff: "Human tissue burdens of halogenated aromatic chemicals in Michigan." *JAMA* 1982; 247(15): 2112–2116.
789. *Wood, R. W.: "Stimulus properties of inhaled substances." *Env Hlth Persp* 1978; 26: 69.
790. *Woolcock, A. J.: "Asthma." In: J. F. Murray, J. A. Nadel (editors), *Textbook of Respiratory Medicine*; 1988: 1030–1069; W. B. Saunders, Philadelphia.
791. *World Health Organization: *Indoor air quality research: report on a WHO meeting.* EURO Reports and Studies 103, 1986. An excellent, thought-provoking report which addresses many issues which can be applied to problems in the area of chemical sensitivity disorders. Summarizes special research needs in three areas: physical characterization through chamber studies, chemical analysis and biomedical research. Worth looking at is their summary of division of responsibility for healthy indoor environments.
792. *WTMJ radio (Milwaukee WI): *Terry Meeuwsen Show,* transcript of interview by Dr. Samuel Epstein, June 17, 1986.
793. *Yagi, K.: "Assay for serum lipid peroxide level and its clinical significance." In K. Yaki (editor), *Lipid Peroxides in Biology and Medicine*; 1983: 223–242; Academic Press, San Diego.
794. Yamato, N.: Concentrations and chemical species of arsenic in human urine and hair. *Bull Env Contam Toxicol* 1988; 40(5): 633–640.
795. *Yodaiken, R. E.: "Problems of communicating with the at-risk worker." In *Annals of the American Conference of Governmental Industrial Hygienists: Protection of the Sensitive Individual.* 1982; 3: 99–102; Cincinnati OH.
796. Young, B. B.: "Neurotoxicity of pesticides." *J of Pest Reform*; 6(2): 8–10.
797. *Zahner, G. E. P., et al: "Psychological consequences of infestation of the dwelling unit." *Am J of Pub Hlth* 1985; 75: 1303–1307.
798. Zamm, A., R. Gannon: *Why Your House May Endanger Your Health.* 1980; Simon and Schuster, New York.
799. *Zatz, C. J., J. K. Sherwood: "Defending speculative injury claims." *Toxics Law Reporter* 1987; June 17: 76–80. Discusses *Stites vs. Sunderstrand Heat Transfer,* DC W Mich (No. K84 299 CAC8), which dismissed (on a motion for summary judgment) all risk of cancer claims for exposure to trichloroethylene (-012 ppm TCE in February and March 1983) and half ot the plaintiff's fear of cancer claims. According to Michigan law, claims of future injury are compensable only if the injury is reasonably certain to occur. Points of debate included 1) whether TCE is a human carcinogen at any level of exposure, 2) what the level of risk was, 3) whether the immune system plays a major role in monitoring and fighting the development of cancer cells, and 4) whether the route of exposure was by ingestion, inhalation or both. Levels which constitute unacceptable risks in a regulatory setting do not demonstrate a reasonable certainty that the affected plaintiff will get cancer.

The court also correctly noted the differing purposes and burdens of proof in rule-making procedures and tort suits. The former are geared toward the absolute elimination of risks and normally take an extremely precautionary approach as required by statute. The standards they set include enormous margins of safety and say little or nothing about the extent or causation of risks to any particular tort suit plaintiff.

800. Zeidner, R. L.: "$20 million suit filed over EPA's Air." *Federal Times,* Nov. 26, 1990; p. 4.
801. Zeiss, C. R., C. L. Leach, D. Levitz, N. S. Hatoum, et al: "Lung injury induced by short-term intermittent trimellitic anhydride (TMA) inhalation." *J of Allergy Clin Immunol* 1989; 84(2): 219–223. Significant immunologic damage from short-term TMA exposure.
802. ______, ______, L. J. Smith, D. Levitz, et al: "A serial immunologic and histopathologic study of lung injury induced by trimellitic anhydride." *Am Rev Resp Dis* 1988; 137(1): 191–196. "Immune response to inhaled TMA occurs parallel with the development of lung lesions, and antibody levels in bronchoalveolar lavage fluid and serum are highly correlated with lung injury."
803. ______, D. Levitz, R. Chacon, P. Wolkonsky, R. Patterson, J. J. Pruzansky: "Quantitation and new antigenic determinant specificity of antibodies induced by inhalation of trimellitic anhydride in man." *Int Arch Allergy Appl Immunol* 1980; 61: 380–388.
804. ______, ______, C. L. Leach, N. S. Hatoum, H. V. Ratajczak, M. J. Chandler, J. C. Roger, P. J. Garvin: "A model of immunologic lung injury induced by trimellitic anhydride inhalation: antibody response." *J of Allergy Clin Immunol* 1987; 79(1): 59–63.
805. ______, J. Mitchell, P. F. Van Peenen, J. Harris, et al: "A longitudinal study of workers exposed to trimellitic anhydride TMA 1976–1987." Forty-fifth annual meeting of the American Academy of Allergy and Immunology, San Antonio, Texas.
806. ______, ______, ______, ______, D. Levitz: "A twelve-year clinical and immunologic evaluation of workers involved in the manufacture of trimellitic anhydride (TMA)." *Allergy Proc* 1990; March-April 11(2): 71–77.
807. ______, R. Patterson, J. J. Pruzansky, M. M. Miller, M. Rosenberg, D. Levitz; "Trimellitic anhydride-induced airway syndromes: clinical and immunologic studies." *J of Allergy Clin Immunol,* 1977; Aug. 60(2): 96–103.
808. ______, P. Wolkonsky, J. J. Pruzansky, R. Patterson: "Clinical and immunologic evaluation of trimellitic anhydride workers in multiple industrial settings." *J of Allergy Clin Immunol* 1982; 70(1): 15–18.
809. Zielhuis, R. L., A. A. Wibowo: "Work, chemical agents and offspring." *Ned Tijdschr Geneeskd* 1990; July 21 134(29): 1395–1398.

809a. Ziem, G.: "Multiple chemical sensitivity: Treatment and follow-up avoidance and control of chemical exposures" (unpublished paper).

Legal Aspects

810. **Bandura vs. Orkin Exterminating Co.,* tried 4/21/86: "Product Liability—Consumer Fraud—Overspraying Termites (11)." Source unknown, issue No. 29, Vol. BB. Verdict of $625,000 determining that defendant violated Consumer Fraud Act causing injuries. Exposure was to chlordane and heptachlor, and injury was listed as "profound immune depression."

811. **Brandt vs. St. Vincent's Infirmary*, 85-142, Supreme Court of Arkansas, Dec. 16, 1985, cite as 287 Ark. 431 (1985). Case of a psychiatrist who claimed that St. Vincent's Infirmary had unreasonably, capriciously, and arbitrarily restricted her right to prescribe and administer megadose vitamins therapy and Candida antigens. Decision in favor of St. Vincent's.

812. *"*Fitzgerald vs. Mallinckrodt, Inc.*, Fungicide Exposure." *Toxic Chemicals Litigation Reporter*, Jan. 6, 1988; 7,939–7,940; 7,959–7,963. U.S. District Judge ruled that the plaintiff's state common law tort claims based on negligent labelling and failure to warn were preempted by the Federal Insecticide, Fungicide and Rodenticide Act (FiFRA).

813. Inlander, C. B., E. I. Pavalon: *Your Medical Rights*. 1990; Little, Brown and Company, Boston.

814. **Rea, W. J., et al. vs. the Aetna Life Insurance Company and the Prudential Insurance Companies of North America*, Civil Action No. 3-84-0219-H, U.S. District Court for the Northern District of Texas, Dallas Division, filed Feb. 25, 1985. Denial of a motion to maintain a class action suit against the defendants for conspiring "to deny insurance claims for services rendered by physicians who practice clinical ecology in order to destroy the ability of such physicians to compete in the marketplace." Motion denied on the grounds that the "Plaintiffs have not met their burden with respect to defining the class of the specific elements of numerosity, commonality, typicality and adequate representation."

In the decision Judge Sanders notes that Dr. Rea has said that clinical ecology is a "point of view" rather than a "field of medicine." While Dr. Rea stated there were 3,000 clinical ecologists in the country and 5 environmental units, Judge Sanders ruled that the plaintiffs failed to establish specific requirements for class certification.

Appended to the decision is a letter from allergist Dr. Tim Sullivan to Dr. Salvaggio (January 30, 1986) stating that the judge has also "thrown out forcefully" the concept that there was a class of patients with so-called ecologic diseases that were not recognized and under the proper jurisdictions of disciplines such as allergy, immunology, toxicology, infectious diseases and the like. "Dr. Sullivan said this was good news for the Academy, encouraging it to develop position statements on debunked, unproven, unscientific medicine . . . in particular . . . clinical ecology."

815. **Rea, W. J., et al. vs. the Joint Committee on Allergies and Immunologies, the Aetna Life Insurance Company and the Prudential Insurance Companies of N. America*, Civil Action No. 3-84-0219-R, U.S. District Court for the Northern District of Texas, Dallas Division, filed Feb. 10, 1985. In this suit in which clinical ecology is called a "method of practice," insurance claims have been denied based on the determination that the method of clinical ecology is unscientific, unproved and not accepted by the medical community. The suit states that clinical ecology is a "viable, succesful and appropriate method of treatment." Alleges that the Joint Committee on Allergies and Immunologies combined to engage in predatory business practices and improve its market position through means other than lawful competition. Rea suffered actual damages in excess of $1 million in lost payments for services and lost business. The suit also alleged tortious interference with contractual relations, breach of contract, as well as libel and commercial disparagement.

816. **Schickele vs. Rhodes*, No. C-451843, Motion in Limine Re Alan Levin, M.D., Superior Court of the State of Arizona in and for the County of Maricopa,

filed June 23, 1986. Arizona Rules of Evidence require that "an expert's opinion . . . be both helpful to the jury and based on the type of facts reasonably relied upon by other experts in the field." Dr. Levin's testimony that the plaintiff's immune system was disrupted by one exposure to Nitrosulvapor was thus disallowed. (Nitrolsyl is ammonium polysulfide.)

817. *_Sterling vs. Velsicol Chemical Corp._, No. 86-6087, U.S. Court of Appeals for the Sixth Circuit, filed May 24, 1988. Judgment on a class action for personal injuries and property damage resulting from a landfill contaminating the local water supply. The appellate court found that the district court "probably held Velsicol liable . . . but erred in the nature and amount of the damage awards," and emphasized that individual particularized damages still must be provided on an individual basis. In Tennessee, damages for fear arising from an increased risk of disease are recoverable. The court reversed the district court's awards of damages for impairment of the immune system and for post traumatic stress disorders.

818. *_Viterbo, J. R., et al. vs. Dow Chemical Co._, No. 86-2806, U.S. Court of Appeals, Fifth Circuit, Filed Nov. 11, 1987. Discusses the question of "whether it is so if an expert says it is so." The experts opinion was determined to lack "the foundation of reliability necessary to support expert testimony. . . ." "We do not hold, of course, that admissiblity of an expert opinion depends on the expert disproving or discrediting every possible cause other than the one espoused by him. . . ." In this case, the doctor's testimony is "no more than Viterbo's testimony dressed up and sanctified as the opinion of an expert."

Newsletters

819. *_The Chemical Sensitivity Connection_, P.O. Box 81, Baldwin MD 21013; Sept. 1988.

820. *_Ecological Illness Law Report_, E. S. Davis, editor, P.O. Box 1796, Evanston IL 60204.
Vol. I, No. 3, March/April, 1983
Vol. II, No. 3, May/June, 1984
Vol. II, No. 6, Nov./Dec. 1984
Vol. III, Nos. 1 and 2, Jan.-April, 1985
Vol. III, Nos. 3, May/June, 1985
Vol. III, Nos. 4 and 5, July-Oct., 1985
Vol. III, No. 6, Nov./Dec., 1985
Vol. IV, No. 1, 1986
Vol. IV, Nos. 2 and 3, 1986
Vol. IV, Nos. 4 and 5, 1987
Vol. IV, No. 6, 1986–87

821. *_The Human Ecologist_, 7330 N. Rogers Ave., Chicago IL 60626.
No. 3, June, 1979
No. 7, Feb., 1980
No. 9, June, 1980
Nos. 11 and 12, Oct.-Dec., 1980
Nos. 15 and 16, March, 1982
No. 22, Summer, 1983
No. 25, Spring, 1984

No. 26, Summer, 1984
No. 27, Fall, 1984
No. 28, Winter/Spring, 1985
No. 29, Summer, 1985
No. 30, Fall, 1985
No. 31, Winter, 1985–86
No. 32, Spring, 1986

822. **Institute for Comparative and Environmental Toxicology (ICET) News*. Vol. 4, No. 1, 8 pp., winter 1988.

Index